25·00

Portraits of
Homoeopathic Medicines

Volume 1

Portraits of Homoeopathic Medicines

Psychophysical Analyses of Selected Constitutional Types

Volume 1

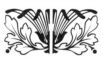

Catherine R. Coulter

Quality Medical Publishing, Inc.

ST. LOUIS, MISSOURI
1998

PUBLISHER Karen Berger
BOOK DESIGN Paula Morrison
COVER DESIGN Diane Beasley

Printed in the United States of America

Quality Medical Publishing, Inc.
11970 Borman Drive, Suite 222 • St. Louis, Missouri 63146

ISBN 1-57626-089-5

CT/WW/WW   5 4 3 2 1

To my family

The author wishes to thank

The National Center for Homoeopathy

for providing financial assistance while this
book was being written

Contents

Preface

Two hundred years after its discovery, homoeopathy is still under cover, and that for good reason. Even if we ignore the controversy about the efficacy of the ultramolecular dosage of a potentized substance, the epistemological implications of homoeopathy are too staggering for ready acceptance. They challenge some of our most cherished post-Cartesian beliefs about the nature of biologic and psychologic functioning and their interrelationships.

The paradigm of a healthy body espoused by biology and medicine is still largely that of a physiochemical machine responding and successfully adapting to external threats to its functioning. When this machine partly or wholly succumbs to such external interference or runs down from age, illness is assumed to ensue.

Yet, the experimental and clinical evidence of homoeopathy makes it quite evident that what we call health and illness are mutually inclusive of one another. They are changing faces of one and the same entity, two sides of the same coin: the individual constitutional state, or archetypal form pattern. The same dynamic fields inherent in the various substances call forth illness as well as health.

These fields are, moreover, intrinsic to the very organismic process, our own as well as the planet's. The dynamic of every existing substance, whether it be mineral, plant or animal, hence every constituent of our bodies as well as of the universe in which we live, is able to call forth illness patterns in its own likeness (as in a "proving") and of healing through that likeness when used in therapeutic dosage. The tendency to illness is "built in" to physical existence. Illness is an aspect of being alive, an aspect of the constitutional inherency of a particular person. But so is also healing. They both are elements of the "principium individuationis," the urge to individuation; and this in quite specific psychosomatic terms.

By and large psychology and psychoanalysis have been viewing the psychological makeup of a person primarily, if not exclusively, in terms of environmental conditioning and developmental influences, foremost among them of inadequate or outright destructive parenting. Yet the fact is that specific constitutional states (which are also potential illness patterns)—inclusive of psychological features—are inherent and, hence, a priori "given" (when, for instance a constitutional prescription is called for and proves effective in a newborn baby). This makes it evident that also psychological patterns are at least to some extent inherent as parts of an overall constitution—notwithstanding the fact that they may also, to varying degrees, be subject to environmental modification.

A child's personality is then not only structured by parental and environmental influences, but also, selectively, in its own individual ways, evokes and responds to "like" or corresponding parental and environmental influences. In its own way it will also constellate and call forth environmental factors that a child of a different makeup will not. A *Natrum muriaticum* or *Lycopodium* child may stoically withdraw, even sever communications, where a *Sulphur* child may respond with overactivity or a *Hepar* or *Arsenic* type with fury or anxiety respectively. It is, of course, also to be considered that environments that encourage anxiety or withdrawal may also help produce corresponding *Arsenic* or *Hepar* constitutional states. In either case, the somatic indications for a particular remedy can alert the experienced prescriber to the potential presence of specific psychological predispositions as yet dormant and unrecognized.

I need not elaborate upon the implications of such somatopsychic constitutional understanding for education and psychotherapy. It may alert us to propensities and limitations otherwise yet unrecognizable. In concert with educational or psychotherapeutic measures it can also help us to avoid pathogenetic extremes through homoeopathic medication free of side effects, in contradistinction to psychotropic drugs.

Lastly, if particular somatopsychic features and their exacerbations are individually predetermined as part of constitutional structuring, one can be healed only within and "into" the limits of one's individual pattern. There can be no average standard or definition of health that would fit everyone. One person's normality may be another's pathology and vice versa. Health and illness are not more than relative standards of comfortable adaptation or survival.

In listing mental (or emotional) symptoms as important criteria for the selection of an indicated remedy, homoeopathy has, in the past, implied the above considerations. Any systematic exploration in depth is still in its infancy. In William Gutman's essays on *Calcarea carbonica* and *Silica* and in my own *Psyche and Substance* the somatopsychic interrelations, as such, of some substances have been explored. Catherine Coulter's book is the first psychological description that widens the personality picture of the substance patterns beyond the hitherto standard enumerations (frequently overlapping) of relatively single criteria such as jealously, fear, desire to be alone, etc. Her book deserves to be studied by every homoeopathic prescriber as well as by the practicing or research psychotherapist. To the former it offers widening of perspective for remedy selection, while the latter can gain new insights into constitutional data and the possibilities of a new typology that bridges the gap between psyche and soma. Here is a view of therapeutic possibilities beyond the limits of a purely psychological approach to personality problems.

It is to be hoped that this book will also stimulate new research into the relation of constitutional and environmental factors as well as verifications of the clinical data offered here.

Homoeopathy bridges the Cartesian body-mind split. The body-oriented physician in the past has tended to gloss over psychological determinants and their fine points in the genesis of illness. The psychologist on the other hand has lacked adequate specific data for linking biological factors with psychic dynamics. This book is primarily (though not exclusively) descriptive of psychological features. Therein lies its virtue as well as a deliberate limitation; familiarity with the basics of the homoeopathic *materia medica* is taken for granted. For this reason I cannot conclude without a general caveat to the homoeopathic beginner and the less experienced prescriber. An adequate selection of a remedy cannot safely rely upon a psychological picture alone. There are still too many inadequately defined lines of demarcation, possibilities of temporary shifts in moods and overlappings. No matter whether one tries to help somatically or psychologically, the leading somatic guiding symptoms and modalities must also be considered.

Edward Whitmont, M.D.
Former Chairman,
C.G. Jung Training Center, New York

Introduction

Homoeopathy was founded by Samuel Hahnemann (1755-1843), who was born in Meissen, Saxony, the gifted son of poor but educated parents (his father was a painter of porcelain in the porcelain works for which Meissen is still famous to this day). After completing his education, he started on a career as physician but became progressively more disillusioned with what he had learned. Finally he renounced medicine altogether and for some years made a living by translating works on chemistry and other subjects from English, French, and Italian to support a large and rapidly growing family.

While translating William Cullen's *Materia Medica* he made a discovery that was to completely change and redirect his life. Dissatisfied with Cullen's explanation of how Peruvian bark (quinine) acts to cure malaria, Hahnemann decided to test the substance on himself and observe its effect. He found that he was developing the symptoms of malaria: chills, drowsiness, heart palpitations, trembling, prostration through all the limbs, pulsation in the head, redness of the cheeks, thirst, rigidity of the joints, etc. This discovery acted as a catalyst to his medical thinking and gave birth to the science of homoeopathy.

If quinine *(China),* which caused the symptoms of malaria in a healthy person, could cure malaria, this signified that it acted as a *similar medicine,* curing the sick by virtue of its ability to produce the same symptoms in the healthy. After repeating the same experiment with other substances, Hahnemann generalized this observation into the "law of similars," i.e., that *all* substances—animal, vegetable, and mineral—cure their similar conditions. Hence the name, "homoeopathy," from the Greek *homoios pathos,* meaning "similar disease."

Hahnemann had then to devise a method for ascertaining the curative powers of medicines (in order to use them as similars). This is where his genius came particularly to the fore. He discovered and elaborated a method known as the "proving" (from German *Pruefung* meaning "test" or "trial") by which substances are administered on a systematic basis to healthy persons over a period of days or weeks. The "provings" have revealed that each substance in nature has the power to bring out a set of symptoms peculiar to itself when given in this way to the healthy.

Once the homoeopathic physician has a complete and exhaustive listing of the patient's physical, emotional, and mental symptoms, he compares them with the listings of symptoms in the homoeopathic books of "provings," or *materia medica,* and selects his remedy on the basis of the *totality* of the patient's symptoms. Cure will take place in due course, even in chronic disease, when there is precise correspondence between the patient's symptoms and the symptoms of the medicine administered; the one which acts curatively is called the *simillimum,* the "most similar" remedy.

In other words, the homoeopathic physician does not treat the disease entity but rather the symptom complex of the *individual* who has heart disease, arthritis, migraine headaches, colitis, cystitis, influenza, dysmenorrhea, insomnia, or the common cold. And this ability to make distinctions among patients and among superficially similar disease processes—that is, to "individualize" every case—is the natural corollary of the concern for the whole person which lies at the core of homoeopathic practice.

In homoeopathy the expression, "constitutional remedy," signifies the medicinal substance which encompasses the sum total of the individual's physical, emotional, and mental picture. Homoeopathy denies any inherent or qualitative distinction between these, assuming that all processes within the organism are interdependent. Physical illnesses (apart from accidents and injuries) have a mental aspect, while mental illnesses have a physical aspect, and the prescription of medicines must be based upon a consideration of both categories of symptoms. A patient is said to be a *Phospho-*

rus, a *Silica,* a *Pulsatilla,* or some other type, according to the constitutional remedy which most closely approximates his total picture. To find this constitutional remedy the physician not only records painful sensations, symptoms, pathology, and the like, but also how the patient looks and behaves when in health, what he says, how he responds, his temperament and disposition, strengths and weaknesses. After collecting, arranging, and evaluating these characteristics, he matches them to the remedy which most expresses this "wholeness" of the patient. Espousing this truly holistic approach, each chapter of this work describes the relationship between a given type's physical, emotional, and mental patterns when viewed in their dynamic interaction.

To ensure that the individual features of a case are preserved in all their purity, Hahnemann urged the physician to take down the symptoms and sensations in the patient's own words, not in neutral "scientific" language. Following his precepts, this text seeks to record in "layman's" language those details of a given homoeopathic medicine that best conveys its individuality, that makes its "personality" more easily recognizable by the physician, and that deepens his understanding of its nature.

The remedies are the building blocks of the homoeopathic discipline, and their pictures remain forever valid. Their contours have been delineated by the masters of old in the records of provings and cures which constitute the foundations of homoeopathic literature. But, like all classics, they must be reinterpreted by succeeding generations. This book explores the behavior and psyches of nine constitutional types in health and illness, as manifested by the patient's manner, voice, speech, gestures, expressions, thoughts, feelings, hopes, fears, tastes, and common or idiosyncratic physical symptoms.

The word, "Portraits," in the title is used deliberately. A portrait-painter selects certain features to reveal his subject's true character. The same is true for these descriptions of the homoeopathic remedies. They are selective rather than comprehensive presentations. Certain features are emphasized, certain themes developed, and certain nuances brought to the fore, because they appear quin-

tessential to the type. Of course the characteristics of various remedies can and do overlap, as witnessed by the frequent cross-refer-
ences in the text—particularly the sections which compare and dif-
ferentiate the remedies; also, there are no absolutes in the remedy
pictures: a *Silica* patient need not be chilly, a *Sepia* one can sparkle with cheerfulness and mirth, *Natrum muriaticum* can dislike
salt, and *Arsenicum album* may be quite unconcerned with his
health. But in any constitutional type certain features stand out.

To clarify and illustrate these points examples have been taken
from history and literature. Famous persons, or what we can know
of them, and well-known characters in fiction, often seem to portray constitutional types in concentrated form, and because they
are familiar parts of our cultural heritage, any allusion to them suggests to the reader a host of associations which bring the remedy's
specific personality into clear focus. Thus they serve as archetypes.
A prime example is the *Natrum muriaticum* type of loyalty in
friendship illustrated by the relationship of Dr. Watson to Sherlock
Holmes. Ultimately every prescriber forms his own associations.

Yet few individuals are pure types. Few are covered by a single remedy throughout a lifetime. In treating Samuel Hahnemann
as a *Sulphur* and choosing to emphasize those traits in his personality, we necessarily simplify a complex nature that also displays
features of *Arsenicum, Lycopodium,* and others.

The prescriber must pay close attention to the relationship
among remedy-patterns within the individual patient. Most persons
oscillate among two, three, or four remedies during the course of
their lives, exhibiting their various characteristics in alternation.
The body and personality are affected by external stresses—physical or emotional trauma, job or vocation, the stresses and strains of
marriage or lack of it—which leave their imprint and promote
change and modification in the individual's physical, emotional, or
mental life. Genetic endowment and childhood development must
also be considered, as well as racial or national background. They
all affect the total constitutional picture. These complex questions
are raised and discussed at appropriate points in the text below.

The material presented in the following pages should be useful to others besides homoeopathic physicians: to a wide range of healers and medical practitioners who, *with the proper training,* can employ the remedies as helpful adjuncts to their specific techniques for relieving humanity's physical or mental ills. They help make surgical operations less hazardous and facilitate recovery. Osteopaths and chiropractors have reported that their treatments are made more effective by concomitant administration of the appropriate remedy, as have dentists and veterinarians. Pediatricians and family physicians consistently find that prescribing the constitutional remedy when the patient is in good health helps prevent future acute or chronic illnesses. Particularly in the psychiatric field, psychotherapists, as well as clinical, analytical, and behavioral psychologists, will find that the homoeopathic remedy brings about a profound inner change in the patient beset by fears and neuroses, anxieties of conscience and moral turmoil, or suffering from mania, depression, suicidal impulses, and even "borderline" mental illnesses. He may start to relinquish his anxieties and other disorders within days or weeks, rather than months or years.

The time is at hand for a more general acceptance of homoeopathic principles by physicians and public. This approach to healing, which uses botanical, biological, and chemical substances singly and in very small quantities, which stresses the need for holistic treatment of the individual and which reinforces his inherent defensive and recuperative capacities, has tremendous appeal at a time when orthodox medicine uses ever more potent drugs in ever larger doses—often many different ones at the same time. All those practitioners who desire "the highest good" for their patients, and who want "all parts of the organism in admirable, harmonious, vital operation, as regards both sensations and functions, so that our inherent reason-gifted mind can freely employ this living healthy instrument for the higher purposes of existence" (Hahnemann, *Organon of Medicine,* Sec. 9), will find their efforts enhanced by application of the homoeopathic simillimum.

Portraits of
Homoeopathic
Medicines

Volume 1

Phosphorus

THE homoeopathic remedy is made from the luminescent element, phosphorus, the only non-radioactive substance capable of producing its own light. The name originates from the Greek words *phos,* meaning "light," and a form of *phoro,* meaning "to bring" or "to bear"—hence "bringer or bearer of light." Both the etymology and the associations evoked by the element provide fitting keys to the *Phosphorus* personality.

Anyone who has been by the ocean at night has seen the flecks of sparkling phosphorus dancing in the foam or gleaming in the swells. This restless element captures the attention, and the *Phosphorus* individual has a similar eye-catching impact. He attracts by his sparkling appealing manner and his bright intelligent face.*

He is usually of slight build. The woman is slender and graceful, the man spruce and dapper. Both sexes have neat, refined facial features and a clear, delicate skin that flushes easily from strong emotion or excitement ("is seized with heat when grasps an idea vividly": Hahnemann). Occasionally the complexion has "the pallor of porcelain" (Borland) or even a translucent quality. The hair is fine and soft, with natural highlights. If brown, it has glints of chestnut; if blonde, it has glints of red; and, if black, it appears glossy. Redheads are quite often *Phosphorus.*

The eyes, however, are the type's most striking feature. Framed by well-shaped eyebrows and long lashes, they shine with a soft luminous quality or captivating sparkle that draws another closer. These arresting or enveloping eyes sometimes have a mischievous, humorous glint, as they eagerly notice everything around them or virtually dance with excitement.

---

*For stylistic purposes and to avoid cumbersome phraseology, the masculine gender has been employed throughout the text to denote both sexes, except when specified otherwise.

Sensitivity

Emotionally, *Phosphorus* is sympathetic, responsive, and sensitive to another's wavelength. The whole manner betrays a readiness to establish warm communication with his interlocutor, and he immediately senses how best to establish rapport. Finely intuitive in his dealings with people, he predisposes others toward himself by little verbal kindnesses, warm praise, or touching consideration, and at times by almost undue generosity. When assistance is required, he will drop whatever he is doing and be the first to arrive. A woman will immediately deposit her children in a neighbor's lap, leave her job early, or cancel an important appointment, to be there, ready to help. In fact, *Phosphorus* loves the excitement of rallying round during minor disasters. A busy farmer, whose every minute costs him dollars during the planting season, will stop his own work and offer his equipment and time to help pump out a neighbor's flooded cellar. After spending an hour cheerfully supervising the relief operation, he will insist that the homeowner *be sure* to call him again whenever help is needed.

In conversation he has the same expansive impulses. He is a highly reactive listener, entering wholeheartedly into another's happiness and sympathizing fully with his hardships. He is also a good talker, seldom heavy or overbearing, and invariably supportive: "Yes, I know *just* how you feel. You had no choice but to act as you did. The same thing happened to me when . . . " And he proceeds to contribute something amusing or illuminating that makes the other believe that his own conversation is also interesting and perceptive. In the physician's office he leans forward in the chair, even resting his arm on the desk to get as near to the doctor as possible, while his alert eyes also follow him closely. He may begin by inquiring after the physician's own well-being, work or family. On the conscious level, this sympathetic nature is indeed sincerely solicitous, but by ingratiating himself he also secures the physician's special attention in return. After being charmed, as it were, the latter will respond all the more concernedly with, "But tell me how are *you*? And what brings you here today?"

Phosphorus is gregarious and needs people around to feel whole, well, and happy. He likes to speak of his "dozens of intimate friends" (only the outgoing, ever-responsive *Phosphorus* has dozens of "intimate" friends), and is seldom overly critical of others, being diverted by, and sympathetic toward, their follies, weaknesses, and incongruities rather than censorious of them. Life's setbacks, absurdities, and inconsistencies entertain him instead of being irritating or frustrating. Thus his disposition is cheerful, optimistic, and resilient, provided he is not pushed too far. His (and especially, ''her'') excitable nervous nature may break down under too much stress or hardship. Whitmont likens this type to a delicate blossom that ''thrives in the sunshine of favorable circumstances but wilts in the darkness and coldness of adversity.''

Phosphorus is highly *impressionable* and susceptible to his emotional environment. Since he cannot be happy unless others are also, is sensitive to criticism and fears rejection, he will bend over backwards to accommodate or to preserve a harmonious atmosphere. Disagreeable or unpleasant feelings can make him physically ill, bringing on trembling stomach and head pains, or palpitations. Even pleasurable emotions affect him similarly. He starts quivering or is kept awake by a stimulating conversation, a good novel, or ''from excitement after theatre'' (Hering). To such an extent does he identify with others that he takes on their enthusiasms and adopts, if only temporarily, their tastes, beliefs, and lifestyle. For example, the child or young adult knows *exactly* what he wants to be in life—only he changes every six months, according to his milieu. Or his easily empathizing nature may assume a friend's very ailments. If the latter describes a shoulder ache, soon *Phosphorus* feels the same pain. A not infrequent request of this patient to the physician is: ''I want to stop being so sensitive to everything. I'm being pulled in all directions, reacting to everyone around me whether I want to or not. I am just one exposed nerve . . . ''

Nash claims that no remedy has a stronger action on the nervous system than *Phosphorus* (to this we would add *Ignatia* and *Nux vomica*).

His impressionableness is also seen in his psychic and telepathic abilities: ''clairvoyant state with heightened sensibility'' (Boenninghausen). This is the type who sees auras and experiences the *deja vu* sensation of having previously known a person he has just met, of recognizing as familiar a place he has just visited. Some will sense the illness or death of a relative or friend before being told of it. Or he correctly intuits that a friend has just received some good news and telephones to ask what it is. He often anticipates what another is going to say (*Lachesis*) or surmises the content of a letter before opening it. Some have premonitions both awake and when asleep. Others recount (in wonderful detail) their encounters with the spirit world. If in a house reputed to be inhabited by a ghost, *Phosphorus* will invariably elaborate on the elusive inmate's appearance or behavior, instead of only hearing the creaking floorboards like everyone else.

Any constitutional type may experience psychic feelings, correct intuitions, and brushes with the supernatural, but *Phosphorus cultivates* this side of his nature. He loves to consider himself endowed with extrasensory perception. Although he is, upon occasion, remarkably clairvoyant, he is also conveniently forgetful about the times he was wrong.

The physician repeatedly encounters patients with this tendency to read psychic dimensions into every natural phenomenon and aspect of life. For example, there was a college student who suffered from a sour taste and painful burning eructations, or simply much discomfort beginning half an hour after meals. She claimed that the reason for her malady was that the dormitory cook carried sorrow and anger in her soul, which was reflected in her cooking. The patient had never addressed, nor even seen, this allegedly unfortunate person, but she insisted on her interpretation. As it happens, *Phosphorus* evinces this type of digestive disturbance, especially after food has warmed up in the stomach; accordingly, she received a dose of *Phosphorus* 1M, and soon her digestion had improved to the point where she could enjoy meals without paying a penalty for it. But she explained that she had meditated daily on the cook's soul and that her prayers of intercession had produced a profound spiritual transformation in that lady, whose food was now permeated with happy vibrations instead of angry ones.

This emotional sensitivity finds a parallel on the physical plane. *Phosphorus* is "excessively sensitive" (Hahnemann) to his surroundings: to certain odors (particularly the smell of perfume and of tobacco); to incandescent or any strong light (his eyes ache, and he sees halos around objects, black specks or floaters before eyes, red or green flickerings, etc.). With his unstable circulation, he is also highly sensitive to changes in temperature or atmospheric pressure, being known as the "human barometer" (Boenninghausen). His hearing is extra acute, and he is hypersensitive to noises. He startles, with nervous jangling, from sudden bangs, shouts or thunderclaps; he cannot tolerate loud music. If he lives in noisy surroundings, he cannot sleep without a fan whirring in his room all night to drown out other sounds.

The nervous and excitable disposition is susceptible to various fears: of the dark, where he imagines "something creeping out of every corner" (Kent), of illness ("anxiously solicitous about the unfortunate issue of her disease": Hahnemann), of impending misfortune, "as if some accident has happened to her beloved ones" (Hahnemann), of the future, and of death (*Arsenicum, Calcarea*). Sometimes it is more an overall undefined dread: he is worried "without any imaginable reason" (Hahnemann). In his apprehensive state of mind he suffers from insomnia, or he sleeps unsoundly and has many anxious dreams (Hahnemann lists some sixty sleep and dream symptoms). He is also subject to "somnabulism" (Kent).

One key symptom is an extreme fear of thunderstorms. He senses electrical changes in the air as does no other constitutional type; it is as if he were producing enough of his own already, and more throw him off balance. Several remedies manifest the symptom, "worse *before* thunderstorms," when the barometric pressure is falling (*Sepia, Arsenicum, Lachesis, Gelsemium,* and others), but, once the storm breaks, they feel better, even exhilarated. *Phosphorus*, however, is also "restless" (Hahnemann) or worse *during* the storm (*Natrum carbonicum*). He panics from the flashes of lightning and trembles at the sound of thunder. Some patients admit that they crawl under a bed or a table from fright, and one female patient even tried to persuade her grown children to do the same.

All his fears are exaggerated by solitude. Being alone can throw him into a panic ("great anxiety and irritability on being alone": Hahnemann), with trembling and a "feeling of helplessness" (Kent); thus a guiding symptom is marked "amelioration from company" (Boger). His fears, both concrete and imaginary, can be allayed, even physical complaints are alleviated, by the presence of others—from whom he is always "seeking reassurance" (Blackie).

Few respond to reassurance as gratefully and trustingly as *Phosphorus*. A typical case was the patient who, on being told that homoeopathy would probably be able to help his ulcerative colitis (he had the remedy's characteristic bloody diarrhoea and "feeling as if anus remained open after emptying": Hahnemann), promptly exclaimed: "I just *know* that homoeopathy is going to cure me . . . I already feel completely confident in your powers. You know, that gripy crampy pain in my abdomen has just vanished"—and he went on in this way, thanking the physician for his cure, even before receiving the first prescription. *Phosphorus* has a way of making up in trust and confidence what he lacks in knowledge and experience.

Sparkle and Self-Love

There are two distinct *Phosphorus* types. The first possesses a quiet refined personality that emits a gentle luminescence. He is friendly, sympathetic, and somewhat shy or reserved, even while liking people. He is there when needed but otherwise retires into his own world of intellectual and artistic pursuits. The second type is a more projecting, dynamic personality: "lively" (Kent), effervescent, champagne-like, overflowing with spirits. He actually looks as he feels—*glowing:* "good-humored, with agreeable warmth all over the body; everything seems bright to him" (Hahnemann). Just as the element generates light spontaneously, this "sprightly" (Boenninghausen) individual throws off sparks from a seemingly inexhaustible internal source of light. The impression is compounded when *Phosphorus* is artistic, which he often is, either actively or latently. He possesses the artist's nervous sensibility and heightened sensitivity, observant eye and vibrant imagination, which add an artistic flair to any activity or occupation.

This artistic flair may be manifested early. A two-year-old boy came to homoeopathy for repeated chest infections, usually commencing with a sore throat and then progressing to the chest, with a hard racking cough. He was placed in a chair in the office and told not to move while his case history, complicated by a strong tubercular inheritance, was being discussed (*Phosphorus* frequently displays the chest weakness and other symptoms of an inherited tubercular diathesis). Whenever he became restless and made a move as if to slide out of the chair, he was strictly ordered, in the parents' Southern drawl, to "Gi-et, ba-ack!" Without making a scene, he started chanting the syllables, "Gi-et ba-ack," repeating them like a parrot. Next he proceeded to experiment with the different sounds. Then, with the shiniest of eyes and coyest of looks (as he closely followed his audience's reaction), he improvised a tune on the two words, trying out various pitches and rhythms until he came up with a delightful little song. In this creative way he entertained himself, his parents, and the physician according to the gifts of his *Phosphorus* nature.

Phosphorus is made for happiness and may have a highly developed sense of fun. He is easily amused, quick to see the humorous side of things, and ready to laugh at himself. Whereas *Calcarea carbonica, Pulsatilla,* or *Natrum muriaticum* might feel wounded by teasing, *Phosphorus* takes humorous shafts with spontaneous gaiety and fully appreciates the attention. From life he derives the maximum delight and joie-de-vivre ("mirthful, merry, good-humored; sings and trills": Hahnemann). He knows how to enjoy himself and be entertained; he also knows how to entertain, frequently displaying a fine gift for mimicry and an ability to improvise. His imagination can be as unsubduable and his conversation as sparkling as the phosphorus of the sea: an example from literature is Gulley Jimson, the impoverished and roguish painter hero of Joyce Cary's *The Horse's Mouth*, whose bubbling creativity endows his own difficult life and his neighbors' bleak existence with brightness and color.

At times, like the grasshopper in Aesop's *Fables* who chirrups and dances all summer long, giving no thought to the future, *Phosphorus* lives only for the present, as if there were no tomorrow, in contrast to the hardworking *Arsenicum* ant, who, with great foresight, spends his summer storing up winter food. This characteristic contributes to his overall allure, but it also can be a weakness, reflecting the nature's flighty side. Indeed, there may be something light and airy about *Phosphorus*, something frothy and superficially glittering. Yet the absence of mental profundity is frequently offset by the interplay of his impressionable psyche and emotional receptivity. And he is, as we shall see, more complex than is suggested by his seemingly open and transparent nature. Observing him is like peering into a deep pool; everything is quite visible, even in the depths, but the shimmering play of light and water allows for no true clarity.

His innate expansiveness and the pleasure he derives from making others happy lead him to extend warmth and sympathy not only to friends but even to newly formed acquaintances—persons in whom he has intrinsically little interest apart from his overall amicable nature. He has all the tools of sympathy at his command and can communicate his concern to perfection. In comforting or supporting others, he instinctively finds the right words and gestures. He will put a sympathetic arm around the other's shoulder or waist or will hold his hand to help soothe the distress. Or, during the course of a conversation he may simply lay his hand on his companion's arm to establish closer rapport. He constantly addresses others as "Sweetie" or "Dearest" (those sceptical of *Phosphorus'* sincerity claim that is because it is easier than remembering names). At times, his very voice is suggestive, with a low, confiding, sometimes breathless, almost caressing tone that invites intimacy. Indeed, he himself needs physical closeness and is *demonstrably* affectionate.

A cnild will virtually wrap himself around a parent, murmuring endearing words. *Phosphorus* enjoys being hugged and kissed ("kisses everyone": Kent) and is better from being "rubbed" (Hahnemann), touched, massaged. If he cannot get to sleep from nervousness or excitement, a back rub will quiet him better than anything (an equally restless or sleepless *Arsenicum* responds best to a hot drink).

He can also exhibit exceptional comforting and healing capacities, both professional and personal. The *Phosphorus* nurse, for instance, need only enter a patient's room to make him feel better. Her sympathy and cheerfulness, her very presence, are bracing in themselves, not to mention her instinctive sensing of the patient's needs. The type can even be competitive in the desire to help. Yet there is something to be said for such competitiveness, as in the heart-warming case of two *Phosphorus* sisters, each attempting with loving care to be the more dutiful (and favored) daughter to their elderly parents. Accustomed to being the generous, kind, attentive one, he wants to remain the brightest star in the firmament and is prepared to ingratiate himself and work hard to this end "It's amazing how much I do for others!" more than one *Phosphorus* has exclaimed, only half in humor, in the physician's office.

All in all, with his affectionate nature and sensitive manner, his desire to see the best in people and his talent for making others feel positive about themselves, this constitutional type is able to reach out to many, not just to a chosen few. Such is the special talent of *Phosphorus*.

The *Phosphorus* sparkle proceeds not only from eager responsiveness to others and love of life but also from *self-love*. He considers himself more sensitive and refined, more intuitive, more entertaining, more gifted, more spiritual than others. He can be quite fascinated with himself and view his person as the center around which others revolve, or as a latter-day Prometheus whose talents enrich mankind like the fire stolen from heaven. He will tell the physician, "I have a very special way with children. I can charm them into performing better than any other teacher." Or, "I am talented in any art form I choose, but I am most gifted in. . . . " One 75-year-old *Phosphorus* being treated for rheumatic pains, whose chirruping presence raised the physician's spirits whenever he entered the office, said, "One thing I can tell you is that I have been the best of husbands. I am as easy and pleasant a person to get along with as you will ever encounter, and for fifty years I've kept my wife completely happy and our marriage a success. Now, that is an accomplishment!'' And it was, without any doubt. But the physician, who knew his wife, suspected that some of the credit for the longevity of the marriage belonged to her.

Phosphorus does not dominate aggressively yet still manages to divert attention to himself. Usually, however, he does it so subtly that others hardly realize what is happening, or so entertainingly that they do not object — especially as he invites them to join him in having positive feelings about themselves. Furthermore, even when vaunting himself, he may impishly undercut his vanity with humor. Thus, although he can harbor a subliminal conceit (almost unbeknownst to himself), even when boastful he is seldom offensive. His spontaneity, near-innocence, and captivating manner permit him to do and say what in others would be considered conceited or in poor taste.

Liking of self must be considered a healthy characteristic (as the Dauphin in Shakespeare's *Henry V* tells his father, ''Self-love, my liege, is far less a sin than self-neglecting''). But carried to an extreme, it reveals a negative side, a self-limiting narcissism. One such patient was an attractive woman in her thirties, a singer who complained of soreness and dryness in the larynx and a voice that was becoming husky, rough, and whispery from overuse; she also suffered from hoarseness which was worse in the evening. Even if her physical symptoms had not fitted the *Phosphorus* picture so well, her mental ones would have indicated the remedy. During the consultation she mentioned that she had just become engaged. Congratulating her, the physician asked about the fiancé. ''He is a very special person,'' she said, ''so discriminating and discerning! He told me only yesterday that he never believed anyone could be as feminine as I am but still be so dynamic, and that this special combination is even reflected in my singing. What really fascinates him about me is the way I. . . . '' She continued in this way, and while the doctor learned much about her, he discovered precious little about her fiancé.

What she said of herself was doubtless true enough. She had the *Phosphorus* attractively coquettish manner and knew well how to elicit the admiration of men. But with such undisguised egocentrism, it was hardly surprising that the engagement eventually fell through — her third in as many years.

These individuals may be quite vain about their looks, but again in a beguiling rather than an unattractive way. They dress with taste, at times flamboyantly, their clothes reflecting the artistic, Bohemian vein that runs through the type. The child will enjoy wearing bright or unusual clothes to school for effect; the man will be something of a dandy. In a dance or gymnastics class, the woman will take a position nearest the mirror so as to admire herself throughout the drill, thus deriving extra enjoyment from the class. Indeed, the *Phosphorus* narcissism may manifest itself in a liking for mirrors; these individuals, both male and female, will have a number of them distributed around the home. They explain them as enhancing the light or expanding the space, but the unconscious motivation is a desire to admire themselves in any room of the house.

Likewise, *Phosphorus* may be suspected as a component of the constitution of any individual whose house is covered with photographs of himself in various activities, poses, or stages of life.

Another, perhaps subconscious, form of vanity is the way in which an attractive woman will speak self-deprecatingly about being overweight or having some minor physical defect: "I hate my turned up nose . . . my lumpy arms . . . my short legs . . . ," thereby forcing others to notice the particular feature in order to protest her assertion and assuage her concern. A *Phosphorus* woman may be inordinately afraid of growing old. She cannot accept philosophically the diminishing of her good looks. In contrast, a *Lachesis* woman fears aging out of regret for missed opportunities, while *Arsenicum* dreads old age for fear of accompanying illnesses.

The Eternal Child

Whether actively seeking it or inadvertently attracting it, *Phosphorus* from an early age manages to capture notice. He is appealing in both looks and manner, and even passers-by exclaim, "What an attractive child!" "Just look at those eyes!" The cry is instinctive, as they gaze with open admiration at a child whose alertness, grace, charm, and bubbling good spirits compel attention.

The youngster is often aware of the effect he is producing and may glance from under his brow, or out of the corner of his eye, to observe his impact. From his knowing expression it is clear that, while acting in all sincerity, he is still conscious of his winning ways. In the physician's office he will closely observe not only the physician's reaction to his recounting of symptoms, but also that of his parents. He is always sensitive to the impression he is making, concerned to say the right thing in the right way.

Phosphorus can be impatient, desiring gratification at the very moment and, if thwarted, throwing impressive tantrums. But he is easily appeased and snaps out of his anger whenever he pleases, revealing that the act is largely for exhibition. Sometimes he will station himself before a mirror to observe himself crying or raging, genuinely fascinated by his own performance.

He does not allow sadness to last and does not bear resentment. Like a jack-in-the-box he pops up smiling even after being reprimanded. If punished by being sent to his room, he will sing or whistle unconcernedly during the confinement, then emerge cheerful and sunny as if nothing had happened. The sensitive nature feels the disgrace but covers it up, all the sooner to reenter others' good graces. Thus, with a psychological astuteness which may be quite extraordinary for his age, he wins forgiveness by manifesting affection and forgiveness toward his disciplinarian. Even in illness *Phosphorus* can be irrepressible. Despite his indisposition he acts so chipper and bright that parents can hardly keep him subdued. During the office consultation his appearance may belie the severity of his condition. On the other hand, some of these children, when unwell, become clinging like *Pulsatilla*, requiring the reassurance of physical touch and closeness and adhering like a limpet to the parent.

The child also has the happy capacity of transforming work into play. School for him is one long carnival, and he will make a game even out of homework. His elders must remind him to settle down, to stop illustrating his math or spelling exercises, and to study his history lessons rather than acting them out (*Sulphur*). When ordered to do some tiresome household chore, he does not argue or make a scene but just conveniently disappears. Or, alternatively, when he cannot evade his duties, he will approach them creatively: the boy will artistically rearrange the furniture when cleaning up his room, and the girl will decorate with flowers the table she is laying or the room she is vacuum-cleaning.

As concerns his studies the young *Phosphorus* loves anything that captures his imagination, such as having stories told or read to him, but dislikes anything requiring sustained application, anything that is not "fun." At the same time he wants to be best in everything without really working for it. Whatever he is trying to accomplish, he must "get it" the first time. If unsuccessful or thwarted in his attempt, he may react hysterically, stamping, shouting or throwing down his tools in frustration. Because he is quick ("quick memory": Hering) and absorbs things easily, he often does manage to be a good, but not an excellent, student without studying too hard.

When studying a musical instrument, he will practice eagerly—up to a point. Having once acquired the knack of the piece, his concentration lapses, and he trusts his innate musicality to carry him through the lesson or recital. This pattern of insufficient preparation and reliance on inspiration can continue into adulthood. Even though his performance may reveal technical inaccuracies, an improper interpretation, or excess freedom with the material, *Phosphorus charms* his audience into thinking his playing is better than it is. He does have flair, his love of hearing himself perform is contagious, and the audience cannot help but respond.

Phosphorus children are seldom mean and do not bully others. They are not necessarily angels, but they gain the upper hand in a diverting, not a disagreeable, way. Their mischievousness comes out in teasing, playing jokes on others, or tricking their elders. Children less than a year old and still unable to walk, may crawl away to hide in a closet; while others are searching and shouting their names in concern, they sit concealed, gurgling with pleasure at their own cleverness. If an older child answers the telephone, and the caller mistakes him for someone else, he will not pass up this golden opportunity, but in a most convincing manner will act out the role inadvertently bestowed on him.*

In fact, those children who do not wear their hearts on their sleeves

---

* A minister telephoned a parishioner to ask her to take charge of the flower arrangements for Easter and, mistaking her young son's voice for hers, launched into the reason for the call.

"I would be glad to help you out," was the ready reply, "but I think that this year, for a change, we should decorate the altar with something different, maybe with some vegetables."

"Vegetables?" was the dismayed response.

"Yes, our spring onions are out, and the early radishes, and the asparagus is just coming up—I think they would look beautiful in (and the transparently honest individual is often a *Phosphorus*) can be most convincing simulators. When they must weasel out of tricky situations, they look you directly in the eye while fabricating a complete untruth. With their ready imagination, they are adept at twisting facts or concocting spur-of-the-moment explanations why they didn't do their homework or their chores. Sensing another's credulity, they will get away with the most outrageous lies—in contrast with the *Natrum muriaticum* child who looks guilty even when he is not, and who always gets caught in the slightest fib; he just does not have that *Phosphorus* aura of truthfulness. You feel that he *must* be telling the truth, with those wide clear eyes gazing straight at you. But by no means! The more innocent *Phosphorus* looks, the guiltier he usually is. He has simply practiced his act and raised it to the level of art.

The child can be mentally resourceful. A notoriously insecure sixth-grade teacher assigned a *Phosphorus* girl a spontaneous five-minute speech on the topic, "Why did my teacher take so long to like me?" The sharp-witted girl, immediately grasping the absurdity of the topic, fraught with embarrassment for either the teacher or herself, replied, "Can I refuse the topic, M'am, and get a lower grade? Although I really cannot understand why my attractive personality did not appeal to you from the beginning, it is not for me to question your judgment or taste." It was brightly and charmingly done, in typical *Phosphorus* manner, giving offense to no one while maneuvering herself out of a tight corner.

Older children are the kind of people to whom wonderful things are always happening. There is so much in life they want to enjoy and experience! The class queen will frequently be a *Phosphorus*, as much for her outgoing personality as for her appealing looks. Boys are popular without necessarily being leaders; they are just friendly, vital, and enthusiastic. In recounting his adventures the adolescent may exaggerate in his own favor, but his willingness to share with others the exciting

---

church."

"But, my dear friend, what are you talking about? We can't have radishes and onions as Easter decorations!"

"I don't see why not. Vegetables are also God's creations. And it's time we broke with tradition. People get tired of the same lilies every year."

The deeply concerned minister was only enlightened when he heard laughter at the other end of the line.

things, as well as the tribulations of his life, is always beguiling. Friends
and strangers alike respond to his expansive charm, and many a dreary
life has been brightened by the antics of a lively *Phosphorus.*

All this excitement and stimulation may undermine his health,
however, and the adolescent begins to suffer from headaches, insomnia, and nervousness; or, more subtly, he loses his emotional stability
and mental cohesion (discussed in a later section). The younger child
may even fall ill from anticipation or excitement: of such happy events
as Christmas, participating in a school play, or a birthday party. Or he
remains sleepless and overwrought from elation long *after* the pleasurable event.

Even the adult may retain some of the uninhibited spontaneity that
is usually found only in children. He is the free spirit ("freedom of
spirit": Hahnemann) who blithely and light-heartedly flits through life,
the Peter Pan who refuses to grow up. This emotional youthfulness finds
a happy parallel on the physical plane: both men and women can look
remarkably young for their age, retaining the shiny eyes, glowing skin,
good hair color, and the alert and sprightly manner of a younger person. And, like the *Phosphorus* child, they can be cheerful and look well
even during the most serious diseases.

However, the adult can be "capricious" (Hahnemann) or childishly
aware only of himself, his passing needs and moods, and unable to bear
any responsibility. The type is not emotionally superficial; his feelings
run strong and true. What he professes he genuinely feels—at the
moment—but he may lack the emotional steadfastness to sustain those
feelings under stress. Nor is he deterred from doing what he wants by
excess consciousness of duty or feelings of guilt.

A woman in her early thirties came to the physician for chronic
low-grade vertigo associated with faintness and periodic neuralgic
headaches. Since her condition had several possible remedies, and as
she was otherwise healthy, the physician concentrated on obtaining
a good mental picture as a guide to the simillimum. The woman was
open and trusting, and soon confided to him her boredom with her
family and household obligations. "Nobody wants me to do what *I* want
to do, and everyone wants me to do what I *don't* want to do; I want
to feel free to do what I want when I want," was her mock spoilt-child
cry, and yet her mother and husband constantly helped her with the

housework at the expense of their own interests and obligations. Then she added perceptively, "I really would make a much better grandmother than I do a mother. I would have the children brought to me, not to be disciplined, educated and cared for, but to be pampered, loved and enjoyed. Then they would be taken away until I wanted them back again." Homoeopathic *Phosphorus* not only cured the patient's physical problem but—despite the tug of her free spirit—enabled her more easily to accept her maternal and wifely responsibilities.

Such reluctance to feel shackled, or to be curtailed in the enjoyment of life, was manifested quite differently in an eleven-year-old boy. Highly popular among his peers, he was always being nominated for class president, yet each time would refuse to run for office. His reason was that he enjoyed above all being liked. The presidency would involve disciplining his classmates for poor behavior, which he was reluctant to do. He preferred to remain popular and the target of no one's envy or resentment. Also, he loved having fun, and, as president, would have had to relinquish opportunities for mischief. Altogether, he preferred remaining a child to assuming the responsibilities of adulthood. There was no arguing with such self-knowledge. Some *Phosphorus* individuals who are less in tune with themselves will not decline the honor of public office even if they dislike the attached responsibility. Wanting to dance but not to pay the fiddler, they will then fall down on the job.

Curiously enough, those around *Phosphorus* not only indulge him, but almost seem to conspire to keep him immature. His enjoyable company, his overt gratitude toward, and attractive response to, those whom he graciously allows to spoil him, encourage them to humor and care for him, at times to his own detriment. What is appealing in a youth may lose its charm with age. Others may weary of the adult who moves through life with a child's solipsistic awareness and counting on others to bail him out of any difficulty.

Phosphorus can be *unreliable* about keeping appointments or showing up at a rendezvous. With the best will in the world, somewhere along the way he becomes distracted, or a more pressing matter captures his impressionable mind, and he forgets his original commitment. He is also incapable of carrying through a task. Although marvelous at initiating projects and inspiring others (it is surprisingly difficult to refuse to go along with *Phosphorus*), all too frequently his initiatives come to nothing ("little staying power": Whitmont). Either he loses interest and concentration, or he will claim that there was not enough time to complete the work begun, supporting this with convincing arguments. But as everyone else realizes, he always finds time to do what he really wants to do; it is merely a question of his priorities.

This same pattern recurs throughout his life: the initial enthusiasm, the strong start, the impressive gesture, then the withdrawal halfway through, with the good intentions only imperfectly realized. He habitually promises more than he can deliver, leaving the followers and supporters he has swept along with him in the lurch. He also unrealistically assents to whatever is asked of him, because he *does* intend to carry through. His heart is in the right place. Yet, despite the most generous impulses, he may remain remiss in practice ("actions are contradictory to intentions": Boenninghausen).

Sometimes, however, he can be manipulative, conveniently using his image of good will to gain advantage without any intention of fulfilment. Typically, the individual will say, "I *really* would like to help you, and you can count on me any other time. But today I just cannot. I *must* go to . . . and so on." When this happens repeatedly, the true nature of the individual's kindness becomes apparent. Or the unreliable *Phosphorus* is so carried away by wishes and good intentions that he claims to have performed some task which has manifestly never been done. A patient who desperately wanted to support a benefit performance for a favorite cause reserved twenty-five seats insisting that this number of persons were already committed to attending; but on the day of the concert he arrived with two companions—and twenty-two seats went to waste.

The homoeopathic remedy, however, can help to moderate this unreliability. One patient habitually forgot to meet her young nephews at the train station on their way home from boarding school, although she had willingly volunteered to do this. The young boys were left stranded in an unfamiliar city, not knowing what to do or where to go. After constitutional treatment with *Phosphorus* for recurrent insomnia (described by her characteristically as: "I can't sleep if I'm happy, and I can't get to sleep if I'm sad; and I can't get to sleep if I'm in between and can't decide which I am"), she became almost as trustworthy and punctual as an *Arsenicum*.

Another form of *Phosphorus* unreliability is over money—his own and others'. He himself will be spontaneously generous with both money and his possessions, freely giving the coat off his back to an admiring friend, a needy relative, or even a stranger. The limit of his largesse is, in general, set only by the size of his purse, as he does not care about money per se. If he has it, he spends it like water and shares with others. If he doesn't have it, he borrows it. If he can't borrow it, he somehow manages without. He may also forget to repay borrowed money but believes that others should be as carefree or unconcerned as he is. In fact, he may be scornful of the lender for remembering ancient history. "How uncouth to recall such petty, mercenary details when there are so many wonderful things going on in life!"

The individual may go out of his way to return favors, often with some endearing or dramatic flourish. One woman owed her physician a substantial amount of money. Since she was the family breadwinner and, as a free-lance artist, carried no medical insurance, the physician did not press her. One day she landed a good job, and the money started coming in, but rather than paying off her debts, she invited the physician, together with some other friends (presumably those to whom she owed money), to a lavish dinner at a good restaurant followed by an evening at the theater. Thus her money was spent as fast as she earned it while her debts remained unpaid. In this she exhibited the *Phosphorus* penchant for gestures. It is far more effective to splurge on friends and be regarded as a "Lady Bountiful" than drearily to repay one's debts — and also cheaper; *Phosphorus* can be shrewd at sensing what is both enjoyable and expedient.

The Performer

He has a performer's temperament. Beneath his genuine sociability lies the need for an audience, whether of one or of thousands, for whom he is prepared to supply entertainment and affection and to give his all. For he needs others' appreciation and attention to bring out the best in his own nature and to feel alive.

"Snoopy" from the *Peanuts* comic strip is a born *Phosphorus* entertainer, with his serial improvisations as athlete, author, scout leader, attorney, World War I ace pilot, etc. *Phosphorus* also is his infectious self-love. For example, after completing one of his primitive short stories, Snoopy the Author is shown wriggling his toes in delight as he beamingly exclaims, "It's exciting when you've written something you

know is *really* good," or "Wow, how do I do it!" Even when entertaining others, *Phosphorus* is his own most appreciative audience.

This performer mentality was displayed in a seven-year-old girl
emerging, with the aid of homoeopathic *Opium*, from several weeks
of unconsciousness after sustaining a severe head injury. Her first words
were, "Look at me! Look at me!" as she smiled and excitedly clapped
her hands while the doctors and nurses around her bed were peering
down in concern. Even in her critical condition, she derived inspiration from an audience, and from then on she remained the star of the
hospital ward. This behavior indicated to the physician that *Phosphorus*
would be the principal remedy to start and sustain her on the long road
to recovery.

A high proportion of actors and other performers in the arts have
Phosphorus characteristics. They excel not only through their innate
artistry, natural stage presence, and love of an audience, but also because
they never tire of performing. Other constitutional types with equal
talent eventually weary of hearing themselves act, sing, play, and being
applauded. They give up their draining careers as performers to go into
teaching, directing or management. They may even remain amateurs
because they cannot take the glare of life behind the footlights. Not
so *Phosphorus*. His energy is refueled by applause and, like *Arsenicum*,
he stays on to dominate the stage and screen.

There was much of this remedy in the great pianist, Artur Rubinstein, who graced the concert hall for over seventy-five years and finally
retired only because of blindness. His ebullient and entertaining nature
is graphically revealed in his autobiography where, with undisguised
self-fascination, he describes in loving detail what seems to be every
gourmet meal, every wine, and every woman he ever enjoyed throughout an amazingly productive life. While he talks of his many loves, the
reader quickly senses that this great performer was most in love with
himself. The *Phosphorus* in him makes for lively comments and fascinating anecdotes, but the book also reveals the typical *Phosphorus*
weakness: the bubbling flow of gossip, famous names, and humorous
incidents, while eminently entertaining, leaves the reader with the sensation of having consumed too much tea and pastries—surfeit without
nourishment.

In the person with a strong urge to entertain one method of attracting an audience is *self-dramatization*. We have already noted how

these children dramatize their tantrums; the adult also infuses with drama and romance, or magnifies into near-disasters, even such every-day occurrences as milk boiling over on the stove, while the more important events in his life become endowed with cosmic signficance. The lovable and expansive Mr. Micawbar in Dickens' *David Copper-field* is a comically dramatic *Phosphorus*. Ever on the verge of certain financial collapse, ever promoting some new and grandiose scheme, with his high-falutin' language and irrepressible nature (calling himself the "ruined vestiges as yet remain of a fallen tower"), he is invariably either confronting some new crisis or sinking into dramatic despair. It does not matter which: whenever he appears, the spotlight is always on Mr. Micawbar.

On the negative side, the *Phosphorus* penchant for histrionics can degenerate into hysterics, exhibitionism, and the courting of difficulty and danger to exploit the attention and sympathy of others. The individual is secretly proud of his untoward behavior and its power to cause commotion in others' lives. One teen-aged girl was subject to just such periodic, hysterical outbursts. When feeling ignored, she would erupt in impassioned weeping, "Oh, I am so selfish and difficult, so utterly hopeless. No wonder nobody likes me. But I *do* want to change and improve. I hate the way I am . . . " She would cry and run on in this way, exciting herself more and more, until others had to rally around and give her the reassurance she was demanding. Eventually these continued outbursts became tiresome, as she came from a large family and was receiving more than her share of attention. One dose of *Phosphorus* 1M virtually eliminated her selfish histrionics. While she remained a *Phosphorus*, and would still occasionally come rushing into the house, doubled up in real or imagined pain, moaning, "I'm poisoned! I'm going to die! I must have eaten at least a gallon of chocolate ice-cream [one of the remedy's strongest cravings], and now my whole liver is on fire! I can just picture those big black holes the chocolate must have made in it—if that's what *does* happen to the liver . . . ", now she was dramatizing in the spirit of play and was a pleasure to have around (her parents reported) instead of being draining. Although still exuberant, she was in every respect more emotionally controlled.

The homoeopathic physician does not seek to *change* a patient's character with his remedies but rather, by modifying its tone, to *enhance* it. The notes remain the same, but the piece is now played well instead of badly.

Phosphorus is thus kind, intuitive, charming, magnetic, and artistic; he loves people and life and has a sense of humor. Yet, for all these qualities, the one who is so eminently capable of helping and pleasing others may be unable to put his own house in order.

Sometimes he seems to spread himself too thin or extend himself too much. Other constitutional types, even those of a giving nature, instinctively learn how to husband their resources, leaving something for themselves. But the impulsive *Phosphorus*, in his anxiety to please, knows little of emotional moderation: constantly giving out and over-extending himself, he leaves little time for taking in.

In one of the striking parallels between physical and mental symptoms often encountered in homoeopathic practice, the *Phosphorus* overflow of feelings and emotions is correlated with a tendency to hemorrhage (the "overflow" of blood). The remedy is thus effective in epistaxis (nose-bleed), menorrhagia (profuse menses), hematochezia (rectal bleeding), hemoptysis (blood from the lungs), hematuria (urinary bleeding), as well as in hemorrhage from inflamed hemorrhoids, uterine fibroids, and gastrointestinal ulcers. Boericke suggests that it has benefited in hemophilia, and it has proved invaluable for post-operative bleeding. It cured the case of a child with hemorrhage after a tonsillectomy which conventional drugs could not control: he was given *Phosphorus* 200x in water, and his lips were wetted with it every twenty minutes for two hours until the bleeding was arrested.

The *Phosphorus* individual with a better-developed sense of self-preservation knows how to rest and refuel. He balances gregariousness with solitary pursuits and quiet moments. But others feel a constant need to be charming, likable, and responsive, to live in perpetual social motion. Hence, although they may appear successful enough in the eyes of the world, they deplete their energies and all too often become physical or emotional wrecks, living on sleeping pills and tranquilizers (also *Ignatia*).

One such case was a middle-aged actor who suffered from a protracted jaundice, having never recovered his strength, color or spirits since an acute hepatitis attack many months before. This was not surprising since, in addition to his stressful career, he pursued an intense social life, while his atrocious eating and drinking habits were concurrently undermining what little health remained. Yet he claimed to need that stimulus to nourish his art and to be psychologically "up" for performances. In a diverting slip of the tongue, he said one day that his liver had "just given up on me." He meant to say "given out," but one could easily envisage the exhausted, exasperated, maltreated liver deciding, in mute protest, to stop functioning. Unlike the stronger *Sulphur*, who can be socially indefatigable and professionally productive without apparent adverse effects, *Phosphorus* is constituted more delicately and, when burning the candle at both ends, begins to pay a price for too high or too irregular living.

Constitutional treatment with the remedy in ascending potencies slowed the patient's social pace somewhat, permitting him to direct the bulk of his energy into his art. He did not become a recluse, but the edge was taken off his nervous, depleting need to socialize, without in the least dimishing him as an actor.

Intellect and Understanding

Phosphorus is seldom a bookish academic. Although his initial grasp of intellectual matters is as good as anyone's, and better than some, his mental cast is predominantly intuitive and artistic. Unless heavily alloyed with the deep intellectual bent of *Sulphur* or *Lycopodium*, the solid, dogged intellect of *Natrum muriaticum*, or the critical acuteness of *Arsenicum* or *Lachesis*, *Phosphorus* can be an intellectual lightweight ("devoid of mental firmness": Whitmont). Like a butterfly, flitting from flower to flower, he skims the surface of things, tastefully sipping here and there, in contrast to the true scholars, the caterpillars who for long periods of time grub away in the academic soil searching for a new idea and then assiduously weave their own intellectual cocoons (*Sulphur*). Generally speaking, this constitutional type is weak in disciplines requiring subordination of inspiration or intuition to conceptual understanding; and, other than in the performing arts, where he can take certain liberties, he dislikes subjugating the freedom and spontaneity of his imagination to any rigorous method or system.

Some display a catchy eclecticism, attractively parroting the thoughts of others, which makes them seem more intelligent than they are. The mind is so agile and responsive, so sensitively tuned to the wavelengths of others, as to obscure the fact that the individual's basic comprehension is defective. However, the *Phosphorus* of stronger intellect, while remaining a popularizer of ideas, will inject his own intuition to come up with something original, playing the role of Engels to the *Sulphur* Marx.

He is often an excellent teacher, receiving enthusiastic comments on student evaluation forms. Inspired by the audience, he inspires it in return, infecting others with his own enthusiasm. He possesses that invaluable quality of a teacher—the gift of *suggestion* with which he stimulates thought. Performer that he is, he communicates with his whole personality: eyes, gestures, and tone of voice, in a way that transcends mere words. Even when his teaching is not illuminated by logic or intellect, even if, as sometimes happens, the thoughts are muddled and refractive, some instinctive and intuitive quality in him remains right and true; the audience senses what he is trying to convey and what he really means.

Despite his intuitive brightness, *Phosphorus* may have severe limitations of understanding. Trusting and somewhat naive, he is misled by surface appearances, unable to learn from experience, and repeatedly misjudges people and situations.

This is partly because he is headstrong, willful, and heedless of advice. He rushes into impractical ventures and does not tolerate efforts to restrain him ("flies into a passion when opposed": Hering). He exhibits what has been called a "whim of iron"—a strong wishfulness combined with an unrestrained determination to act upon impulse ("I will do what I want to do, and no one is going to stop me!").

Wildly optimistic about some new project one day and abandoning it the next, easily influenced by the latest fashion to come down the pike or adopting too easily the enthusiasms or ideas of someone he particularly likes, he jumps from one interest to another. He does not lack discernment in his own particular field or vocation—it is when he plunges into foreign waters that his judgment flounders woefully. His impressionable psyche is excited by too many different stimuli, and his generous nature sees too much good in too many things. For instance, the patient will espouse first one medical therapy, then another, some legitimate, some verging on quackery. *Arsenicum* also has this tendency, but his more systematic mind leads him to stick with whatever he finds satisfactory. *Phosphorus* plunges into any and all cures, from faith-healers and laying-on-of-hands to fig juice and almond diets, insisting (with enormous conviction) that whichever one he is currently espousing cures all illnesses—"from the common cold to cancer." Each therapy he embraces becomes, in turn, *the* answer to all human ills rather than just *an* answer to some.*

Thus, *Phosphorus* enthusiasms are strong and contagious but, like many enthusiasms, may not endure ("easily enthused, but without perseverence": Whitmont). Living, feeling, experiencing primarily for the moment, he embraces the evanescent present or his transient feelings as the entire truth. He does not employ the faculty of memory to gain perspective or as the intellectual ballast to the emotions that it is meant to be. Completely forgetting his previous fads, he hails each new one as a revelation and pursues it with the same abandon. This type does not easily learn that instincts, impulses, and enthusiasms must sometimes be controlled rather than encouraged.

The patient under psychiatric treatment demonstrates another facet of *Phosphorus'* inability to learn. Despite years of therapy he may remain as confused as ever, with little progress in self-knowledge or understanding. Maybe he perceives the psychiatrist as an audience rather than a source of enlightenment, an opportunity to talk about himself rather than to change. Or perhaps he is just not willing to tarnish his glowing self-image with unpalatable truths. No one likes to face these truths, but *Phosphorus* responds with total denial (*Lycopodium*). At the same time, since his actions and manner are quite open and transparent, and he seldom tries to hide his nature, he ends by deceiving himself far more than others.

A diverting example of the individual's dislike of admitting weakness or failure was a minor-circuit concert pianist who had regular homoeopathic constitutional treatment to keep himself, as it were, finely tuned. While talented, he was a temperamental performer and could

---

* The philosopher William James, whose charming mercurial nature exhibited a strong *Phosphorus* streak, was just such a medical enthusiast, not to say hypochondriac. He travelled the world seeking different cures for his elusive ailments. Yet it was this same open and eclectic *Phosphorus* quality that prompted him to speak out against the closed allopathic mind and to defend homoeopathy in an address before the Massachusetts legislature. While he did not understand it fully, his fine intuition sensed its profound truth, and he urged physicians to investigate it (see Harris L. Coulter, *Divided Legacy*, Vol. III).

never confess to a poor recital. When he could not ignore an unfavorable review, he blamed it on the piano (out of tune or of poor quality), the orchestra (underrehearsed), the conductor (off tempo). Or (as a final resort) the audience and critics were blamed for inability to appreciate his innovative interpretation.

But the homoeopathic remedy can broaden the individual's understanding and encourage his self-awareness. A case in point was the woman being treated for a persistent bronchial inflammation and who presented with what she called her "graveyard cough"—deep, hollow, gasping, and sounding as if it indeed came up from the depths of the underworld. *Phosphorus* is only one of several excellent remedies for clearing up long-standing chest conditions (some others are *Tuberculinum, Sulphur,* and *Calcarea carbonica*). Her physical symptoms fitted each of these remedies to some extent, but when she started discussing her recently dissolved marriage, the simillimum became apparent. She recounted most convincingly what a good wife she had been to her difficult husband, how generous and attractive he (and other men) had always found her until he so inexplicably departed. There was little self-searching about possible reasons for his desertion. As the other symptoms suited *Phosphorus* well enough, she received a dose in 1M potency and was told to come back in three weeks. When she returned, the cough was gone and her health improved, but above all, her understanding had grown. She said she had done some *serious* thinking (adding, with a rueful smile, that it was perhaps for the first time in her life), and concluded that she, too, had not been so easy to live with. Now she realized that in a subtle way she had put too many demands on her husband. Gone were the recriminations and the self-justifications. She had transcended her egocentricity and was able to see another's point of view.

In *Phosphorus* mental confusion can arise from an over-impressionable imagination. Not only does he too readily believe whatever he is told, but he persuades himself that his fantasies are true. His own version of reality is so much closer to his feelings and desires that it becomes irresistibly plausible, and he confuses it with fact.

A patient was being unsuccessfully treated with *Arsenicum* and *Natrum muriaticum* for hay-fever symptoms when, at the third visit, he mentioned owning an electronic gadget which purportedly counteracted harmful radio waves in the air. So healing was it (he said) that when he carried it to work on the subway in the morning, people crowded around him, unconsciously attracted by its healing rays. This was highly interesting! But he seemed oblivious of the fact that on the subway during rush hour people would have crowded round him if he had been carrying a ripe Limburger cheese. After hearing this story the physician started him on *Phosphorus*, with much more gratifying results.

Sometimes *Phosphorus* is carried away unwittingly by his active or "excited imagination" (Boenninghausen). At other times he embroiders reality deliberately. He cannot resist making some incident just a little more colorful, to give others greater pleasure or to make a statement more interesting. One patient sometimes maintained that he "never slept a wink all night" and, at other times, that his sleep was "so deep and death-like as to be almost frightening." He gave different versions on different visits. The obvious fact that he alternated between sleeping well and sleeping badly was just too pale a rendition of reality. Nor is the individual loathe to employ his supposed telepathic sensibilities in a convenient manner. It is much more dramatic to ascribe one's inclinations and actions to clairvoyance, inner voices, and the prompting of spirits, than to say that one does or does not do something merely out of desire. Whatever the underlying motives, when facts fail him fancy, waiting in the wings, is ready to step on stage.*

---

* What should the physician do when the patient does not tell him the truth? Since homoeopathic prescribing relies on an accurate account of the patient's symptoms, the inaccurate reporting of symptoms would seem to be a bar. The usual assumption that the patient comes in to be helped, so why should he *not* tell the truth? — is inadequate, in view of the propensity of *Phosphorus* and some other types (especially *Lycopodium* and *Natrum muriaticum*) to conceal facts from the physician. All that can be said is that the physician learns to take this into account and use it as an indication, since the different constitutional types conceal or distort for different reasons. *Natrum muriaticum* conceals *deliberately*, for personal and protective reasons (he does not want the physician to probe the inner recesses of his mind); *Lycopodium* dissimulates out of determination to maintain his image of strength or virtue, i.e., to save face; *Phosphorus* is frequently simply confused or unaware of the truth in his own mind.

Not surprisingly, the individual of strong intellect, with his vivid fancy, heightened imagination, and artistic talent, makes a good fiction writer. In English literature alone, such female authors as Jane Austen, Emily Brontë, Virginia Woolf, and Katherine Mansfield; such male authors as Charles Dickens and Joyce Cary; and the poet John Keats, all display a strong *Phosphorus* streak (poetic geniuses, who tend to mature early and draw inspiration from their own intuitions and emotions rather than from intellectual development and experience, frequently exhibit characteristics of this remedy). In fiction, where the confusion of imagination and reality is sublimated in a higher reality, the *Phosphorus* imagination—which in everyday life may depart from veracity—is brought into the service of artistic truth.

To take but one example, the physical and emotional picture of Jane Austen (from the little we know of her secluded life) well fits the personality type. Contemporaries commented on her refined physical appearance and delicate features, her extraordinarily lustrous eyes and vivacious manner. She was a born mimic and storyteller, entertaining her family with dramatic readings from her novels. She exhibited the *Phosphorus* tendency to faint from sudden emotion (as when she learned that her family was moving from her beloved home to Bath). Moreover, she died of Addison's disease, for which *Phosphorus* has always been one of the principal remedies (Boericke).

Elizabeth Bennet in *Pride and Prejudice* is the most prominently *Phosphorus* of Austen's heroines. Her liveliness and brightness, energy and charm, reflect this element at its best, as do her mental refinement and wit, her wholesome optimism, and her buoyant refusal to be depressed by vexing relations or circumstances. The author's own comment on her heroine is also typical of the nature's self-appreciation: "I must confess I think her as delightful a creature as ever appeared in print, and how I shall be able to tolerate those who do not like her . . . I do not know."

Furthermore, the language of *Pride and Prejudice* is true to the type: spirited, vivacious, effervescent, the wit anchored in that special luminescent style. Austen herself remarked in self-critique: "The work is rather too light, bright and sparkling: it wants shade, it wants to be stretched here and there with a long chapter of sense." In actuality, the novel's emotional subtlety and depth, the effect of its many layers of irony, exemplify the *Phosphorus* imaginative talent raised to the highest genius.

Love Life

Loss of perspective, lack of proportion, confusion of mind, and overdevelopment of the imagination are sometimes revealed in the *Phosphorus* love life, especially in women. Their willingness to be carried away by enthusiasm finds ample scope here, and *Phosphorus* has a notorious tendency to perceive in those she loves more qualities than they actually possess. Like Titania in Shakespeare's *A Midsummer-Night's Dream* who has received a love potion which makes her see beauty even in an ass's head, she credits the love object with what she *wants* to see in it. Although this is hardly an unusual characteristic of persons in an enamored state, the emotionally susceptible *Phosphorus* nourishes more extreme illusions than most.

These patients recount their current lover's attributes with a sincerity that is never quite matched by accuracy (he speaks eight or nine languages, plays with virtuosity on a dozen musical instruments, exerts a major, though clandestine, influence on world events, etc.). And the same goes for relationships other than romantic: *Phosphorus* will often choose to be impressed by a friend, colleague, relative, or child, projecting onto the beloved all her own benevolence, generosity, and talent. Incapable of seeing his defects, she then harbors expectations impossible for the other to meet, and these exaggerated expectations can ultimately have an adverse effect on the relationship.

Phosphorus in love possesses little remembrance of having previously felt the same way about another. Each time is the first time, the "real thing," and each time is forever. The young person has an appetite for emotional stimuli and physical thrills and is prone to strong crushes, at times getting involved early in romantic adventures. Even the older individual is a romantic (*Tuberculinum, Ignatia*) and cultivates the idea of being "in love," with its accompanying emotional soarings and plummetings, as he seeks to sustain the intensity of passion. A history of multiple marriages (three or more) or numerous liaisons immediately suggests this remedy, as does a tendency to adolescent-like infatuations, an erratic love life that keeps the patient in a state of turmoil, or being perpetually in a state of "spring fever."*

---

* During a lecture on *Natrum muriaticum*, which emphasized the strongly monogamous nature of this type, a young *Phosphorus* girl stu-

"Nymphomania" and "satyriasis" are words used in the materia medica to describe the sexuality of *Phosphorus*; also, "wildly passionate," "violent sexual excitement, seeking to satisfy his sexual instincts on no matter whom," "shameless, erotic mania" (Hahnemann, Hering). These terms are too strong for most cases encountered in everyday practice (although one male patient did claim to be a "veritable fiend" in bed), but elements of what Hering pithily calls "excessive amativeness" can be detected in *Phosphorus* patients ("Some part of me desires to run away with every attractive man/woman I meet").

The girl can be a regular honey-pot, attracting men like flies with her openly enticing manner. The pretty fluffhead, Katie, in Ring Lardner's *The Big Town*, with "welcome embroidered on her pan" and who falls in love with every young man she meets, is a comically superficial *Phosphorus*. A more serious portrayal of the type's sex appeal is Natasha Rostova in Tolstoy's *War and Peace*. The author beautifully captures her spontaneity and sexuality, whether playing with her doll as a young girl, admiring the stars at night, attending her first ball, or responding to the overtures of a practiced seducer. This appeal is, to be sure, not limited to females; *Phosphorus* males can have the same inviting manner and responsive look, which is immediately felt by the opposite sex.

Yet the sexual drive is only partially responsible for the marital instability of this type and its search for new gratification. Egocentrism and self-love also play a role: how better to satisfy a need for admiration, and be the center of another's life, than in a love relationship? However, when the admirer's initial all-enveloping infatuation wanes, when love necessarily takes its place among the other elements of daily life, *Phosphorus* may rebel against the emotional sameness of marriage and seek to regain the former emotional excitement through a variety of new stimuli (Flaubert summed up the romantic dilemma of his *Phosphorus* heroine, Emma Bovary, when he wrote: "She found in adultery

---

dent came up to the speaker and eagerly said, "Now I *know* I am *Natrum muriaticum*, I am completely monogamous by nature." "That's strange," he replied, "I've known you for five years, and during that time you've had easily as many boyfriends." "Yes," she replied, her expressive eyes alight, "but it has always been only one at a time."

all the platitudes of marriage").* Patients will admit to the subliminal thought: "I'm so attractive, affectionate, and giving that it's a shame to limit myself to just one person. I want to give myself to many." Of course, the performing arts—particularly the theater and the screen— offer a perfect sublimated outlet for such feelings.

The "Shadow" Side

The impressionable nature, so capable of rapture and elation, is also prone to depressions. And surprisingly, in view of what has been said of his sparkle, *Phosphorus* is also subject to *ennui* (which remedy should be added to the Kent *Repertory* under that rubric). His very ebullience and joie de vivre, and the continual need for company, some-

---

* In *Anna Karenina* Tolstoy explores his heroine's *Phosphorus* love mentality in even greater depth. Her attempt to preserve the intensity of romantic love is doomed to disappointment. When her lover, Vronskii, no longer responds with his former passion, when she is no longer the only focus of his thoughts and life, she is unable to shift down to a quieter level of love. She magnifies Vronskii's (to him) natural loss of passionate adulation into rejection, her despondency grows, and she begins to vacillate between loving abandon and unreasonable demands in an overwrought way that resembles *Lachesis*. All the while she tries to keep intact their original all-consuming passion and resents Vronskii when she fails. Yet, being an affectionate *Phosphorus*, who needs to give as well as to receive love, she cannot live with the emotional discord she herself creates (in contrast to *Lachesis*, who can), and her subliminal emotional instability emerges with her disappointment. Losing control over her feelings and behavior, Anna plummets into despair. Distraught and hysterical, she takes her own life by throwing herself under a train. Although the picture is complicated by the illicitness of the relationship, her guilt vis-a-vis her beloved son, and the heavy moral and social opprobrium that overwhelms her, Anna's conduct throughout the affair and her response to her dilemma are *Phosphorus*.

A pertinent element of literary background is that Tolstoy's original intention, as seen in his notebooks, was to depict Anna as an evil seductress who rightly suffered for her moral transgressions. But, as he wrote, her warmth, charm and kind impulses (i.e., her *Phosphorus* nature) began to take over and acquire a life of their own; and she ends by eliciting sympathy and compassion rather than censure.

times seem subconscious defenses against the grimly hovering spectre of boredom.

This may be why *Phosphorus* is one of the finest remedies for adolescents. Its mental picture precisely reflects their roller-coaster emotions, inability to concentrate on studies, and unfocussed, undirected energies. The remedy also suits the adolescent's strong but short-lived enthusiasms, and need for emotional excitement, to escape the boredom that too easily descends on him. Physically, as well, it befits the thin, drooping, narrow-chested, delicate or anaemic youth whose strength cannot support his fast-growing frame, but who is restless and fidgety despite his weariness. He craves ice-cream, chocolate, and anything with a zesty or salty flavor (this is true for *Phosphorus* at any age); he desires cold, sweet drinks for quick energy and to relieve his hot, burning feeling inside (*Sulphur*). Occasional doses of the remedy administered to this type throughout the difficult adolescent years can help make this period considerably less stressful.

The *Phosphorus* "down" may be a natural reaction to his "up." Living, as he does, in a state of exaltation ("ecstasy and excited imagination": Hering) and, like Aesop's grasshopper, consuming all the happiness and life around him, he must at some point descend. And when this happens, he sinks into the depths of "loathing of life," "deep despondency," and "suicidal despair" (Hering), "sadness and dejection; surfeit of life; disconsolate sorrowfulness" (Hahnemann). Other constitutional types also suffer from low spirits and intense depression. But, whereas *Natrum muriaticum* still puts on a brave face when depressed; *Lachesis* retains some vital quality despite his troubles; *Arsenicum*, although despairing, still knows best and tells the doctor what to do; and *Nux vomica* is seldom too "down" to cease being angry and irritable, or *Sepia* to complain—*Phosphorus* becomes withdrawn, reluctant to attend the social gatherings that he previously loved so much ("misanthropy": Boenninghausen), is "indolent, not disposed to do anything" (Hahnemann); or, losing all ambition, falls into "apathetic indifference" (Hering).

Although we have concentrated on the lively extroverted *Phosphorus*, the homoeopath must remain aware of this "other side of the coin" so often encountered in the polychrests. These major constitutional remedies are so rich in symptoms, so broad in function, that they embrace their opposites (what Jung called the "shadow" side). Sometimes the polarity is distributed among different patients; at other times it is found in the duality of a single individual: today strongly inclined in one direction, tomorrow inclined equally strongly in the opposite. Age is definitely a contributing factor to the *Phosphorus* polarity. With hardship and degenerating health, the effervescent, sparkling side becomes dim, and the despondent "shadow" side emerges.

A woman in her mid-forties came to be treated for intensifying cardiac symptoms. She had palpitations accompanied by anxiety about impending death. She was worse lying down at night, especially on her left side. At times her chest felt oppressed as if by a weight; at other times there was violent throbbing as if (to use her words) wild horses were galloping there and she was trying to rein them in. This was all typically *Phosphorus*. But then the mentals were so unlike!

She acted sour (*Sepia*), imagined wrongs (*Natrum muriaticum*), and whined (*Pulsatilla*). So the physician asked her husband about her youth. Indeed, she had been a happy bright-eyed youngster and, when older, a "life-of-the-party" type, ebullient and highly attractive to the opposite sex. Little of this remained now. The spirited *Phosphorus* personality was buried somewhere deep beneath the crust formed by her hard life and developing illness. But, predictably, as her cardiac symptoms improved with the remedy, she became more cheerful and regained some of her former buoyancy.

Another case was slightly different: a self-centered and garrulous middle-aged woman being treated with *Lachesis* for arthritis of the fingers. The remedy had cured most of her pain and discomfort but was unable to eliminate the stiffness and pain of the last two fingers of her left hand. She obviously needed a different constitutional remedy. On the following visit she walked into the office and announced to the young (female) physician in charge of her case, "Good morning! My love life is terrific! I have two boyfriends who, although together they do not entirely satisfy me, still make me feel wonderful! Now, tell me all about *your* boyfriends!" This was a completely new side to her character. A lighter, easier-to-be-around, layer of her personality was emerging, and for the first time she could listen to others. The *Lachesis* had worked its way back to her younger *Phosphorus* years, as the layers of her accumulated troubles peeled away. All signs now pointed to *Phosphorus* which did indeed resolve the case.

Confusion of Identity

Like the restless element from which the remedy derives, the *Phosphorus* individual may appear volatile and unsettled, without a grip on reality (ungrounded). Wanting focus and direction, his mind seems to wander around at some more rarefied level of the atmosphere. Even his eyes sometimes have the far-away expression, the ethereal gleam, of one who sees above and beyond ordinary mortals or to whom some special revelation has been vouchsafed.

This *instability* may stem from the lack of a well-defined center to the *Phosphorus* nature, that core or field of gravity in the psyche which sifts, sorts, and interprets information and impressions so as to make them meaningful. In labile *Phosphorus,* constantly responding to his environment, the essential "I"—the selecting, binding, unifying principle—is not solid. The individual is a psychic sponge, his heightened responsiveness soaking up, almost at random, the various impressions that invade and bombard him from the external world. To him everything is equally exciting. There is no *center* to which impressions can be referred; they remain diffused throughout his entire being without coalescing into a structure ("abundant flow of ideas which she finds difficult to arrange": Hahnemann), and he gives the impression of being out of rapport with himself.

Certainly, any constitutional type undergoing stress, trauma, or change can be, or appear, unstable, but with *Phosphorus* the condition tends to be chronic. He is a bright child whose intuitions are too quick for his mind to control and whose impressions have no conceptual structure to give them meaning. Thus he can be overwhelmed by his intuitions and emotions before he has had time to put them in intellectual order. Whitmont describes him as "a drifting straw, an almost helpless victiim of outer influences and inner emotions."

In many an unsettled or uncentered patient the *Phosphorus* guiding symptom has been the time-of-day modality. Twilight, that ambiguous interval between day and night, is the emotional low point of the day for this type: "many anxieties in the evening; sadness at twilight" (Hahnemann), "restless at twilight" (Hering); it can provoke anexacerbation of physical symptoms as well—although the opposite modality, marked "amelioration of symptoms at twilight" (Kent), is occasionally encountered.* Whitmont has likened the *Phosphorus* mental state to "inner twilight"—a semi-anesthetized mode in which the individual is not wholly in the conscious world but hovers between consciousness (light) and unconsciousness (darkness). This mode provokes the surfacing of such instinctive ("twilight") states of consciousness as clairvoyance, clairaudience, and ecstasy.

Accordingly, *Phosphorus* is the classic remedy for "ill effects from anesthesia" (Guernsey), the "twilight zone" of consciousness. It relieves the vomiting, headaches, and mental derangement that may follow. It also aids the patient who cannot fully emerge from under its influence.

The type's instability is accentuated by his tendency to overempathize with—even to assume—aspects of his environment, to reach out and respond to others or, in his attempts to gratify everyone, to go through life playing different roles. His search for ever more novel spiritual and emotional stimuli, the effort to ascertain who he really is, may involve him in continual psychological ambiguity, leading to chronic "confusion over his own identity" (Kent). Like many a fine actor, he is uncertain which role to play in private life ("I don't know who I am . . . I don't really know what I think or feel . . . I am such a chameleon that I can never get my own act together . . . I have such a tendency to relate to others' personalities that I lose contact with my own . . . What is reality? Am I living in a fantasy world? . . . " are characteristic remarks). The prominent *Phosphorus* symptom, "desires company" (Boenninghausen), could thus be viewed less as a *Pulsatilla*-like need for everyday support than as a dread, when alone, of losing his conscious identity (his Ego). The presence of others grounds him and "helps to strengthen the accustomed reality against invasion from the darker [unconscious] strata [the Id]" (Whitmont).

The short-story writer, Katherine Mansfield, who herself had a many-faceted personality that lacked cohesion (in her Bohemian existence she experimented with a variety of life-styles and flirted with different religious paths) put in a nutshell the dilemma of the *Phosphorus* identity. In response to the famous advice of Polonius to his

---

* Tolstoy's unerring instinct had the *Phosphorus* Anna Karenina's despondency and hysteria escalate to a daily pitch at twilight, and this was also the time when she committed suicide.

son, Laertes (in Shakespeare's *Hamlet*), "This, above all, to thine own self be true . . . " Mansfield wrote, "True to oneself—which self?"

To be sure, not all who are part actors, part spectators observing themselves perform, or of a mercurial, "artistic" temperament, are subject to confusion of identity. A case in point is Benjamin Disraeli, twice Prime Minister of England and long-time leader of the Conservative Party, who embodies many of the *Phosphorus* traits described in this chapter.

His temperament was as volatile as the element itself—"An enigma to his contemporaries and an enigma to us today," as one historian has remarked. This was due in part to the multiple facets of his personality and in part to his constant acting out of roles. He started life as an author, writing several fashionable novels, and later in life seemed almost to act out the roles of his own characters.

He wooed the staid and stolid Queen Victoria with flamboyant gallantry, exaggerated hand-kissing, acknowledging the bouquets of wild flowers she sent him with tender notes in which he called the little round tub of a woman his "faery queene." Yet she responded to this flattery and flirtatiousness with unprecedented tolerance and affection.

At the same time, while laughing at his own performance, he always knew where he stood on the larger political scene. He thus left others bemused and unable to distinguish between political genius and mere surface sparkle, while he himself played out his roles in full seriousness.

His personal life also exhibited typical *Phosphorus* characteristics. He was a notorious dandy, dressing in frilled shirts and flashy waistcoats, self-consciously and even narcissistically cultivating his own mannerisms and external appearance; even as a mummified octogenarian he remained vain of his looks, dying, waxing and elaborately curling what little remained of his hair. He exhibited the nature's sparkling wit (of his lifelong political rival he said, "Gladstone has not one redeeming defect") but appeared to be intellectually superficial—mostly froth and little substance. In youth he indulged in a series of romantic affairs, but then, finding that they interfered with his political ambitions, married a widow fifteen years older who was neither beautiful, clever, nor even particularly rich. When asked by his amazed friends the reason, he ascribed it to gratitude, "that rarest of human virtues." Indeed, earlier in his career she had helped him financially and with her political connections, she had a kind heart and, most important, she absolutely adored Disraeli. They were happily married for thirty years because she gave him what *Phosphorus* most craves: continuous, complete, and unequivocal adulation. Other types may think they want to be catered to but, unlike *Phosphorus*, often become dissatisfied once they achieve it.

Disraeli's political and personal stability despite his phosphorescent disposition undoubtedly reflects the presence in his constitution of *Arsenicum*—a type that is always aware of its own interests and identity. These two remedies, in fact, were used by the homoeopathic physician who treated the venerable statesman's severe asthma during the last few years of his life.

At times the *Phosphorus* confusion of identity leads to self-delusion, described in the homoeopathic literature as "exalted opinion of self," "exaggerated idea of own importance," or, in an intensification of the above, "egomania and megalomania." Traces of these symptoms are commonly seen in the patient who, because he senses in himself a myriad of possible achievements, overestimates the significance of success in some minor enterprise, magnifying one swallow into a whole summer.

He feels himself talented ("How is your self-confidence?" asks the physician. "No problem," is the reply. "I have plenty of that"), often rightly so, but mistakes this potential for accomplishment, confusing the fantasy of what he could do with the reality of what he has done. Thus, when he gives the impression of being foolish, this is not due to slowness or simple-mindedness (*Calcarea carbonica*) but to overestimation of his own capacities. Likewise, when a gifted *Phosphorus* fails in life, it is likely to be from overreaching and not, as with *Sulphur*, from doing nothing while expecting the world to fall into his lap. He acts with resolute energy to achieve his desires and is fertile in ideas, often displaying considerable ingenuity, but he lacks system and may not persevere. Although he senses his own capacities, he does not know how to manage them, how to follow up methodically on an initial success or correct intuition.

This is why a gifted *Phosphorus* sometimes leaves an unsatisfactory impression. He is the firecracker that takes off with a tremendous explosion and much promise but then—while all are in expectation of a dazzling display of colors—gives off a few empty bangs and an anticlimactic smoky hiss. However, as the remedy takes effect on the physical plane, the patient's attitude may slowly change. He comes to view his ventures more soberly and undertakes more realistic steps to accomplish them.

A man in his mid-thirties was treated for a burning pain in the left hip which he experienced upon walking even short distances. In one significant respect the physical symptoms of this remedy differ from the qualities of elemental phosphorus: the latter emits light without heat, while the patient often exhibits symptoms associated with "burning sensations" in affected areas of the body—head, stomach, joints, throat, chest (*Sulphur* and *Arsenicum*). He did not know how it arose and stated, "It just happened." *Phosphorus* has an affinity for the bones and is used homoeopathically in such ailments as rickets, bone pains in growing children, and sharp burning nocturnal pains in adults; it has applications in arthritis, jaw pains, bony spurs and exostoses, osteomyelitis, and tuberculous affections of the bones—all of which are well repertorized in the classic texts. Thus it naturally came to mind as a potential remedy. Furthermore, the patient was typically *Phosphorus* in appearance and manner: trim of build, with neat features, sprightly and articulate. He even had the elfish quality sometimes encountered in this type. While he worked in a government office, his true interest was photography, and he planned to be a movie cameraman.

This seemed a reasonable ambition. He apparently had talent, and one of his photographs had been selected for display in a local art show. But then, with eyes dancing, he went on to describe how he was planning to demand full artistic control over any movie on which he was working, and would insist on writing the screenplay, playing the lead, directing, as well as filming it. In the meantime he had invested much of his savings in self-promotional expenses which he thought would reap him millions but which, in fact, merely served to accrue larger and larger debts. The *Phosphorus* "exalted opinion of self" became evident, corroborating the physical symptoms, and this was the remedy he received.

Several weeks later his hip was much improved; now he felt pain only after walking long distances, and it disappeared in due course. Even more gratifying, however, were the clear signs that his labile character was stabilizing. When offered a job as assistant to a small TV documentary producer, he accepted it instead of turning it down (as he might have done formerly). From that point he continued to make solid headway toward his goal of cinematographer.

Possibly a similar outcome would have been attained over time even without the remedy, but it would probably have taken longer and been less far-reaching. As it was, this case was a graphic demonstration of the subtle but profound action of the homoeopathic remedy on a patient's psyche.

The confusion in the *Phosphorus* psychic core may be detrimental to his relations with others. For, despite his sensitivity, responsiveness, and warmth, despite his "tenderness" (Hahnemann) and talent for friendship, he is surprisingly prone to edgy personal relationships and may estrange friends, relatives, and well-wishers.

Often the rupture will have no discernible cause, and no one concerned can understand why it occurred—least of all *Phosphorus* himself who will be genuinely upset, even to the point of physical illness (headaches from "excitement of the emotions, anger": Kent). Yet, although eager in theory to do his share in maintaining relationships (in part because he is reluctant to hurt people's feelings), he subtly shifts the burden to others. He demands that they accept him on his own terms: "I am the way I am. I can't change, and others must take me as is." Only *Natrum muriaticum* equals *Phosphorus* (albeit for quite different reasons) in this uncompromising insistence on being loved and accepted for himself, defects and all.

He can also exploit the confusion attending the breakdown of a relationship, playing on the guilt, weaknesses, and feelings of the other to get his own way without appearing to do so. A spouse in a disintegrating marriage, for instance, will complain: "For fifteen years I have put up with my husbands' [or wife's] whims and self-centeredness, yet *I* am the one who feels guilty and compelled to meet all his [or her] demands, no matter how unreasonable. Why is that?" The answer is that he is confronted with the fine intuitive ability of a *Phosphorus* to maintain the psychological advantage. This often involves confusing the issue instead of calmly discussing it, constantly contradicting himself, or saying one thing and acting quite differently, so that the other does not know where he stands.

As mentioned earlier, *Phosphorus* is an expert at eliciting assistance and (like *Pulsatilla*) arousing the instinctive solicitude of others. As long as they remain under his charm and are willing to dance to his tune, he is grateful and obliging, warmly praising their character, clothes, children, looks, and tastes. But once they stop dancing, *Phosphorus* becomes argumentative, quarrelsome, capricious, "demanding and ungrateful" (Hering). If thwarted in his desires, he may resort to lies and slander, exhibiting the element's destructive potential ("incensed; when annoyed he falls into furious anger and malignancy": Hahnemann). He becomes "malicious, vindictive" (Kent), creates enemies, then vociferously trumpets his victimization, being especially liable to bring accusations against anyone to whom he is indebted. Ironically, this eminently grateful type is also unable to tolerate indebtedness (we recall that he likes to be the helpful one, to whom others are indebted) and may quarrel or sever relations with others to feel absolved of this obligation . After all, one has no moral obligations toward an enemy.

But, except for such extreme cases, *Phosphorus* does not bear grudges (unlike *Natrum muriaticum*) and will not permit ill-will to be prolonged after a disagreement. Nor does he usually break with people once and for all. Being naturally affectionate and wanting to return to the other's good graces, he will respond happily to overtures of reconciliation. Or he himself will initiate them, maintaining sincerely that he bears no hard feelings and trying to prevent a past friendship from dissolving into nothing.

The constitutional type is recognized in the patient who is likable and attractive and displays the warm and extroverted manner of one who wants to be liked and can make himself liked; who has developed and put to good use his wonderfully positive approach to people and life. He may possess a quiet charm or a brighter luminescence but will always evince that special *Phosphorus* sympathy and responsiveness that ranks compassion before justice and generosity before truth.

Yet he may also suffer from a tendency to emotional excess, lack of restraint, confusion of fantasy with reality, and uncertainty about his own identity. His imagination outweighs his understanding, his instability overrules his judgment; he believes only what he wants to believe, is governed by caprice and cannot see beyond himself. So that for all his promise and fine talents his life falls short of its potential.

The homoeopathic physician, however, is confident that many of these patients can learn, can change, can stabilize. To assist them in finding a solid basis for their lives and cohesive direction, he prescribes the homoeopathically prepared and potentized *Phosphorus*.

Calcarea Carbonica

*C*ALCAREA *carbonica* is the potentized carbonate of lime, taken from the middle layer of the oyster shell. Several images are evoked by this mollusc. First, there is the animal itself—cold, pale, moist, limp, inactive. Second, there is the shell—thick, impenetrable, fixed to a rock, protecting the completely defenseless creature within. Third, within this otherwise undistinguished creature there grows a pearl of polished and delicate beauty, born through steady concretion around an irritating grain of sand. Keeping in mind these three images: the oyster itself, the shell, and the pearl, let us examine how they relate to the *Calcarea* individual.

The Oyster

In outward appearance *Calcarea* is what is known as the "leucophlegmatic" type (Hering), described in the homoeopathic literature as unhealthy looking, chalky or pasty-faced, fair-complexioned, lymphatic, tending toward a flabby or unwieldy type of corpulence with little muscular power. The face may be pudgy or bloated, with the thick skin and puffy cheeks causing the underlying bone structure to be all but invisible. His handshake is characteristic. There seems to be no bone, no firm responding grip, as the patient offers his limp, clammy hand to the doctor.*

---

* Some experienced physicians such as Margery Blackie have claimed that the handshake alone helps to spot the constitutional remedy. She mentions the firm grateful grasp of the *Lycopodium* who has been helped, the cold dry grasp of *Arsenicum*, the *Silica* hand which is rough and cracked, with overgrown nails, the *Hepar sulphuris* hand which is as cold and damp as *Calcarea*'s but not as limp, and the sweaty *Thuja* handclasp.

The individual is chilly, sometimes extremely so, despite his fat which should keep him warm. Or he is cold in isolated or "single" (Nash) parts of the body. But it is a cold felt from the outside that merely is uncomfortable, and which can be warmed by clothes and a warm room, in contrast to the *Arsenicum* coldness which can be incapacitating, and so penetrating that he feels "as if ice-water is running through his veins" (Hering) and that he will never get warm, no matter how much clothing he wears or how closely he hugs the fire (*Silica, Nux vomica*). *Calcarea*'s skin is often lacking in tone, or moist with copious perspiration around the neck, head, and upper parts of the body, sometimes with a sour smell. After sleep the child's damp head may smell mildly of cottage cheese or more strongly of old cheese.

Indolence or "inertness" (Hering) is a key characteristic. Recall the inactive oyster, the most passive member of the mollusc family, only opening and closing its shell to take in food or to reproduce. This same sedentary nature is manifested in the *Calcarea* individual, who is lethargic and placid, neither easily aroused nor easily moved, and content to do the barest minimum. In fact, "exertion produces a jaded state—mentally and physically" (Boericke).

On the physical level, *Calcarea* has a slow metabolism, a sluggish circulation, and an overall lack of endurance and resilience. He is worse from any lifting and straining (*Rhus toxicodendron, Arnica*), and even mild physical effort leaves him perspiring and out of breath. Children, for example, suffer from car, sea, or air-sickness, as if rapid movement in a vehicle were tantamount to physical effort. Especially the least exertion in an upward direction—ascending stairs, hills, ladders—causes dyspnoea, palpitations or a copious sweat quite disproportionate to the actual effort involved. He "cannot stand or walk long; he has to sit in a chair and slides down because he is so flabby" (Gutman). "There is simply little bounce to the ounce," said one such patient of herself—who was exhausted by sweeping floors, raking leaves for ten or fifteen minutes, or by walking up two flights of stairs. This may be due to using the body wrongly: the person is often inagile, with uncoordinated movements, and consequently tires easily. Tyler sums up the picture pithily: "In *Calcarea* everything is slow and late and heavy and weak." This is hardly surprising in view of the fact that the source of much of the constitutional type's troubles lies in a pituitary and thyroid dysfunction (Boericke).

A peculiar aspect of *Calcarea*'s inactivity is that he feels better when constipated. There is no urge, but he appears quite comfortable, even when the bowels move only once a week. Conversely, after a bowel movement (a form of exertion!) he may perspire, feel tired and drained ("weak": Kent), or experience aggravation of a specific symptom such as a cough, headache, vertigo, or pain in the chest or back. Exercise can actually intensify his costiveness: often his bowels function best when he is leading a sedentary life.

Another "worse from exertion" symptom in the *Calcarea* male is extreme weakness and/or irascibility after coition. While having no problem during the act itself (in fact, sexual desire can be "very much increased" [Hahnemann] or even "excessive" [Hering]), the subject is left not only physically exhausted for a day or more, but also unaccountably depressed and irritable.* In a woman, exertion or excitement can produce early onset of menses: "least excitement . . . endangers return of menses or causes metrorrhagia . . . [or] . . . dysmenorrhoea" (Hering). In general, the female *Calcarea* exhibits a picture of too early, profuse, protracted, and/or painful menses, with a tendency to fibroids.

Even *Calcarea*'s tastes run to the non-stimulating. He prefers his food bland and may dislike strong-tasting or spicy dishes. He likes starchy, creamy and dairy foods, such as potatoes, all forms of pasta, bread and butter, peanut butter, whipped cream, ice cream, milk and cheese (although these last four may not be well tolerated), and is often "averse to meat" (Kent)—the symbol of energy and stimulation. Hence, he can be a natural vegetarian whose palate is satisfied by sober (what others might consider tasteless) foods. As one patient said, "I consider baked squash and boiled millet with tamari sauce an exciting meal."

Yet this type also includes those of eccentric tastes, like the child who craves and eats strange foods such as chalk, clay, lead pencils, raw potatoes, the solid cores of cabbages, and other "indigestibles" (Kent). One of the commoner peculiarities is the child who eats sand, stuffing handfuls of it into its mouth, spitting out some but swallowing the rest with every sign of enjoyment (*Silica*).

The strong moon modality encountered in *Calcarea* offers inter-

---

* Other constitutional types (*Kali carbonicum, Lycopodium*) have post-coital weakness; *Selenium* experiences irritability, while *Sepia* and *Natrum muriaticum* feel depressed. But *Calcarea*'s prostration or out-of-sorts feeling is unusually prolonged.

esting symbolic associations. Ailments such as worms, bronchial coughs, enuresis, eczema, and epilepsy are aggravated primarily at the full moon (Boger), when it emits most light (i.e., exertion), and secondarily at the new moon (Boenninghausen), the time of exertion for new growth.

In a characteristic polychrest polarity, the opposite of indolence and inactivity—excitation—is encountered in *Calcarea*'s affinity for convulsions and seizure disorders (hyperelectrical activity or hyperexcitation of certain brain cells). It is well-known that "calcium insufficiency leads to restlessness, muscle twitchings, and ultimately convulsions" (Gutman), and the homoeopathically prepared calcium is therefore invaluable in treating both children and adults for grand mal, petit mal, and other seizures. It can be given alone or, together with others suggested by the patient's immediate symptoms, as an intercurrent constitutional remedy (see the numerous references to epilepsy in Hering's *Guiding Symptoms*, Calcarea, under the sections, "Mind" and "Nerves"). While there are other excellent remedies for epilepsy (e.g., *Sulphur*, *Silica*, *Oenanthus*, and *Lachesis*), in our experience *Calcarea* is the one most often indicated.

On the mental level, as on the physical, any exertion easily fatigues him. This emerges in such symptoms as "drawing in the right side of the head from thinking" (Hering); "with a very short exertion in speaking, he felt as if his brain was paralyzed" (Hahnemann); "after exerting mind, trembling spells" (Hering); reading and writing can bring on waves of heat to the head, palpitations, headaches, or a temporary impairment of vision (*Natrum muriaticum*). These last two symptoms are also brought on by watching a movie or television program, even if the patient's eyesight is satisfactory. Apparently, this too is sometimes a form of exertion for *Calcarea*.

At times mental indolence is reflected in his studying and working habits. It may take him a day or more to accomplish what others do in a couple of hours. The remedy is suited to young adults who are forever changing schools, never finding one suited to their particular needs. Patients admit to having attended as many as *six* undergraduate colleges without adapting to any one. Some take off a year or a semester in the middle of their studies, not for any specific purpose but because of inability to complete any course of instruction ("intellect dull; unable to progress in studies": Hering). Others, from lack of perseverance, continually switch areas of study, while a third group drops out of college altogether.

In general, *Calcarea* may retain a certain immaturity or undeveloped quality, even in adult life. He usually empathizes readily with children, and sometimes he is more comfortable with them than with adults. He can remain callow, naive, constantly duped yet still trusting, and sometimes unworldly to the point of simplemindedness. In fact, he often wants to remain a child—preferring its slow, protected, tranquil existence to the striving competitive world of adulthood. Thus, the theme of "the child" runs through the whole analysis of this type.

This is not to suggest that he does not possess a full range of intellectual capacities. There are brilliant *Calcareas* as well as slow ones. But even the brilliant ones need a prod to get going; otherwise a childlike unworldliness or dreaminess or an inability to follow through may prevent them from fulfilling their potential. The type suffers less from lack of ability than from what Hering calls a "disinclination for work" and Hahnemann an "indisposition or aversion or repugnance to all work . . . even while conscious of his powers" (i.e., laziness).

Calcarea's inertia is traceable to "lack of determination" (Hahnemann) and the absence of such other qualities as ambition, energy, and drive. The individual is rendered inactive by being too easygoing, too resigned, or he may consider striving and work to be as unnecessary for others as they are distasteful to himself. He may thus be a failure by ordinary standards (leaving aside spiritual or moral worth) because he will not push or compete in a world where a certain amount of pushing and competition is required.

Inability to sustain mental effort is a well-known *Calcarea* symptom and has been fully described by Kent, but the more subtle variant is also found: inability to *begin* mental work. This is an interesting distinction. The type puts off, is easily distracted, tarries, and fiddles with little things, unable to get down to the serious business at hand. He wears himself out with minutiae, so as to postpone undertaking the larger task. But once his imagination has been stimulated by the job and he catches fire, then, like an enthralled child, he cannot tear himself away and sticks to his last with unwearied pertinacity.

In any sphere of activity, then, *Calcarea*'s major problem is to muster up the energy to get started. Aware of this weakness, the housewife, for instance, works relentlessly all day for fear of being unable to resume her chores once she stops. One patient, aspiring to be a writer, would habitually start the day by wandering around the house, picking up dishes and rinsing out ashtrays, making unimportant phone calls, sorting out old papers or pottering around the garden, until he had so depleted his energy that the whole day was wasted as far as serious writing was concerned. Following a prescription of the remedy, however, he was able to focus his mental energies sufficiently to work the whole day through on his writing, barely stopping for meals.

The momentum, however, usually has a subdued quality and is not as eruptive or contagious as the enthusiasm of *Phosphorus, Sulphur,* or *Arsenicum.*

Calcarea can also present the polar opposite of the traditional picture of indolence—manifesting such typically *Arsenicum* or *Nux vomica* symptoms as "steady inclination to work"; "ill-tempered, restless, nothing pleases as soon as he ceases to work"; or, "better as soon as he undertakes mental pursuits; aversion to everything as soon as he sits idle" (Hering). Even some headaches are "better from mental occupation and from his attention being engaged" (Hering). Thus *Calcarea* is sometimes lethargic, apathetic, and phlegmatic, and at other times an immoderate worker who perseveres in order to overcome, or overcompensate for, his fundamental slowness and inertia. Indeed, this diligence can sometimes reach the point of "exaggerated" or "insane industry" (Kent), where he works day and night without letup.

The remedy has even been successfully prescribed for "anorexia from overwork" (Boger). This is different from *Arsenicum*'s ideological or competitive anorexia, in which the thin patient wants to be thinner yet, or his hypochondriacal anorexia, in which he has convinced himself that, "This does not agree with me . . . That is bad for me . . . ". It also differs from the neurotic anorexia of *Natrum muriaticum,* which arises out of general protest and self-punishment, or the desire to prove something to the world. Finally, it differs from the *Ignatia* anorexia which follows upon emotional trauma or after fright (Hering). *Calcarea* becomes anorexic from mental pressure, from the feeling of being intellectually pushed. Thus, the fatigued mind, the worn mind, the stressed or overworked mind, might well require this medicine.

The words, "stressed" or "overworked," are relative, however. What is stressful to *Calcarea* might be a part of another's normal routine. To this inactive individual even the slightest additional exertion is too much effort, and anything may seem too much trouble. Inviting close friends to dinner or a pleasant social outing only leads to apprehension about how much work will be entailed and raises the question, "Is it worth the bother?" In fact, he sometimes cannot imagine others even wanting to do that which is an effort to him.*

On the other hand, *Calcarea* is also called for in true emotional trauma. Along with the better-known *Natrum muriaticum, Ignatia,* or *Staphysagria,* it is one of the best remedies for the "results of sorrow and grief" (Hering) and is also useful in "complaints from prolonged worry" (Kent). Just as the individual is physically slow to rebound from stress and illness, so he lacks the ability to overcome emotional shocks, to snap back after a hurt (an ability possessed in abundance by this remedy's close relatives, *Sulphur* and *Lycopodium*).

At times *Calcarea*'s mind becomes confused. He cannot collect his thoughts, or finds himself "confounding words or using wrong expres-

---

* A caricature of this aspect of *Calcarea* is seen in the person of Lady Bertram in Jane Austen's *Mansfield Park.* She is a kindly, gentle, well-disposed woman, but with a trifling mind, and her whole existence centers on how best to keep from exerting herself, even on behalf of those she loves. In her placid selfishness she approaches every situation from the exclusive point of view of the trouble it will cause her. When her niece-in-attendance, Fanny Price, receives her first invitation to dinner, all Lady Bertram can think about is whether she can spare Fanny for the evening.

"'But why should Mrs. Grant ask Fanny?' said Lady Bertram . . . 'I cannot spare her, and I am sure she does not want to go. Fanny, you do not want to go, do you? . . . I will ask Sir Thomas [her husband] as soon as he comes in, whether I can do without you . . . Sir Thomas, stop a moment—I have something to say to you . . . Mrs. Grant has asked Fanny to dinner.'

'Well,' said Sir Thomas, as if waiting for more to accomplish the surprise . . .

'But can I do without her?'

'Indeed, I think you may.'

'She always makes tea, you know, when my sister is not here . . . '"
and so on.

sions" (Hahnemann), such as saying, "I am living in New York" when he means "Boston" (*Lycopodium, Medorrhinum*). He cannot comprehend what others are saying, nor what he is reading; with his poor concentration he cannot "recollect what was spoken" (Hahnemann) or "any details of what he has read the moment he puts down the book" (Borland); or he comes up with a different number every time he adds up a column of figures (Kent). It may take him a while to understand a question put to him, and in his reply he may stop in mid-sentence, losing his train of thought ("his ideas flit away; his memory is short": Hahnemann). One person cannot recall what he has to do or where he has put things; another enters a room and forgets why he has come. In the consulting room, the patient cannot remember the dates of his illnesses, and sometimes he does not answer a question directly. The confusion is also reflected in his rambling mind and meandering conversation, in which he branches off into areas only marginally related to the question asked. Or he takes a long time to get to the point.

Calcarea may sense (or fear) that he is mentally below average ("she is afraid people may notice the confusion in her head": Hahnemann), and this concern is often a guiding symptom to the remedy. As one patient said of herself disarmingly, "Few persons would ever accuse me of being quick, bright, or intelligent" (in more severe cases, he "fears that he is losing his senses": Kent). Yet, just as a child may seem to be off in his own world, not following the drift of conversation, then suddenly make a comment of startling or original insight, so the adult, with his somewhat crab-like mind, eventually works around to the point, his perceptive comment revealing an unexpected understanding. The seeming simpleton in fairy-tales, who surprises everyone by coming up with the solution to a problem that has baffled wiser heads, is *Calcarea*.

A definite slowness or even deficiency may exist, however, and then *Calcarea* laughs foolishly (Boenninghausen lists the remedy under the rubric "foolish, silly"; and in Kent's *Repertory*, it should be added to the rubric, "laughing; silly"), makes irrelevant comments, or speaks whatever first comes to mind, altogether giving the impression of being simple-minded. A woman can listen to a discussion of how homoeopathic remedies may affect the body's electromagnetic field and respond with a digressive monologue about how vitamin C helped the winter colds of her sister-in-law's child. "Nothing going in; everything going out," was one listener's comment.

The *Calcarea* nature is *vulnerable* (think of the vulnerability of the oyster's soft body). He is sensitive to criticism ("weeping on being admonished": Hahnemann) and full of anticipatory anxiety about the future or about impending misfortune. Many of his fears are health-related: "in despair about his shattered health" (Boenninghausen), "apprehensive about his heart and fears heart disease" (Hering), "she is afraid of losing her reason" (Hahnemann). These ever-present concerns can bring on a "despairing mood, with great anguish and palpitations" (Hahnemann). Usually, however, although his anxieties about sickness and ill-health resemble those of *Arsenicum* in substance (often a *Calcarea* layer underlies *Arsenicum*'s fears), they are less frenzied in style. He is not *driven* by them (like *Arsenicum*) but flusters about in a perpetual flurry of small insecurities ("anxious about every trifle": Hahnemann). At times these arise from lack of confidence in his own capacities. The student in school is so fearful of failing that he is unable to study, and his worst apprehensions are confirmed: the incompetence he fears becomes a reality. A man worries about performing adequately at his job. One patient, a columnist with fifteen years experience and good work behind him, was still fearful of criticism each time his editor called him in—until the remedy abolished this particular insecurity.

Calcarea also displays a fear of succeeding. When things are going well, the student in law school, the man thriving in business, the woman rising in her profession suddenly throws it all over and drifts away: "right in the midst of his success he quits his business . . . and leaves all" (Kent). He either loses sight of the larger ambition or is overwhelmed by the responsibility and backs out. Or he gives up when the challenge is too great (*Silica*).

His fears and feeling of vulnerability are even expressed vicariously. He does not like hearsay or newspaper accounts of violence ("fear excited by reports of cruelty": Hering), and a man of the world will refuse to look at war movies or read a book depicting cruelty. This is even more true of the *Calcarea* female, who will not listen to the news on radio or television and refuses to read the daily paper; if she hears something upsetting, she cannot get to sleep at night, immediately identifying with the victim of violence and fearing that it will affect her next. *Calcarea* may avoid sensationalism in any form and, instead, seeks out sober, understated intellectual or artistic stimuli.

The other side of the coin is the patient who "thinks and talks of

nothing but murder, fire, rats" (Hering)—i.e., things that frighten her
most.

The Shell

We turn now to the hard protective shell in which the oyster's soft
defenseless body is encased. The principal defense of this weak and
vulnerable creature against an intrusive or inimical environment, or
against the stronger beings that surround him, is to withdraw into himself. And this, indeed, is one of *Calcarea*'s principal defensive reactions.
To protect his sensitive psyche he retires into his shell, closing off the
world and ignoring it. He sees how the world is but decides that it is
not for him and refuses to compete. The outcome may be a failure of
adaptation or psychological isolation from others. However, it can also
contribute to his particular autonomy—which is a source of his strength.

Yet he is not a true loner; a number of his physical symptoms are
actually "aggravated while alone" (Kent) and ameliorated by talking to
or being with others (*Pulsatilla, Phosphorus, Arsenicum*). If too long
in solitude, he may begin to talk to himself or imagine voices and people: "imagines someone is walking beside her; that something hanging
over back of chair is a person sitting there" (Hering). Also, although
withdrawn, he is not as closed or introverted as *Sepia* or *Natrum
muriaticum*. Nor is he necessarily shy or timid. He has an intrinsically
sociable disposition and can possess a quiet philosophic assurance and
stolidity. "Diffident" or "retiring" are more accurate terms for him.

Sometimes, however, he should learn to act more boldly, to venture forth emotionally from the shell of his restricted life.

A middle-aged woman with a pleasant moon-shaped face and a
phlegmatic manner, but somewhat bewildered and overwhelmed by
life, came to homoeopathy for treatment of her early, heavy, protracted
menstrual periods, also for a strong tendency to chapped hands, lips,
and skin. But her mental symptoms interested the physician even more.
For many years she had been married to a disagreeable man who criticized her relentlessly. After the divorce her ex-husband continued to
exert moral pressure on the patient in order to keep her in emotional
subjugation, but she nevertheless managed to find an agreeable gentleman friend, deeply devoted to her and a suitable potential husband.
What did *Calcarea* do at this point? She began to be overcome with
remorse, even with affection for her ex-husband, wondering whether

she should not return to him; whether it would not be better for the children, and so on.

Why at this point? Why not during the two or three years she was on her own? This was obviously the *Calcarea* fear of a new challenge, of an enterprising new start. Her old life may have been restricting, even difficult, but was at least familiar and thus less psychologically intimidating than the challenging new love. But the remedy helped her overcome the "inability to meet a challenge" (Whitmont), and she ventured into the new marriage.

Calcarea's emotional restrictiveness is occasionally exhibited in a need for the physical proximity of home. An extreme example of this was a two-month-old baby, a contented and placid child who had hardly ever cried from the day she was born. When taken on her first weekend visit to friends, however, she took one look at the unfamiliar surroundings and broke out in such uncontrollable screaming that the parents had to take her home. The pediatrician attributed the incident to coincidence or to being frightened by something in the new house. No baby of two months, he claimed, could realize she was away from home. But two weeks later, when the mother tried to leave her at the house of a sitter, the same scene was repeated. She was howling inconsolably even before her mother had left the room. Yet at home she was fine with any sitter. When sent off to summer camp ten years later, the child was so homesick that she came back within a week. And this was repeated twice more. No amount of *Ignatia*, *Silica*, or *Capsicum* (the best homesickness remedies) was of any avail. The following year a course of *Calcarea* commenced months before departing from home enabled her to withstand the first two unhappy weeks of camp until the new locale became familiar.

The disorientation of these individuals when away from home resembles the oyster which is unable to survive without its protective shell; even adults get restless, unhappy, ill or out of sorts. One patient joked about his *Calcarea* wife, "Whenever we are away from home and driving back, she is in such a hurry that I can hardly persuade her to stop for gas!" In families with a heavy *Calcarea* component the members like nothing better than to sit around enjoying each other's company (*Pulsatilla*). They do not go out and *do* things but are content with a uniform, uneventful life, and for weeks or months on end simply appreciate the closeness of being at home together.

In fact, *Calcarea* must cling to everything related to home. He wants to gather his family and pets around him (the type is often extremely fond of animals, as they do not challenge his low self-confidence) and can be uneasy at even the temporary absence of a member. In the home he finds the security and support that nothing else can begin to supply. The often-encountered physical modalities of the remedy—better from warmth, closed stuffy rooms, heat of the fire, warm drinks, and worse from cold in every form—all serve to reinforce the symbolic association with the home. And yet, in a characteristic "shadow side" of the picture, *Calcarea* is one of the few remedies listed in the Kent *Repertory* under the rubric: "aversion to members of family."

Although Kent lists this remedy under the rubric, "avaricious," it is more accurate to state that *Calcarea* tends to *hang on to his own*. He is not usually materialistic or accumulative except as concerns food—where he does need to "take in" and "accumulate." He is the type who is always eating snacks; he does not suffer from overwhelming cravings or a desire for uncontrollable binges but has a constant need for oral gratification. Or he stocks the refrigerator and freezer full to bursting, seeking security in the knowledge that there will always be enough for his family. Sometimes, like a dog that will not eat but buries his bones, he keeps a mass of supplies in a closet or in the basement, prepared for any eventuality (*Arsenicum*).

Another *Calcarea* protective technique against too much external pressure is *"obstinacy"* (Hahnemann). A quiet stubbornness of disposition can be found in even the best-natured individual. *Calcarea* husbands of domineering wives and wives of overbearing husbands tend to exhibit this kind of intractability. Even the apparently mild and docile individual may be impossible to move: he simply balks or goes his own way. As one woman said of her endearing, roly-poly husband, "Sure, he looks like a cream puff, but *no one* pushes him around!"

Something in the apathetic unyielding nature does invite criticism and incite others to push or change him. But in his impassive and lethargic way he resists even the strongest pressure, holding steadfastly to his position. At the extreme, he refuses even to help himself or cooperate with those trying to help him. Attempts to make him respond are like prying open a reluctant oyster and may lead only to further withdrawal into the shell. Sometimes the pressured *Calcarea* turns peevish, grumpy, querulous, or childish, but he is rarely nasty.

His stubborness may be manifested in a petty self-assertiveness. For example, an employer will tell his *Calcarea* secretary to type letters in a particular way. Doggedly, and without arguing, she will continue typing them the same way as before. Her employer can rant and rave but to little avail. He is quite helpless confronted with her *passive resistance*. This non-aggressive but determined obstinacy at times looks like slowness or denseness, but it is merely the weaker individual's defense against more powerful forces.

An extreme example in fiction of the impassive bland *Calcarea* woman is Catherine Sloper, the lackluster tongue-tied heroine of Henry James' *Washington Square*. Troubled by self-doubt and a sense of inferiority vis-a-vis her brilliant but cold and forbidding father (who considered her merely "as good as good bread"), she can oppose his influence only by putting up a mute and passive resistance. Her stolidity and placidity give the impression of unresponsiveness, even of insensitivity (the shell), but as the author says of her, "in reality, she was the softest creature in the world" (the oyster) and "an impression once made on her is made forever." When a former suitor who had heartlessly deserted her for mercenary reasons returns after many years and seeks to make amends, she resolutely turns away with the simple words: "I felt it very much. I felt it for years . . . Impressions last when they have been strong. But I can't talk."

Calcarea's dislike of outside pressure may be revealed physically in a definite preference for loose comfortable clothes. He wants nothing that presses, squeezes, or binds him. While *Lachesis* is most sensitive around the neck, *Calcarea* dislikes tightness around the waist (like *Lycopodium*) and in the hypogastric area, and may prefer suspenders to a belt.

His outlook is often limited, with an inability to see beyond the shell of his own petty concerns ("tendency of the mind to dwell on little things": Kent). The woman, for example, is incapable of raising her sights above complicated and all too frequently trifling social relationships: who quarrelled with whom or what one family member said to another. She then communicates her agitation over these tiffs (or other pet concerns) to anyone who will listen, even to total outsiders.

She does not offer solutions or consider any effective course of action, but harps on what she has seen or heard in a helpless, hopeless way. At times, in her fluster, she repeats the same sentiment in some identical phrase, such as, "Oh, I wish such and such had [or had not] happened!" (pointlessly, since it already has, or has not, taken place). She does not let go even at night and lies awake churning over some one worrying thought in her mind (*Pulsatilla*).

Altogether, the constitutional type tends to magnify the personal and the particular. He observes an act of meanness and decides that the whole world is full of meanness and cruelty (*Natrum muriaticum*). But he does not (like *Phosphorus*, *Lachesis*, or *Sulphur*) exaggerate events for effect. There is no desire to astound. He only magnifies their importance to himself. When, as Kent noted, the physician feels like admonishing a fretting patient: "Why don't you put that aside? That doesn't amount to anything," the patient is often *Calcarea*. But his instinctive response to such a charge would be, "What *is* more important than personal relationships and the small things that make life either pleasant or disagreeable?"

Part of this "littleness" stems from a basically *conservative* mentality. He dislikes change, is afraid of upheavals, clings to the status quo, and prefers even a monotonous existence to venturing forth into the unknown.

The following two patients caricature *Calcarea*'s conservative tendencies. The first was a mild, middle-aged man of apprehensive expression and timid behavior, rotund in build and with pleasant but indistinct features in a flabby face. If ever a person resembled an oyster without its shell, it was he. Emerging from the consulting room he commented with a sigh that the lateness of the hour prevented him from buying some picture hooks he needed. "I always patronize a hardware store near here, which closes at six."

"There is another hardware store nearby which is open till nine," the receptionist assured him.

"Oh, but I wouldn't *think* of shopping anywhere but in that particular store," he confided. "The salesmen there are so nice and polite. Also, I know them and they know me! I guess I will just have to wait until the next time I come." With his proclivity for familiar surroundings and mistrust of unfamiliar ones, this *Calcarea* required an homelike environment for even his simplest purchases, or preferred to go without.

The other vivid example of *Calcarea*'s lack of enterprise and willingness to remain where life plunked him down was a dyspneic elderly
gentleman who had been a bank teller his whole life. He had remained
at the same bank, almost at the same window, for more than fifty years,
never receiving a promotion or even a raise in salary (beyond automatic
increases). He was perfectly content with the job and had stayed on
well beyond retirement age.

Calcarea's foreshortened outlook is also seen in his readiness to
become absorbed in detail for its own sake, without it leading to anything particularly significant. The mature mind, wrote Aristotle, does
not seek greater precision than is inherent in the subject matter. In this
respect *Calcarea* may well be immature. Time and again he attributes
greater importance to a problem than it warrants and devotes disproportionate mental effort to its solution: how many steps it takes to walk
from the Capitol to the Lincoln Memorial, precisely how *few* grams of
steel would be contained in a ten-inch model of the Eiffel Tower, or
why the letter "q" in English is always followed by "u." He has difficulty with broad concepts and tends to get bogged down in inconsequential minutiae.

A memorable example of the *Calcarea* philosophical intent falling
short was a young man being treated for emotional complaints following his father's demise. He produced a free-verse poem to his father's
memory whose gist was: "As I elevate and contemplate this potato
[*Calcarea* has a great love of potatoes] which I am about to peel, I am
reminded of human frailty and of my all too fleeting manhood. For,
in just this way, my lately departed father would denude this vegetable
of its skin—which act has now taken on for me a new and more profound significance . . . " and so forth. He was obviously trying to instil
life and death symbolism into the act of peeling a potato but could not
quite pull it off (so to speak). John Keats could formulate an aesthetic
philosophy from contemplating a Grecian urn, but the *Calcarea carbonica* potato was simply incapable of conveying so much symbolic
meaning.

Ponderous strivings, however, do not make *Calcarea* a fool, even
when they amount to little. He may be unenterprising, unworldly, at
times of small outlook or unimaginative ("weakness of the imaginative
faculty": Hahnemann), but not foolish, because he does not nurse un-

due pretensions about his own intellectual capacities. He senses his limitations, knows when *not* to discuss matters about which he knows little, and does not overestimate his abilities; thus he escapes the *Sulphur* kind of foolishness. Self-conscious about saying something inappropriate or silly and insecure about his intellectual powers, he may be reluctant to join a conversation unless well-versed in the subject. He is seldom boastful and, as likely as not, feels thoroughly uncomfortable in the limelight, even when it is deserved.

With feelings that are deeper than he is willing to express, *Calcarea* is fair-minded, often displaying a low-key wisdom. In group situations he plays the role of the passive and non-judgmental observer to whom others gravitate for support. Even when disapproving of others' behavior, he is quickly resigned to whatever he cannot alter. His serene acceptance is a precious possession, but when carried further, this quality can develop into a fatalism which is reinforced by his inherent indolence. "What is fated to be will be. What is the use of opposing destiny?" he reasons, refusing to make any effort to improve a situation.

A fine portrayal of *Calcarea* withdrawing into his shell is found in the Russian novel *Oblomov* by Ivan Goncharov. The hero, Ilya Oblomov, is a plump, sensitive, and quietly charming gentleman, unexciting but gentle-natured and pleasant-mannered, who takes 200 pages (one third of the novel) just to get out of bed in the morning and put on his bathrobe. This slow-paced opening scene symbolizes the nature of the man and of his subsequent life. Resisting all the energizing efforts of his active friend, Stolz, Oblomov prefers to sleep and dream rather than get up and take an interest in the world. Also, as the flashbacks in the novel reveal, he is attempting to recreate his happy childhood and the leisurely, peaceful, carefree contentment he knew growing up at his mother's knee.

Through apathy, procrastination, and refusal to rise to an emotional challenge Oblomov (in whom sexual passion is still undeveloped) loses the woman he loves, and who loves him, to the energetic Stolz. But he accepts the loss with typical *Calcarea* resignation and lack of resentment, sinking back into his habitual inertia. For the rest of his life he remains ensconced in his pleasantly stagnant morass of a home, as passively content with his limited and rather empty existence as an oyster on a rock.

Isolating himself in his own thick shell, *Calcarea* may grow out of touch with the outside world and lose a sense for what is or is not socially acceptable. He may begin to exhibit childlike or *eccentric* behavior. A child can stand up in a public place and loudly announce "I like everyone here!" or, as the case may be, "I do not like all these people," and everyone will smile at his uninhibited candor. But in an adult such lack of self-consciousness—for instance, entering into a long conversation with some total stranger who has stopped him to ask directions—such deviations from conventional behavior, provoke a different response.

One patient, a retired navy man, had the habit of rushing into the kitchen at any time of the day with bucket and mop and energetically washing the floor, gleefully exclaiming throughout this ritual "Swab the decks, mates! Swab the decks!" The old sailor was obviously reliving with relish his former service days. Such behavior was tolerable at home, but when after a meal at a friend's house, he performed this ritual with the same enthusiasm, his wife pleaded for help. He received a dose of *Calcarea* 200x and could thenceforth be dissuaded from swabbing the kitchens of friends, although nothing could deter his zeal at home. The remedy supplied just the necessary additional degree of social awareness.

Another patient was being treated for a long-standing twitching of the eyelid which, while neither painful nor alarming, was extremely irritating over a period of months. He demonstrated a good grasp of homoeopathic principles even though it was his first encounter with this discipline; but every few minutes he would pull out an old pocketwatch and comment on the time, "Hmm, it's just past five o'clock" or "It's almost five-fifteen," half to himself and half to inform others of this interesting fact. It was not a serious aberration, just a harmless peculiarity which in a child with a new toy would be considered normal. In his case it provided the mental symptom needed to confirm the physician's choice of *Calcarea*. On the return visit, not only had the twitch disappeared, but he pulled out his pocket-watch only once, toward the end of the consultation, even though his absorbing interest in the exact time had been a long-standing habit.

Sometimes the eccentricities are localized, manifested as some quirk of the personality (as in the above two cases). At other times eccentricity pervades *Calcarea*'s entire being. Or he may be one of those individuals commonly described as "a character," in the sense of being different or unusual in some endearing way. Alternately, he is merely too simple or naive in worldly matters. "Pogo," the endearing opossum hero of Walt Kelly's famous comic strip of the 1950s and 1960s, is *Calcarea*. Naive, unworldly, non-instigative, but not unaware, he stands at the center of the action in his comic-strip world. He is *Calcarea* in his blandness, his appealing modesty, placid sensitivity, and quaintly original or resignedly philosophical outlook. When he has been coerced to run for President, he announces, "If nominated I will not be elected; if elected I will not run," (paraphrasing General Sherman's more acid remark, "If nominated I will not run; if elected I will not serve"). Typical of the *Calcarea* non-heroic hero, Pogo's main role in the Okefenokee swamp life is to resolve the interminable conflicts and passions seething around him by inviting everyone over to his house to eat (this type can be exceptionally hospitable, and enjoys serving up food at every opportunity).

Of course, other constitutional types can possess eccentricities, *Natrum muriaticum* and *Lachesis* coming first to mind, but they are different from *Calcarea*. *Natrum muriaticum*, for example, is *aware* of acting strangely. He knows the norm but is not capable of observing it, seemingly compelled by some contrary force to act differently. Afterwards he suffers mortification at the memory of his own "strange, rare, and peculiar" behavior; however, occasionally he is proud of being different and cultivates it. *Calcarea* is like a child, unconscious of his departure from the norm and therefore free from embarrassment. *Lachesis* can partake of either state: sometimes he is overcome with shame at his own unconventional behavior, at other times he is quite oblivious of it; and usually his eccentricities are more pronounced or intrusive than *Calcarea*'s.

A final childlike trait, again reminiscent of the shell which shields *Calcarea* from the world's pressures, is an *undeveloped sense of time*. Unconcerned with punctuality, he can be chronically late, or, if engrossed in something of interest, may lose track of time altogether. "I'll *just* finish this article," he thinks, "and then I'll run that errand." Then he "just" forgets. Or he wants to stop by the post office on the way to an appointment but starts chatting with a friend there . . . and the time passes faster than he realizes.

He is a procrastinator, postponing what he knows must be done.

The adult puts off writing thank-you notes and just cannot get to the telephone to make necessary calls. The child delays and delays doing the dishes or mowing the lawn, even though, once on the job, he does it well. The otherwise responsible youngster puts off sitting down to his homework and, with the best will in the world, cannot finish a test or assignment in the allotted time. Older students are chronically unprepared in class and unable to submit papers on time, asking for deferments. They have had as much time as anyone else and are just held back by inertia. The housewife procrastinates with her chores, the husband with his house repairs, until completely overwhelmed by the accumulated responsibility and unable even to start. Then they worry about all the things they should have done and develop a flustered and unproductive guilt over their lack of accomplishments in life. Or they tire themselves out worrying about the things they should be doing but are not. These individuals just cannot adhere to timetables, cannot exert themselves sufficiently to plan their time and meet deadlines. They then find themselves in the invidious position of having to operate under pressure and end by doing things in a slipshod manner.*

Calcarea is habitually late to the theater, to weddings, religious services, classes, concerts, etc. One patient stated that in a long marriage he and his wife arrived on time to an event only once—the opera *Rigoletto*. The *Arsenicum* in him took many years to be reconciled to this constant irritation, and he only half joked about it as grounds for divorce. But the wife's easygoing nature finally wore down his anxious punctuality. Now he resignedly shrugs his shoulders saying, "I've come to realize that it is not the end of the world to be late for an evening or a performance"—then adds, with a wistful sigh, "But I do hope that *some* day before I die I will be able to see the first act of *Hamlet*, hear the first movements of my favorite piano concertos, and learn exactly *what* happens in the first half of the ballet *Giselle*. I've seen her resurrect three times and still don't know why she died." Thus, the irritable impatience of the *Arsenicum* husband was easier to change with homoeopathic remedies than the lethargy of his *Calcarea* wife.

---

* In an old *Punch* cartoon an elderly *Calcarea* couple are sitting placidly in their home, half-packed suitcases suggesting an imminent journey. The husband is stating to the wife in an unhurried manner, "Ten more minutes, and *then* we will have to rush."

In general, these individuals are difficult to change. The inherent slowness of the process is further compounded by the requirement that the remedy be used very cautiously in adults: not too frequently (many months should elapse before it is repeated) and not in too high potency. As for elderly persons, Hahnemann himself instructed: "In affections of persons of advanced age, *Calcarea*, even after other intermediate remedies, can scarcely be repeated with advantage; a dose which is given after another without previous intermediate remedy, is almost always prejudicial . . ." (*Chronic Diseases*, Volume I).

Just as *Calcarea* is the last to arrive, so he is the last to leave. Once settled at a gathering, he sees no reason to depart and stays on and on. There is a saying that some individuals leave without saying "good-bye" (*Natrum muriaticum*: from awkwardness or embarrassment; and *Sulphur* from haste: once he is up, he wants to get going), while others say "goodbye" and do not leave. *Calcarea* belongs definitely to the latter class: in his enjoyment, and quite oblivious of the time, he will stand in the doorway for an hour bidding his host adieu.

Phosphorus is another constitutional type that can be late, but she (this is especially true of women) does it for effect, realizing that her entrance will be more dramatic if others are kept waiting. She does not want to seem eager — let others be eager. Thus she is aware of time and uses it, while *Calcarea* is unaware of and unable to respond to the exigencies of time.

The Child

We have seen that *Calcarea* retains a childlike quality throughout life, and it is probably the most useful homoeopathic children's remedy — the child's constitutional *par excellence*. Many children start out life as *Calcarea* before they are transformed into other constitutional types by their circumstances and experiences; and most children call for it at some point during their early years.

The child looks fit, with golden curls which later straighten out and become darker, a chubby face, and bright pink cheeks. Yet he lacks energy. The head is large and moist, the torso pear-shaped or pot-bellied, and sometimes the upper lip is swollen or protruding. There is a tendency to swollen tonsils and enlarged cervical, mesenteric, axillary, and sub-mandibular glands (*Silica*). During winter months these children have an unending series of colds, earaches, and attacks of bronchitis.

Their bone development may be poor, with occasional visible curvature of the spine (*Calcarea phosphorica*), irregular formation of the long bones, crooked fingers, or poorly developed teeth and jaw, and the typical high narrow dental arch indicating a need for future orthodontic work. The irregularity of their bodily structure parallels that of the oyster's stubby and asymmetrical shell, contrasting with the smooth and mirrored symmetry of other bivalve molluscs.

Calcareas frequently have chronic snuffles or a runny nose, caused partly by narrowness of the nasal passages and partly by poor assimilation of dairy products. Altogether, the picture is one of imperfect calcium metabolism and "impaired nutrition" (Boericke). The potentized lime encourages the healthy growth of bones, teeth, and nerves by promoting the proper assimilation and utilization of calcium and other nutrients.

The youngster can have a capricious appetite, being extremely picky and limiting himself not only to little food but also to a very restricted variety. One three-year-old patient had only two acceptable dishes: a hot-dog on half a bun one day alternating with a hamburger on half a roll the next. Another young patient would eat only cheese, a third only drank milk, a fourth only fruit juice. That was virtually all they ever touched, although most remained plump. In each case, however, *Calcarea* broke them of their limited diets and expanded their culinary horizons to include some fruits, vegetables, eggs, chicken and other basics.

The infant is frequently a "floppy baby": soft, fat, lymphatic, and muscularly weak, in whom everything operates in low gear. This can be seen physically in delayed fontanelle closure and late or difficult dentition, in slowness to lose his cradle cap, to develop motor skills (especially to walk), and to acquire bladder and bowel control. Every new skill learned, every new effort, can cause a relapse of some particular weakness. A graphic example was a mentally slow twenty-month-old boy suffering from repeated ear and throat infections which invariably developed into bronchitis and occasionally into pneumonia. Every few months he went through the same pattern, with the cycle of physical ailments commencing at each new stage of development: when he learned to turn over at six months, to sit up at eight, to crawl at ten, to pull himself up at twelve, to spoon-feed himself at fourteen, to walk at sixteen, to pronounce his first words at eighteen, and so on. After each such achievement he relapsed into a long bout of infection. Once *Calcarea* was given, however, there were no more bouts of pneumonia, and only a few yearly relapses into bronchitis, while his mental development proceeded nicely apace.

Calcarea's slowness in talking may be self-imposed. The knowledge is there, but he simply does not want to be *hurried* into talking. Sometimes the hitherto inarticulate youngster will start to speak in complete phrases or even sentences, showing that the words were only waiting to be brought out. This differs somewhat from the true slowness in talking of *Natrum muriaticum* and *Calcarea phosphorica*.

In school the child might be "slow," sometimes in all subjects, sometimes in only one; for instance, he likes math (there is something secure in the predictability of numbers) but is poor in reading. He may be ultra-responsible and try conscientiously to keep up, yet real success still eludes him. If he does succeed, it is by spending a disproportionate amount of time on his work—far more than other children. Or he may give up easily; he has too little energy for the effort of concentrating or lacks the drive to complete a distasteful task.

If unsure of himself, he will not open his mouth in class, not even to ask the teacher for clarification, with the result that he may eventually find it difficult to keep up. If pressed, he immediately feels overwhelmed and is incapable of performing at all. In retracing the history of children who are unable to make progress in their studies, the cause is often found in the pressure of a too challenging school situation. The child may be well-adjusted socially, but the learning process exerts no appeal, and he closes himself off from the academic requirements pressed on him by his superiors. Unable or unwilling to compete, he silently turns inward and gives up the struggle. A not uncommon physical manifestation of *Calcarea's* fear or dislike of school is an inexplicable stomachache coming on just before school or during the day.

Parenthetically, *Calcarea* is frequently indicated in brain-damaged and emotionally disturbed children. It has helped those with cerebral palsy and been useful in all gradations of reduced mental capacity, from dyslexia, learning disabilities, and the mildest lack of initiative and perseverence, to severe cases of mental retardation (*Baryta carbonica*). Even when it is not the only indicated remedy, it must often be invoked to keep the case progressing.

This is also one of the first medicines to be considered for children who are bright and intelligent but do not perform up to capacity (the other is *Sulphur*). Either they dislike the teacher or the mental effort, or they balk at the confinement of rules and regulations. The *Sulphur* child fights authority, but *Calcarea* balks. Boys often oscillate between the two remedies during their earlier years and later, with maturity, move on to *Lycopodium* — thus completing Kent's well-known constitutional triad: *Sulphur/Calcarea/Lycopodium* (which is encountered especially in males). For the rest of their lives they may gravitate among these three remedies.*

Typically, the *Calcarea* child is even-tempered, pleasant, and unaggressive ("of a quiet mild disposition": Hering). The infant is content to stay where he is put, doing nothing or playing with whatever is at hand. The older child is intrinsically less tractable than *Pulsatilla* or even *Phosphorus*, because he is less eager to please. He is more independent than responsive and has a mind of his own. Like the other two, however, he is friendly and basically cooperative.

Calcarea can also be recognized in the child who is remarkably self-sufficient. In the physician's office the infant will look around fearlessly, or stare fixedly at some one object or person. If laid down, he will play contentedly with his fingers and toes. The toddler goes his own way, climbing imperturbably over furniture and the knees of adults, exploring the different rooms, placidly but not unimaginatively entertaining himself while his parents talk with the doctor. The older child is capable of occupying himself quietly for hours at a time but tends to keep his enthusiasms to himself. He disappears into his room to work on some project about which others will hear only when he has finished it. But if he loses momentum, he may have trouble getting started again: the formerly industrious and creative child will loll around for days at a loss what to do.

The type can exhibit an amusing equanimity. Older children or siblings can push the young *Calcarea* around, stuff him in closets, shove

---

* According to Kent, the remedies work best in the above order and should be so administered to avoid a symptomatic imbroglio which might confuse the case (*Lectures on Materia Medica:* Sulphur). Hahnemann before him wrote of *Lycopodium*: "It is especially efficacious when it is homoeopathically indicated after the previous use of *Calcarea*" (*Chronic Diseases*, Volume I).

him into drawers, or even put him in the dryer. Throughout all he remains unperturbed. He does not panic but accepts such treatment with resignation, even fatalistically. If pushed too far, however, he reacts with a sudden vigorous protest and then—sensibly and without a fuss—retires from the scene.

When permitted to roam happily, the *Calcarea* toddler responds to obstacles in a very particular way. Instead of crying, stamping, or demanding adult help, he will push, pull, grunt, and strain, trying by himself to get around or dislodge the obstacle. It is heartening to watch him resolve his difficulties calmly instead of throwing a temper tantrum. The following illustrates this trait.

A child of barely two wanted to attract her resting mother's attention. Being of a considerate disposition, she came up and leaned her head against her mother's bed and softly whispered, "Mommy?" No response. She then changed her tone to a still whispered but more imperious, "Mom-my!" Still no response. She then tried the more formal, "Mother?" Her mother pretended to sleep on, hoping the child would leave but, instead of leaving or shouting for attention, there was a long pause. Then the child tried her mother's nickname, "Becky?" The silence continued, followed by the next query, "Rebecca?" Since her mother kept her eyes closed, she next resorted to the Spanish housekeeper's form of address, "Senora!" Another pause, and finally in a desperate last resort, "Mrs. N__, *please!*" At which point the vanquished mother had to concede.

This physically maladroit and emotionally phlegmatic child who could barely talk had figured out an original way of getting a response without making a scene. Even the parents had no inkling that she was so aware of the various forms of address. *Calcarea* children often solve their problems in such quaintly imaginative ways.

The child's quiet independence is also revealed in his surprising ability, even when very young, to recount his own symptoms (Blackie). A dramatic example was the case of a seven-year-old boy with muscular dystrophy, so advanced that he took half an hour to get out of bed in the morning and fifteen minutes to get up from sitting on the floor (where he used to watch television). At times he could go upstairs only on his buttocks, dragging himself up step-by-step in a sitting position. The vast improvement effected by homoeopathy in this case was due in large part to the boy's capacity to report his symptoms and progress accurately: "The getting up from sitting is about 60% improved, but the going upstairs is only 30%," he would state with an accuracy and maturity well in advance of his years. Thus the physician knew precisely whether or not to repeat a remedy and when to change it: for instance, this patient required periodic series of *Rhus Tox* 30x intercurrently with his constitutional remedies (see *Lycopodium* footnote, p. 112).

Similar excellent results have been achieved in "slow learners"—children with learning disabilities—who can be such precise observers of their own improvement, or lack of same, that the physician is greatly aided in his prescribing. With the correct administration of *Calcarea* and other remedies they begin to catch up in their studies and can eventually rejoin their age-level class.

Sometimes what appears to be "slowness" is actually the type's tendency to operate on a different, less competitive plane—on the level of sensitivities and feelings. For instance, listening to a nursery school lesson on the whale family, a *Sulphur* or *Arsenicum* child will absorb the fascinating details of their enormous size, strength, and food consumption, and later relay them to others. A *Calcarea* or *Pulsatilla* child will also listen wide-eyed and attentive to the information, but later that night, cowering in its mother's lap, might remark in an awed tone, "Mommy, I think there must be whales in the dark!"

He is an autonomous little entity who can grow into an original, independent, and easily contented adult. Both at home and in school, he observes clearly and responds sensitively and appropriately when encouraged to develop at his own placid and deliberate pace ("he does best when left alone and allowed to proceed independently": Whitmont)—but within a *structured* environment. The *Sulphur* child approaches problems directly and responds in a predictable manner, but *Calcarea*, in his own circuitous way, will often come up with a novel contribution, an original twist, revealing that he has understood what is going on, even if taking time to digest it. He is the proverbial tortoise, the plodder who may beat the sprinting hare (*Phosphorus*) to the finish line. Sometimes, however, this independence develops into asocial withdrawal. Cutting himself off from others, he enters a fantasy world with his own "imaginary friends," making up stories that run on from day to day, ignoring the other children in the class, and altogether relying on his own resources for companionship and entertainment.

The "shadow" side of *Calcarea*, suprisingly enough, is the terribly difficult and badly behaved child.

What is the vulnerable child's principal defense against the adults who surround and govern him? He is slower than they, less articulate, physically weaker, more dependent—what can he do to get his own way? One technique is to throw tantrums. The oyster shell is a superlative remedy for curbing the temper tantrums of screaming, ungovernable, disobedient, "self-willed" (Hering) children, whose uncontrollable natures keep them from getting along in school or at home.

Of course, not every child with temper tantrums requires this medicine. Even in misbehavior the constitutional types retain their individuality, and distinctions must be made among them. *Calcarea* throws constant temper tantrums or has periodic series of tantrums, seemingly over anything. If one cause is removed, he finds another to scream about; or he wants a thing, then refuses it, then wants something else (*Chamomilla*). Hence his tantrums are continuous and with little or no discernible provocation.

The unruliness or disobedience of *Sulphur* children is usually combined with an energetic manner and decisiveness. They flare up suddenly, becoming red and hot, yelling and stomping. But the reason is detectable, and, once removed, the tantrum subsides as rapidly as it came on. The incident is forgotten, the bad temper vanishes, and five minutes later the child is back to normal.

Hepar sulphuris is more malicious; the child will be gratuitously bullying or cruel, shoving an unoffending playmate off a chair or table, or even through a window—in cold blood, so to speak, since the victim has done nothing provocative. The *Tuberculinum* child can also be physically violent in his tempers but does not attack without provocation. He is especially prone to using violent language, shouting all the foul words he can think of; even a three- or four-year-old, despite his limited vocabulary, will make a heroic effort along these lines, with audacious references to bodily excretions and genitalia.

The *Belladonna* child loses control of himself during a tantrum, biting, kicking, and sometimes tearing at his clothes; he can even precipitate himself into a convulsion. Significantly, *Belladonna* is the acute complement of *Calcarea*. The *Nux vomica* child will also act wild, kicking the adult's shins, but is less demented than *Belladonna*; he makes life miserable for others by daily demonstrations of an irritable, disagreeable temper that occasionally escalates into a tantrum. While a *Lyco-podium* youngster may be obstinate and rebellious, throwing tantrums is seldom one of his usual recourses for asserting his will: "child disobedient though not ill-humored" (Allen).

Natrum muriaticum manifests extraordinary rage with violent sobbing rather than screaming and shouting; if prolonged, it can lead to full-scale hysterics. The outburst arises seemingly over a trifle but is actually the result of a long accumulation of hurts and offenses, real or imaginary. Hence the severity of the anger which takes a long time to subside. *Phosphorus* tantrums are essentially attention-getting techniques, reflecting the child's over-dramatization of a situation. Even when being most obnoxious he will cast sidelong glances at the observer to judge what impression he is making or to decide how the next scene should be played; he will end the tantrum instantaneously if he feels there is no more mileage in it.

The *Lachesis* tantrum is quite extraordinary to behold. Something suddenly snaps in an otherwise controlled child, and he becomes hateful—clawing at himself and striking out at others verbally or physically (for further discussion of bad behavior, see the appropriate chapters).

The *Calcarea* child can also be an unbelievable pest. In the office he prevents his parents from talking, constantly interrupting, crying, begging, squawking, and causing unbearable noise and commotion. At home his demands are thoroughly unreasonable, and he has absolutely no consideration of others. But most of these difficult children can be brought around to behaving like civilized beings by repeated doses of *Calcarea carbonica.**

---

* It must sometimes be repeated frequently in children to obtain maximum benefit. This is stressed by Borland: "Time can be lost by following the rule of never repeating the medicine so long as improvement is maintained. Originally I would have given one dose of *Calcarea carbonica* 10M and, providing the child went ahead slowly but steadily, with no lessening in its improvement, I could find no reason to repeat the medicine for six months or more. But the average child, free from acute illness, will tend to improve even if it has no medicine at all, and the constitutional drug ought to increase the rate of improvement. I therefore started repeating *Calcarea carbonica* at much more frequent intervals . . . " (*Children's Types*). Hahnemann himself wrote of *Calcarea*, "In cases of children, several doses may be given in suc-

An even-tempered and basically "good" child, however, does not want to throw temper tantrums, so he resorts to that other technique for getting his way—obstinacy. "I want to, and I will!" or "No I won't, you can't make me!" *Calcarea* mulishly insists as he digs in his heels. He will not eat his dinner or get dressed and is impervious to coaxing. If pressured in school, he puts up a quiet but stubborn resistance. One typically *Calcarea* four-year-old boy, with a large damp head, a funny protruding "swollen" (Kent) upper lip, round blue eyes, a little pig-like nose, and a particularly endearing combination of friendliness and independence was brought to homoeopathy because of his uncooperative behavior in nursery school. When asked the reason, he answered simply: "Because of my teacher. She makes me ner-vi-ous!" And, indeed, she was an intense pushy type, quite unsuited to the unhurried, independent boy. More phlegmatic youngsters will get a blank stare in their eyes and become balky. Or, to counteract the pressure of ambitious but insensitive parents and teachers, they will sometimes behave like dunces, standing with hanging jaws and uncomprehending looks, pretending to be slower than they really are. These children defend themselves by "switching off" in various ways.

The *Calcarea* child's sensitivity is expressed in his various fears: of being alone, of the dark, of going to bed. He is subject to "night terrors," waking up screaming from the horrifying faces and frightening creatures he sees in his dreams (Hahnemann). Or he exhibits some highly specific phobia. One child will be afraid of spiders and spiders only, another of ants, a third of caterpillars. The fear is not of insects, rodents or reptiles in general, although this more general fear is also possible ("child is afraid of everything he sees": Hering), but of one particular species. A seemingly stolid little girl suffering for months from chronic diarrhea and anaemia was recognized as needing the remedy in part by her incomprehensible fear of ladybugs. She would walk up fearlessly to the biggest dogs and reach out to pat large animals in the zoo; she could stoically confront snakes and mice but had such an aversion to the innocuous little ladybug that she was panicked even by a represen-

---

cession, provided the remedy continues to be indicated: the younger the child, the more frequently may the remedy be repeated" (*Chronic Diseases*, Volume I).

tation of one. Her parents had to cut the ladybug buttons from her bath-robe and tear a ladybug appliqué from the pocket of her dress because they were giving her nightmares.

In these children the effects of frightening experiences can be felt for a long time. One was thrown into convulsions by having a mouse jump out of a drawer at her ("fear of mice": Kent) and was subject to them for years afterwards. Another's four-year history of petit-mal seizures began with the sight of a snake swallowing a frog. Both cases were cured by repeated doses of *Calcarea* in high potency (if they had been caught earlier before the symptoms became chronic, *Ignatia* might have been the required prescription; it is one of the best remedies for hysteria or convulsions brought on by fright: Kent). Often the child cannot sleep from the lingering impression of some frightening event seen on the screen, read in a book, or simply overheard in conversation; dreadful memories of ghost stories may not only cause nightmares (*Pulsatilla*) but even haunt him in the day-time.

Calcarea also cannot handle violence at one remove; he is distressed by physically disfigured persons or ones in wheelchairs. Even the sight of maimed or misshapened persons in television cartoons or comic strips will upset him, and one older child was willing to accept a lower grade on an English examination rather than discuss a book which described harsh and violent treatment of children. She wrote on the examination paper: "I cannot answer this question because I refuse to read or write about this paltry and dismal novel." Such insubordination required a series of notes to the school from her parents and physician, explaining the normally compliant girl's consistently obdurate behavior where unpleasant reading was concerned.

The child is oversensitive to small upsetting incidents of everyday life that offend his sense of justice and propriety (*Natrum muriaticum*). With his solid principles and sound heart, he cannot understand what motivates others to behave irrationally or gratuitously mean. Nor need their behavior affect him personally. He is terribly upset that Susie did not invite Sarah to her birthday party or that Jamie, who used to be friends with Eric, was nasty to him today. He is more concerned by these trifling fallings-out in the endless feuds of children than are the principals themselves. Jamie and Eric will eventually make up or go on to other things, but *Calcarea* is left behind to worry about these conflicts and unkindnesses. These are the Charlie Browns (hero of the *Pea-*

nuts cartoon strip) of the world: lovable but slow, unworldly, and hence a bit victimized. Often they are the last to "catch on" and are never quite able to keep up with the life that whizzes past them. In one sequence Charlie Brown stares in bewilderment at the frenetic activity of the children's world around him and laments, "I never know *what's* going on!". *Calcarea*'s "failure motif" is also well symbolized in his person: never winning a single baseball game, never gathering up courage to approach the pretty little red-head, never succeeding in flying a kite, and never learning to distrust the machinations of Lucy.

Sensitivity to criticism is another aspect of this child's vulnerability. To the teacher or parent he might seem to take it very well—with the passivity of the mollusc from which the remedy derives—but at a deeper level he has been affected. He is not immediately devastated (like *Pulsatilla*) and does not burst into fits of indignation or self-justification (*Arsenicum*, *Natrum muriaticum*). He is a slow reactor. But the adult's lack of initiative and fear of failure are later seen to stem directly from such early childhood criticism.

At other times, to be sure, he is immediately and visibly upset by criticism and takes umbrage at the least little comment. The child told to pick up his room or chew with his mouth closed considers it an assault on his being. He is also easily intimidated and fears ridicule (Borland). Even when people are laughing *with* him, he will think they are laughing *at* him. Those with the mildest tempers can become furious when innocently teased, whereas types such as *Phosphorus* and *Sulphur* love the attention and join in the laughter. But *Calcarea* senses that he is less quick and articulate than other children and is apprehensive lest others be amused at his expense. His manner is not to cry, cling, or seek sympathy (*Pulsatilla*) but rather to withdraw, bruised and silent, and refuse to try again in the future.

The oyster shell, however, can strengthen the child's ability to function in a stressful or inimical environment. It inculcates in the indolent one the ability to persevere, in the insecure one a sense of accomplishment, in a fearful one a readiness to venture and to dare (*Silica*). It also helps a child to take criticism without being hurt, ridicule without being devastated, and, like *Natrum muriaticum*, enables the excessively vulnerable one better to accept the injustices of life. For some children, then, the remedy acts as a shield against the harshness of the world, while for others it provides an irritant to nudge them out of their fears or sensitivities and encourage them to confront challenges, the better to prepare them for adulthood.

The Pearl

The highest potential of the oyster is to form a perfect, lustrous pearl, but if the critical grain of sand is not introduced into its amorphous organism, the pearl remains unformed. By the same token if the *Calcarea* child is deprived of a necessary irritating stimulus, he may become an undeveloped adult, forever callow and incomplete, or exceedingly slow to find himself: late in completing his studies, settling down to a career, falling in love and marrying, or finding a niche in society.

Some natures—shrewd wily street-urchins—can mature on their own. Throw them into the world, and they flourish. They are motivated, savvy, resourceful, and extract lessons from whatever experience life offers—hardy wildflowers that survive by the roadside or weeds that spring up through cracks in city sidewalks. But *Calcarea* is a hothouse plant that thrives with careful and systematic cultivation. He cannot develop by himself but demands structured, and preferably *individualized*, guidance from outside.

This is seen, in an extreme form, in the education of Wolfgang Amadeus Mozart and Helen Keller. Both were gifted and receptive *Calcarea* types who responded to the steady irritation of outside forces: their relentless *Arsenicum* teachers, Leopold Mozart and Annie Sullivan. The stories are legendary of how the latter devoted their considerable energies during long periods of their lives to developing the talents of their young charges, steadily and inexorably steering them to greatness.*

---

* Mozart's temperament, requiring an especially persistent stimulus for proper development, early showed signs of being a *Calcarea carbonica*. Beginning with his intolerance of all milk, even that of his mother and a wet nurse, which necessitated a diet of gruel from birth and made his very survival a miracle, his inability to absorb and assimilate calcium was reflected in his sickly childhood and later in his physical appearance. His poor bone structure is seen in his misshapen head with its round protruding forehead, receding chin, and unhealthy pop-eyes in their sunken sockets. While of independent disposition as a child, he was still amenable to parental authority and allowed his every step to be guided by his ambitious, forceful father. But by the age of

Even the individual of talent and ambition sometimes reveals a delayed development pattern. As the oyster imperceptibly adds layer upon layer to form a pearl, so *Calcarea* works slowly, "ploddingly and

eighteen Wolfgang had had enough of this surveillance and was ready to break away. By now, however, he was so substantially formed, and had been given such momentum, that he could roll along on his own. In this he may be contrasted with the more *Sulphur* Beethoven's relatively haphazard musical training and largely self-educated genius.

Whatever traits of other constitutional remedies Mozart displayed as an adult, and despite all the various myths about him, he definitely retained the typical *Calcarea* immaturity in the sense of being emotionally juvenile, financially naive, thoughtless of the future, and childish in behavior to the point of eccentricity.

Helen Keller was of stocky build, with a pudgy face, wavy blond hair, and full red cheeks; from an early age she was prone to ear and throat infections and high, *Belladonna*-like, fevers, one of which deprived her of sight and hearing when she was only eighteen months old. During the five years which elapsed between her illness and the appearance of her teacher she manifested no particular curiosity or intelligence, her sole interest being food. She made little progress in understanding the dark silent world she inhabited and not only gave no indication of the genius she was later to display (learning several languages, graduating with honors from Radcliffe College, writing and lecturing around the world—achievements never registered before by anyone both blind and deaf), but was even considered mentally retarded. She was also extremely stubborn and self-willed, and her frequent violent tantrums were notorious. When first taken over by Annie Sullivan, she screamed and carried on for hours and days, resisting her obstinately in every possible way. As is typical of *Calcarea*, she was at first slow to catch on; although nearly seven, she took many weeks to understand the relationship between the outside world and the impressions her teacher was making on her hand. Once launched, however, her steady lifelong accrual of knowledge never halted— under the systematic guidance of the driving Annie Sullivan.

Obviously genius does not sprout from a barren seed; talent must be present from birth, and genius results from its cultivation. But the stories of Mozart and Helen Keller reveal the heights the talented *Calcarea* nature can attain with constant surveillance and persistent discriminating guidance.

conscientiously, piling stone upon stone" (Whitmont). A writer will spend his entire life on one novel or a single collection of essays, while some works of promise never come to light at all. Somewhere along the way they are vicitms of their creator's lethargy or sloth. Emblematic of this type is the kindly old headmaster, Dr. Strong, in Dickens' *David Copperfield*, with his childlike simplicity, guilelessness, and interminable "Dictionary of Greek Roots" which, *Calcarea*-like, never gets written beyond the letter "D". Characteristic also is his handshake which Dickens ingeniously describes: " . . . and then he gave me his hand which I didn't know what to do with as it did nothing for itself."

Predictably, this constitutional picture is regularly encountered in the off-spring of very strong or famous personalities who have over-shadowed them and (even if unwittingly) prevented them from develop-ing their own characters or finding their own paths. The son who auto-matically succeeds to his father's business or profession, whether or not he has any natural aptitude for it, or who is content to live in his father's shadow, is frequently a *Calcarea*.

An engaging example of this type is found in O. Henry's story, "The Emancipation of Billy," in which a charming old *Lycopodium* ex-gov-ernor—a long-time dignitary of the small town in which he lives—continually upstages his intelligent but mild-mannered attorney son who has never married and, in fact, turned down an important government position to take care of him. With O. Henry's typical twist, the situa-tion is finally rectified when the ex-governor is presented to the U.S. President on a whistle-stop tour as " . . . the one who has the honor of being the *father* of our foremost distinguished citizen, learned and honored jurist, beloved townsman, and model southern gentleman—the Honorable William B. Pemberton."

He is often content to remain a man of "activities" in lieu of becom-ing a man of action, a dabbler who refuses to enter a profession because of the rigor of its demands. He may take up one thing after another, never applying himself seriously to any one. Or he has an untrained and *sui generis* mind that has never been disciplined or directed; his talent is frittered away on the passing moment, never applied to any large or lasting enterprise. He is the spontaneous and unselfconsciously creative child who extracts freshness from everyday life and contributes in a small way to the world's happiness. However, and this is a prom-inent feature of *Calcarea*, he is indifferent to not fulfilling his potential. Other types would fight frustration, but he is resigned, lacking the drive to start making a pearl from his inherent talents. Left to himself, he is not motivated to strike out and stretch his mind, to seek new forms and experiences as the development of talent requires, but is content to fall back on his "givens."

The remedy, however, can alter this picture. A man in his thirties was being treated with *Calcarea* for eczematous eruptions. He was a gifted painter and actor and sang well enough to appear in an opera troupe, but had rejected all of these paths out of aversion to the discipline of training ("I have always been allergic to formal education!"). Instead he made a living hanging draperies for an interior decorator, catering for parties, and dabbling in small carpentry. During treatment he suddenly decided to go to architecture school where he worked hard for the first time in his life. While still a student, he won a statewide competition to design a church. Possibly his decision to resume his education was only a coincidence, but enough of these "coincidences" have occurred during homoeopathic treatment to confirm this remedy's capacity to elicit and creatively channel the *Calcarea* individual's potential.

Even in the absence of a homoeopathic remedy acting as the irritant grain of sand, this type, sensing the need for more formal guidance, may deliberately subject himself to a strict systematic discipline. A middle-aged woman was suffering from frequent palpitations and chronic chest congestion; the symptoms were oppressed breathing and a lingering dry hacking cough at night. Many of the physical symptoms suggested *Calcarea* but seemingly none of the mentals. She was motivated, businesslike, high-powered, and energetic. Finally, she was asked if she had ever interrupted her education or dropped out of school. She must have thought that the physician was clairvoyant, since it turned out that she had left college after the freshman year and worked for sixteen years at menial jobs, allowing her considerable native talents to go to waste. Finally, craving some intellectual structure ("After having been a drifter for thirty-five years, I suddenly realized that I knew nothing from nothing"), she went back to school, found her true vocation, and completed the undergraduate and M.A. degrees in record time. With this background, typical of the *Calcarea* slow developer, the physician felt justified in prescribing the oyster shell as her constitutional remedy.

This sudden craving for rigorous discipline and an ability to impose structure on himself is even encountered in the young. One ten-year-old patient, whenever he was unpunished for a misdemeanor, would solemnly hand his parents a hairbrush, saying, "You spank me—AND HARD—I know I was bad and shouldn't get away with it like this." Another, slightly older, *Calcarea* boy who usually ate deserts and candy in large quantities, decided to give it up for Lent just to see if he could. A part of him was obviously yearning for a challenge for, when Lent was over, he confessed to having enjoyed the self-deprivation and announced his intention of undergoing it the following year. And a girl of fourteen, whose appearance and behavior suggested a *Pulsatilla/Calcarea* constitution, had a recurring tendency to nocturnal enuresis, attributed by the parents to late-night study. She herself explained that the late hours were spent writing sonnets, sestinas, rondolets, and mock epics in heroic couplets for her English composition course. When asked if she was *assigned* these difficult verse forms, and if all her classmates had to do the same, she replied that they were allowed to write in any form they chose: "Most of the class writes in modern or blank verse. I used to also, but it was too easy. I now choose these highly structured forms to make it *harder*." Then she volunteered this perceptive remark: "By trying to find rhymes and adhering to the rhythms, I find myself looking for new ideas and new words, and this makes me discover thoughts that I *never knew I had!*" *Pulsatilla* would have been most unlikely to subject herself voluntarily to such strict and trying discipline. While any child benefits from a structured environment, *Calcarea* is one of the few to actively seek it (also *Natrum muriaticum*; while *Arsenicum* has an inbred self-discipline), and this girl's resolved enuresis attested to the correctness of the physician's selection.

The remedy is traditionally, and rightly, considered long-acting ("has a long-continued action": Hahnemann); the physician will usually wait at least two months before considering another prescription. The following case, a woman of sixty being treated homoeopathically for pituitary tumor, is illustrative. The tumor, pressing on the brain, was causing constant and violent headaches, various noises in the ears, and a gradually encroaching dimness of vision which was likened by the patient to a veil over her eyes. Fortunately she had undergone no allopathic treatment, since the tumor had been considered inoperable

and impossible even to irradiate. Although the overall mental picture
was not markedly *Calcarea*, a specific fear of snakes kept surfacing in
her dreams. As soon as she fell asleep she had horrible dreams, even
hallucinations, of large, fat, aggressive snakes who crawled all over her
bed; and, if she got out of bed, there were dozens more on the floor,
writhing about and ready to attack. Of course, with such dreams *Lachesis* (Boger) and *Lac caninum* (Kent) first came to mind, but the patient did not fit either of those types in her other symptoms. The next
remedy to consider was *Calcarea* (see Kent, *Repertory*, "Delusions")
which better fitted her physical symptoms: history of enuresis in childhood until adolescence; dysmenorrhoea with too early and too profuse bleeding, terminating in a hysterectomy for fibroids; a slow metabolism, requiring her to take thyroid extract for the past twenty years;
and the veil before her eyes ("dimness of vision: with feathery appearance before eyes; as if looking through gauze": Hering). One dose of
Calcarea 200x diminished the noises in her ears and brought a vast improvement in her headaches and general well-being. The dimness of
vision remained unchanged, but the snake hallucinations had substantially altered. "Now the big snakes stay down below," she informed
us. "They no longer crawl up on my bed." Because she was still improving, at the second visit she received placebo, and when she returned
four weeks later, she reported that the snakes, although still on the floor
near her bed, were now smaller and not frightening. The headaches
had disappeared, although the "veiled" vision was unchanged. She was
again given placebo.

     At the next visit she announced that there were no longer any
snakes around her bed at night. "And even if I do meet them in my
dreams, they scurry off out of my way. Now *they* are afraid of *me!*"
She was given placebo for the third time and after another six-week
interval reported: "If I ever do dream of snakes, they are no larger than
snails, perfectly harmless, and I am not bothered by them at all." But
her vision, although stabilized, had not improved. Since she was no
longer having headaches, the physician presumed that, at the least, the
tumor had stopped growing, and had possibly shrunk. But the ocular
nerves appeared irreparably damaged and did not improve under further administration of *Calcarea* and other remedies. When seen several
years later, she was still well and in stable condition. Probably the first
long-acting dose of *Calcarea* accomplished the most that could be

achieved.

Interestingly, the horrifying snake illusions had commenced some months before the headaches and blurry vision, suggesting that the medicine, if administered at this point, might have arrested the tumor's growth and the subsequent damage to the ocular nerves.

Although the remedy is also traditionally considered slow to produce its effect, the powers of the homoeopathic polychrests transcend the labels attached to them, and *Calcarea*—even on the chronic or constitutional level—can occasionally act with startling speed. The aforementioned, fixed-to-his-window bank teller exhibiting dyspnoea, high blood pressure, chronic constipation, and various aches in his back and legs, had an attack of diarrhoea within fifteen minutes of receiving the remedy, and, in fact, while still in the office. At the same time he experienced a disturbing tingling of the fingers and toes, a symptom he had not felt for years. Afterwards he felt better in every way and continued to do so for months.

The low-key *Calcarea* picture in the patient can easily be obscured by more forceful remedies. But closer investigation reveals the quiet *Calcarea carbonica* beneath the surface, counterbalancing the aggressiveness of *Sulphur*, the nervous irritability of *Nux vomica*, the tenseness of *Arsenicum*, the overstimulation of *Lachesis*, or the flightiness of *Phosphorus*.

Even a thin, wiry, dark, quick, and energetic individual may well need this remedy, which sometimes lies concealed in the highly motivated and efficient person who manifests its typical physical symptoms without the characteristic mentals. How is this to be explained? In the first place, *Calcarea* (like *Sulphur*) is known to be capable of acting at a deeper level than other polychrests, helping with the cure of other constitutional types. It can reach back to the beginnings of the patient's troubles—to unresolved childhood fears and adolescent anxieties—and bring out latent *mental* symptoms in a way that *Sulphur* does not (the latter's powers often being limited to eliciting latent *physical* symptoms only). An examination of the patient's childhood may indeed reveal a clear *Calcarea* picture underlying, for example, today's *Sulphur* or *Lycopodium* (in the male), or *Phosphorus* or *Natrum muriaticum* (in the female). Further questioning may reveal a history of dropping out of school or college; or it may show that, at some later point in his life, the patient undertook a self-imposed course of study or some rigorous discipline which his nature craved. Finally, Constantine Hering (who was himself of Czech origin) has claimed that most Slavs need this remedy.*

Thus the physician must remain alert to the underlying *Calcarea* picture. Otherwise it is not hard to identify in the diffident, somewhat indolent, slow, easily tried, at times mentally passive, occasionally ec-

---

* Prince Myshkin, the hero of Dostoyevsky's *The Idiot* and a quintessentially Russian personality type, embodies many of the characteristics discussed in this chapter. It is a tribute to Dostoyevsky's powers of artistic observation that the epileptic Myshkin should reveal such pronounced *Calcarea* characteristics. Although intelligent and sensitive, he is too naive in his goodness, too unconventional in manner, and too eccentric in behavior (in the opening scene he strikes up a philosophical conversation with an astonished footman, speaking to him as an equal). He is mild, agreeable, charming in a typically *Calcarea* way, but ambiguous and unformed. No one knows what to make of his simplicity, which is combined with an undeniable perceptiveness. He is also childlike, his physician telling him that he will always remain a child in soul and character despite a man's face and figure. Although Myshkin laughs at this, he acknowledges feeling comfortable with children and oppressed with adults. He is also childlike in his moral innocence and especially in his lack of understanding of the force of sexual passion as an essential factor in human relations. For Myshkin, like some slow-to-develop *Calcareas*, is basically without passion or incapable of deep sexual experience, which brings tragedy to the two women he loves.
    It also befits his *Calcarea* nature that his artistic sensitivity focuses on the beauties of the minor discipline of calligraphy. For instance, he discourses at length on the subject of "flourishes":
        A flourish is a highly perilous thing! A flourish demands extraordinary taste; but if it should be successful, if the right proportions should be found, why such a script is beyond compare, so much so that one could fall in love with it!
    Susceptibility to the seductive power of beauty is certainly not peculiar to *Calcarea*, but Myshkin's disproportionate response—choosing as love objects the flourishes at the tops and bottoms of letters—attests to the *Calcarea* in him (also *Silica*).

centric individual. And when the impression made by the patient is indeterminate, either because of vagueness of personality or amorphousness of type; when his perceptiveness or sensitivity are combined with a definite simplicity of manner; when his character is undeveloped and his potential unrealized; when his whole being cries out for guidance, structure, and discipline in order to become less lethargic, less unformed, and more fulfilled, the physician should consider the potentized carbonate of lime. When administered correctly, as instructed by Hahnemann and the other masters, the modest gray shell of the lowly oyster can rightly be regarded as one of nature's greatest homoeopathic gifts to humanity.

Lycopodium

*L*YCOPODIUM is the club moss whose spores are shaped like a wolf's paw; hence the origin of the Greek name: *lyco* (wolf) and *podos* (foot). Moss is one of the oldest surviving plant life forms on earth, having existed since the Silurian period some 350 million years ago. Yet it has survived essentially unchanged despite all the intervening geological and climatic cataclysms and upheavals. The associations evoked by the moss family are serenity and stability. Its lovely green is restful to the eye and soothing to the spirit; its resilient softness is cooling to the touch, and its pertinacious growth throughout the ages suggests an indestructible nature.

As we seek correspondences between the plant and the man (if only for mnemonic purposes), we find that *Lycopodium* possesses a pleasant and self-contained personality, soothing in its composure and reserve and, at least outwardly, cool and restrained. Thus it contrasts with the more heated *Sulphur*, *Lachesis* and others. Furthermore, the nature is viable, displaying the capacity to adapt to changing scenes and varying environments without itself mutating in the process.

The mentality is complex, not always easy to recognize and define, the appearance often having little in common with what transpires underneath. This will become apparent as we attempt to capture the constant tension between the strengths and weaknesses, the image and reality, of this constitutional type.

The following analysis will focus on four prominent *Lycopodium* characteristics: his resilient self-esteem, his unshakeable viability, his imperturbable detachment, and the Achilles heel of this highly capable individual—his tendency to deceive himself. A final section will examine how these traits converge and are reflected in his attitude toward health and illness.

The Divergent Type

The classic picture of *Lycopodium* found in the homoeopathic literature is as follows: the patient is thin, muscularly weak and lacking in vital heat; the hair is prematurely gray or balding; deep furrows (from much thought and worry) line the forehead; the sunken skin of the face is sallow and earthcolored, with premature wrinkles; the worried expression may make him look older than his years; the child will resemble a wizened little old man, while the young man may appear distinguished but somewhat withered. The mind may be developed at the expense of the body. And yet the opposite is also found: mental degeneration, early senility, failing brain power, weak memory. Finally, the individual has been described as melancholy, morose, despairing, defiant, suspicious, inclined to take things ill, excessively irritable, misanthropic, cowardly, and so on. All these characteristics are encountered in the type and must be recognized when present.

The *Lycopodiums* who grace contemporary homoeopathic practice, however, quite often do not fit this picture, either at first glance or upon more extended examination. Hence this chapter will focus (especially in the male) upon what may be called the "divergent type" and present new angles to the remedy.

Lycopodium has been identified in, and successfully prescribed for, a great many patients who are physically strong, attractive looking, and well-built, suggestive of a type of vigor that the subject does little to maintain. In both sexes, the complexion can remain clear and the skin smooth, even into old age. The women are often beautiful and of good carriage. The men possess large and well-defined facial features. "Handsome" and "clean-cut" are appropriate words for *Lycopodium*'s appearance, just as *Pulsatilla* is pretty, *Phosphorus* is attractive, and *Arsenicum* is aristocratic.*

Often these men remain lanky throughout life, but with a leanness that bears the stamp of toughness rather than of frailty (*Arsenicum* and

---

* In this picture of *Lycopodium* the reader will recognize, among others, the peculiarly American type known as the WASP ("white, Anglo-Saxon, protestant").

Phosphorus are the latter). Those who gain weight with age, do so elegantly, becoming portly and distinguished-looking. Weight only seems to add dignity to their bearing and solidity to their being. The frequently strong intellect may be revealed in the prominent brow. This is a compelling feature. The remedy should be considered in any patient with a high-domed forehead or a broad or handsome brow, with or without furrows, or who exhibits the well-attested "disposition to frown" (Kent).

On the mental-emotional plane, *Lycopodium* is usually stable and balanced, with a robust attitude towards life and healthy appetites. He is temperate by inclination and in his essentially measured life style, and seldom indulges in neurotic or hypochondriacal self-deprivation. His behavior, in most respects, is moderate. He seldom over-extends himself emotionally, usually holding something in reserve. An undercurrent of quiet strength can be sensed in *Lycopodium*.

One reason for the seeming discrepancies between the traditional and divergent pictures may be that in Kent's well-known constitutional triad, *Sulphur/Calcarea carbonica/Lycopodium*, the *Lycopodium* temperament shares characteristics with these two flanking remedies. Variations in *Lycopodium* types occur because of a shift in emphasis within the triad. Some lean more to *Sulphur* and project confidence, assertiveness, intellectuality, energy, intrepidness, viability. Others lean more toward *Calcarea* and are apprehensive, slower, with an underlying layer of unresolved insecurities carried over from childhood. An additional factor accounting for the discrepancy in this drug picture is simply age. The basically strong individual remains healthy until middle age or later and thus does not visit the physician until that time. Only when he has tried his constitution too far, and it has broken down, does the weakened physical and mental picture emerge. The man who has ignored his health for four or five decades is now frightened and exhibits all the classic apprehensions and insecurities. Prior to this point he will have carefully avoided physicians.

In fact, *Lycopodium* is apt to be the homoeopathic caboose. What usually happens is that the eager, newly-converted wife (the engine) comes chugging along to homoeopathy, energetically pulling the cars along behind: her children, parents, friends, and relatives. Finally, twenty cars in the rear, comes the caboose—her reluctantly trailing husband. Thus, thanks to the energies of the bulldozing *Arsenicum* or insistently enthusiastic *Natrum muriaticum* or beseeching *Pulsatilla* wives, who drag their sceptical, reluctant, essentially healthy *Lycopodium* husbands to the physician's office, homoeopaths have been able to observe them prior to their breakdown and treat them preventively.

Self Esteem

The first striking *Lycopodium* characteristic is self-esteem. It is seen in the quiet air of one who is self-possessed and obviously has a good opinion of himself. He has confidence in his own judgment, believe-ing that he knows best at all times. Being reserved, he may not always say so, but the thought is still there. The half-mocking lament by a patient — "Oh, what a trying fate it is to be always right, when others are so wrong!" — reveals the true *Lycopodium* mindset.

He considers himself an example of moderation and reasonableness others would do well to follow. He is convinced the world would be a far, far better place if it contained more right-thinking and right-acting persons like himself. *Sulphur* can possess similar self-confidence but is less self-righteous; *Lycopodium* invests moral weight in his "right-ness," while *Arsenicum*'s "I am always right" has an aggressive over-tone which is uncharacteristic of *Lycopodium*.

Sometimes, to be sure, his self-esteem is a facade (what Gutman calls "outward overcompensation") covering a *Calcarea*-like sense of inadequacy. Under the strong exterior lie fears of incompetence ("lack of confidence in his strength": Hahnemann), sometimes justified, some-times unfounded. But even here his insecurity is distinguished from *Calcarea*'s in being overlain with a veneer of assertiveness (sometimes even psychological bullying), while *Calcarea*'s is humble and diffident. In the divergent *Lycopodium*, however, the unequivocal self-esteem is no cover-up. His youthful *Calcarea* insecurities have been resolved, and his air of confidence and strength is the outward manifestation of a truly self-respecting, intellectually and emotionally well-integrated individual.

Indeed, *Lycopodium*'s strength derives largely from his self-esteem, which he uses to gain the esteem of others. His very character, behavior, and assurance all inspire respect, and he is psychologically astute in making himself liked as well as respected. His manner is gracious and courteous, with a self-contained charm (as against the more expansive charm of a *Phosphorus* or *Sulphur*) that almost imperceptibly brings others under his will.

His self-esteem is well-grounded and manifested from an early age, especially in boys, as the following incident illustrates. An artistically talented ten-year-old was being treated with *Lycopodium* for a moist eczema, particularly marked on the hands. He was the son of a rather prominent government official and was himself ambitious for fame. One day his father jokingly encouraged him, "Keep up your drawing, Henry, and someday you will be well-known as the gifted son of the famous Joseph N___."

"No, Daddy, you've got it all backwards," was the cool reply. "*You* will soon be known as the gifted father of the famous artist, Henry N___." The seriousness and self-assurance behind the humor were evident.

In his confidence and ability to deal with situations, the budding *Lycopodium* may be sophisticated beyond his years, maintaining his self-possession even under stress. This trait was exhibited in a young patient whose sixth-grade English teacher, having misplaced the gradebook and believing it stolen by one of the pupils, announced to the class that unless it was found, he would have to decide arbitrarily what grades to give out. The book was not returned and the boy got a C + on his report card. Surprised, he took his compositions and tests to the teacher to show that he had gotten all A's and B's, but the latter, for reasons of his own, stuck by the grade.

After an initial justifiable anger and frustration which, according to his parents, lasted only a few minutes, the boy shrugged his shoulders and said, "Oh, well, what the heck!" and there the matter ended. He later explained to the physician, "*I* know that I got all A's and B's and did well in the course, so what do I care if the teacher gave me a C + ? I suppose it's his way of getting back at me. I certainly was no angel in class this year." He was self-respecting and secure enough not to remain vexed at another's unfairness or nonappreciation of his work. Such a mature reaction was quite the opposite of the fury of a *Natrum muriaticum* at such treatment who, months, and even years, later would still recall with passion and indignation the injustice perpetrated on him.

This student, by the way, was being treated for faulty digestion, specifically manifested as tremendously offensive gas from the starchy and farinacious foods he craved, and it is appropriate to mention here that one of the main constitutional weaknesses of *Lycopodium* is the liver, with concomitant faulty digestion. He suffers from abdominal distension and a distressing postprandial bloating, loud stomach rumbling or gurgling, and a tendency to offensive, sometimes painful, flatulence; an inability to pass wind, burning eructations, satiety even after a few mouthfuls, or a feeling of fulness not relieved by belching. (see Hahnemann's listing of some 300 digestion symptoms). Despite these gastrointestinal symptoms, he may share with *Sulphur* the characteristic of being a hearty, even an excessive, eater ("eating increases his hunger": Kent), or he wakes up hungry in the middle of the night and must eat a snack to go back to sleep. He is better from hot food and may insist on having the plates warmed. He can tolerate very hot liquids, drinking tea and coffee piping hot without burning his mouth. Sometimes *Lycopodium* craves sweets; one three-year-old patient who insisted that sugar be sprinkled over every mouthful of food was only broken of this habit by a prescription of this remedy.

Lycopodium's self-esteem is strengthened by the feeling that he was "born under a lucky star." Life seems to encourage him in this. Being self-disciplined, he succeeds easily in academic endeavors and personal relations, and, generally, in everything he does. He trusts to his good fortune, hopes for the best, and with his innate competence and upbeat mentality his ventures tend to work out well. If they do not, it is no great matter. Resilient and robust, he rises like a phoenix from his own ashes and goes on to something else (*Sulphur*). This all enhances his seeming physical and psychological indestructibility and already high opinion of himself; it also lays the groundwork for the typical *Lycopodium* arrogance which may be disguised early in life but later becomes apparent ("haughtiness": Boenninghausen).

A quite different manifestation of his self-esteem is a reluctance to argue or negotiate. While he can be pugnacious and, like *Sulphur*, enjoy intellectual contention, that is different from arguing on a personal level, with its accompanying loss of dignity. *Lycopodium* feels so obviously in the right that he will often refuse even to discuss a matter. In the middle of an argument, and especially if the other has made a strong point, he gets up and walks away. Like a stately ambassador, ignoring his adversary's challenges, he senses the moment to withdraw from an unproductive situation and retreat with honor. *Natrum muriaticum*, on the contrary, insists upon fighting even losing battles to the bitter end.

When *Lycopodium* does deign to engage in contention, he can be a master of evasion, clever at avoiding direct confrontation on the enemy's own territory. He subtly retreats from hostile ground by eluding the central issue, deflecting the argument, or changing the subject. Thus he pulls his opponent deeper into his own terrain, where he can then more easily rout him (like Napoleon's disastrous 1812 campaign in Russia), while, on the rare occasions when he does admit to being mistaken in an argument, he does not really mean it. His tone conveys a cavalier attitude of "All right, all right, have it your own way if you *do* insist," implying that because the other party is quite unreasonable, he himself is capitulating magnanimously.

One male patient — gracious, intelligent, attractive, and seemingly an ideally supportive husband to any woman — was being treated for gout. After a course of *Lycopodium*, his wife called to thank the physician — not for the cure, but the first *constructive* argument she had had with her husband in years. "I am beginning to realize what a privilege it is for married couples to be able to argue," was her comment. Apparently this strong-minded gentleman had been unwilling in the past to discuss anything which might place him in an unfavorable light or prevent him from doing what he wanted. "This conversation should have ended ten sentences ago, I refuse to hear another word on the subject," he would insist, employing the classic *Lycopodium* tactic of refusing to engage the enemy, and to every convincing argument raised by his wife would oppose a dignified silence. Now he had come down from this proud and unassailable position and was willing to examine their differences, while she no longer felt her former frustration at having nothing to confront or fight against.

Just as *Lycopodium* tries to avoid argument, he will avoid rupturing relationships. Discord or breaking with others is undignified and beneath his self-respect. It tarnishes his image of being able to get along with anyone, of understanding everyone, and of being respected by all. He bends over backwards not to estrange himself from family, associates, friends, and subordinates. Even after a bitter divorce, it is very important for his self-esteem to remain on amicable terms with his ex-wife and in-laws. Contrary to what one would expect, the capable *Lycopodium* employer is reluctant to dismiss incompetent employees; he would rather retain them than sever relationships and create bad feelings. Professionally, also, he will try to patch up relations after any disagreement with an adversary or competitor, by having a friendly drink and talking things over in a tactful conciliatory manner. No type is better at separating personal feelings from professional. He can engage in heated debate with an opponent in the courts, the board room, or the smoke-filled chambers of political life, and be laughing and joking with him an hour later. Calling a cease-fire, he puts aside professional rivalry and honestly enjoys the company of his adversary.

This is an attractive trait. *Lycopodium* is ready to overlook past discord and does not harbor resentments as does *Natrum muriaticum*. Possessing a healthy "That's water over the dam" attitude, he looks forward to starting anew. His conscious or unconscious philosophy is that more is achieved by mending than by breaking, by conciliation than by antagonism. Believing that to forgive is wisdom but to forget is sublime, he makes a point of maintaining social harmony by forgiving and forgetting.

Sometimes his conciliatory impulse leads the self-righteous *Lycopodium* even to apologize—which he does handsomely. *Pulsatilla*, in her desire to avoid discord, apologizes prettily. The difference between the two is that *Lycopodium* is conciliatory partly out of design and remains insistent on his terms, while the naturally peacemaking *Pulsatilla*, conceding from the heart, will sweetly say, "I'm sorry. Do as you want. Have it your own way. I'll go along with you."

Pulsatilla and *Lycopodium* contrast with those constitutional types who cannot apologize at all: especially *Sepia* and *Natrum muriaticum*. It is sheer torture to their sensitive pride. They will withdraw from others or risk breaking relations rather than suffer the humiliation of an apology. It is easier for *Lycopodium* because his apology is less an admission of error than an aspect of his own self-esteem. He apologizes primarily to terminate the quarrel and maintain harmony, not because he believes himself necessarily wrong. Thus, he effectively depersonalizes, or sublimates, his apology into an act of noble sacrifice in the cause of peace. He may also apologize out of shrewdness: to stave off further or more serious criticism on an issue where he knows himself to be not wholly in the right.

Because they confirm his sense of worth, this individual likes praise and compliments. He does not become confused or embarrassed but accepts the tribute with quiet dignity, as his rightful due. He himself is suave and gracious in his compliments and can be extremely flattering when he wants. He seeks flattery in return and soaks it up, no matter how blatant it may be (any spouse of a *Lycopodium* should know that flattery is one way of keeping him or her happy).

Even when given credit he does not deserve, *Lycopodium* is perfectly willing to receive it. He knows the praise is unmerited (he is no fool, after all) but will not object. He thinks somewhat along these lines: "If it gives others pleasure to think me better than I am, why disillusion them? Let them think so. They don't suffer from it, I don't either, and everybody is happier all-around." His acceptance of undeserved credit is thus rationalized as kindness to others. Many individuals will disclaim unearned praise, preferring truth to credit. *Lycopodium* generally prefers credit to truth.

If complimented on some home repair job, for instance, he will come up with an attractively self-deprecating, "I do what I can to help," or "It was nothing difficult, although I *do* have a knack with tools." These are fine answers; *Lycopodium* usually knows exactly what to say and what not to say to maintain a good image. Of course, he may fail to mention that the repair, in fact, did not hold and that a professional had to be engaged. He will not lie, but feels no need to tell the whole truth.

A charming woman was being treated for menstrual irregularities and discomforts of no particular distinction. Her symptoms, physical and mental, alternated between *Natrum muriaticum* and *Lycopodium*. To decide which was currently more prominent in her makeup, the physician inquired about her children's musical careers (knowing that they had always shown promise): "You are such an artistically gifted person [she was a graphic arts designer], all that musical talent must come from your side of the family." He knew very well that her husband was the musical one, but she smiled the loveliest of smiles, implying that his judgment was correct but that she was just too modest to agree, and remarked, "Well, I do play a little" (indeed, she did play "a little" and no more). In the same circumstances *Natrum muriaticum* would in all probability have disclaimed the compliment, insisting that the musicality came from her husband's side of the family. The patient's reply pointed clearly to the remedy, and the subsequent improvement in her periods proved the choice correct.

In dealing with the world at large *Lycopodium* appears full of faith in humanity, but his open and pleasant manner often harbors caution and mistrust, with little faith in anyone but himself ("distrustful, suspicious": Hahnemann). In his heart he is a sceptic who expects little of frail and erring mortals. This mistrust may, in part, be the corollary of his self-esteem. He is convinced that others cannot do things nearly as well as he, and always relies on himself to know or perform better. In fact, the well-known *Lycopodium* "anticipation" symptoms ("fear of breaking down under stress, dread before appearing in public, and anticipatory apprehensions prior to performance": Kent) often reflect threatened self-esteem more than lack of confidence. He knows he *can* and *should* perform well and is prepared, but fears his memory will fail him or that he will in some way lose face (saving face is always a first consideration with him). True conviction of *inability* to perform properly is more characteristic of *Silica* or *Calcarea*. Although the competent *Lycopodium* may ultimately perform beautifully ("he gets on his legs, warms to his work, sails along in blissful self-forgetfulness . . . It is all joy and fluency": Tyler), the next time he is equally apprehensive lest his image suffer.

Yet caution and scepticism do not make him an ineffectual pessimist. On the contrary, they make him *pragmatic*. In dealing with people, he does not aim too high but remains essentially realistic about their limitations (Bismarck, a fine representative of the type's sceptical and pragmatic understanding of the limitations of his fellow humans, commented: "One should never look too closely at how laws and sausages are made"). He tries to work with the material at hand and does not wish for better, subconsciously adhering to the philosophy that "A bird in the hand is worth two in the bush." This is quite different from *Arsenicum* and *Natrum muriaticum* who seek absolutes in their relations with others and have high expectations; holding out for two birds, they may find themselves empty-handed.

Accepting people as they are without being unduly critical contributes to his social resilience. He is not easily disappointed or hurt by others (*Natrum muriaticum*), nor does he hold them up to unrealistic standards (*Arsenicum*). In fact, he is tolerant of mediocrity, and even of inferiority, in those around him. In contrast to *Arsenicum*, he seldom pushes others to do better or to excel themselves and, outside his immediate family, does not try (like *Natrum muriaticum*) to change them. Because of this, others feel comfortable with *Lycopodium*, sensing that he does not expect more than they are willing to give. His lower and more realistic expectations facilitate smooth and easy relationships.

Negatively, however, his scepticism and mistrust can lead him to underrate others' capacities and understanding. That is one reason why this courteous, agreeable type manifests "haughtiness," and an "overbearing" demeanor (Hering). He not only knows best, he wants others to defer to his opinions, at times conveying the message that dissenters are either knaves or fools. He repeatedly underestimates his competitors, peers, family and even friends, while magnifying his own influence or ability. This is one of his consistent intellectual weaknesses. Usually his arrogance surfaces only upon closer acquaintance. Initially he exhibits a social fineness that dilutes arrogance with charm and disguises it with bonhomie. However, it is *Lycopodium* who suffers most from that flaw of the heroes of Greek tragedy, *hubris*: a short-sighted intellectual pride which darkens the understanding.

Finally, his self-esteem is evident in his lenient attitude toward himself. He accepts his own limitations as he does those of others—and he expects them to treat him with the same leniency. Aware that he is not perfect, even though convinced that he is a "good sort," he thinks to himself, "So what? Who is perfect?" and does not linger upon or worry about his deficiencies. The *Lycopodium* God is the forgiving Christ who treats human weaknesses with compassion—not the stern, punitive, biblical Jehovah. Even when a non-believer, he feels that some "Power" up above is benevolently watching over and non-judgmentally inclined towards him. This makes him sanguine and determined to get the most out of life.

However, *Lycopodium* is not necessarily exploitative. Although he can be competitive and jealous of his position, he possesses a keen sense of service and sincerely wants to make a good job of his life. He takes pride in work which is well-done and beneficial to humanity, and will often devote himself unsparingly to this end. In fact, he may derive his greatest security and deepest satisfaction—even his very identity—from it. But the work must be performed on *his* terms, preferably with himself in a position of power and prestige.

Viability

Just as the resilient moss conforms to the configuration of the landscape and the changing environment, while proceeding undaunted along its way, *Lycopodium*'s *viability* ("enormous tenacity for survival":

Gutman) stems from his resolute yet conforming nature which permits him to adapt to fluctuating times and circumstances while pursuing his own policies.

In fact, he commands all the necessary prerequisites for politics and diplomacy. Instinctively espousing the principles of *Realpolitik*, he likes wielding power and, even while wanting to please everyone, needs to be honored or acknowledged as a leader ("speaks with an air of command": Hering).* This need is screened at times by his reserved and courteous manner (the iron hand is well-concealed in the velvet glove), but it is there nonetheless. Moreover, *Lycopodium* knows instinctively how to achieve his desired end by accepting compromise. He also evinces moderation, discretion, even reticence (playing his cards close to his chest), as well as a guarded scepticism.

In addition, this supple mentality allows him to conform to the fluidity of the shifting scene without violating his conscience. When forced to change an opinion, he justifies it with a "What I said yesterday was yesterday. Today is different." Thus he can run with the hare one day and hunt with the hounds the next, for his strongest loyalty is to his own viability. In this way he remains buoyant: when circumstances change, he does not become confused like *Phosphorus*, split like *Lachesis*, or lost like *Natrum muriaticum*.

The French diplomat and stateman, Talleyrand, comes to mind as the quintessential viable *Lycopodium*. A bishop under the Bourbon monarchy, an ambassador under the Girondins, Grand Chamberlain under Napoleon, and Foreign Minister under the restored Bourbon regime, he was hardly a paragon of consistency. It required no common psychic elasticity, not to mention diplomatic ability and tact, to hold leading positions under four different forms of French government without forfeiting his credibility. It was at the Congress of Vienna, after the Napoleonic Wars, however, that Talleyrand best exhibited his incomparable *Lycopodium* gifts of shrewd statesmanship and moderation. Despite much opposition to his very presence, the French envoy insinuated his way into the graces of the other participating countries as they fought each other for power and precedence, convincing them all that

---

* Under "love of power" Kent lists only *Lycopodium*. However, *Arsenicum*, *Nux vomica*, *Lachesis*, and *Sulphur* could also be added to this rubric.

an intact and prosperous France was to their political advantage and thus steering his country through the Congress without loss of territory or prestige. Late in life, when criticized for the apparent elasticity of his principles, Talleyrand would state that he never abandoned any government before it abandoned itself, but he did so just a little earlier than others.

Lycopodium's viability extends even to his style. He is highly conscious of the impression he makes and able to adapt manner and speech to the occasion. Sensitive to the importance of a good exterior, he cultivates geniality, the social graces, and the light touch that influences without arousing antagonism. Whatever else may be faulted in him, few will quarrel with his style and appearance.

In most professions *Lycopodium* rises to the top, achieving social or intellectual eminence. He frankly enjoys shaping policy and working in the front ranks of responsibility and authority. Consequently, these individuals figure prominently as heads of bureaucratic departments, schools, colleges, and other political and social institutions. Nor is this surprising. They inspire trust and confidence; they obviously possess the competence, strength of character, social adroitness, reliability, and adaptability required in these prestigious positions; and their manner is so attractive that their merit is apparent to all. Mankind, on the whole, does not object to being led by *Lycopodiums*.

This type can not only project a good image but also maintain it — if necessary, in the face of adversity. A good example of this was Robert E. Lee, who emerged triumphant and respected even from defeat. History could not have accorded him more honor if he had won the Civil War instead of losing it. This was due not only to his undisputed capability as a general and charismatic leader of men, but also to his noble bearing in defeat. With true patrician dignity, he did not look back in anger and resentment or with feelings of inadequacy that grow out of dissecting the idealized past (as did so many of his fellow Confederates) but intelligently and conscientiously set about adapting to the changed environment. His moderating influence and diplomatic skill helped the South adjust to Reconstruction and get back on its feet once again (ironically, it was the victorious Grant whose life ended in scandal and disgrace). He retained the respect of all and lived out his days in an aura of graciousness.

Lycopodium, then, is viable in the sense of being enterprising and responding well to challenges; he also demonstrates a certain moss-like *indestructibility* that permits him to operate well even in a hostile environment. Experiences and events that would devastate others do not devastate him. This ability to survive where others have failed is exhibited in patients with traumatic childhoods, such as being orphaned, having hostile or alcoholic parents, being the victims of ugly divorces, or living through wars. Although other types bear lifelong debilitating emotional scars from such backgrounds, such early difficulties do not appear to leave lasting scars on *Lycopodium*. They may even strengthen him and equip him to withstand the exigencies of life (for an example see the chapter on *Natrum muriaticum*).

However, one person's viability is often attained and exercised at the expense of another. The more viable trespasses on the terrain of the less viable, causing the latter to suffer. *Lycopodium*, in an unobtrusive way, may oppress weaker persons close to him, particularly his spouse and children. Perhaps he subconsciously seeks out a mate weaker than himself, either in character, talent, or health. Avoiding the stronger organisms he cannot dominate, he will choose a gentle, self-effacing or sickly spouse—who is satisfied to be guided entirely by her husband and prepared to play the role of "the wife" in their married life. He can elicit the most extraordinary devotion of this kind; his wife lives almost solely for his needs, and both partners are content. The woman who was asked how her marrige had survived so long and replied, "It is because we have both been in love with the same man for thirty-five years," surely had a *Lycopodium* for a husband. Trouble begins only when the wife tires of playing second fiddle and wants recognition in her own right.

These wives are often accommodating and compliant *Pulsatillas*, or even more, dutiful and long-suffering *Natrum muriaticum* types. Not to be overlooked, however, are the ones who react to their overly confident husbands or marital stress by exhibiting the opposite side of the *Lycopodium* picture: "insecurity, dependence, sadness with disposition to weep, irresoluteness, and timidity" (Hahnemann and Hering) or "alternately weeping and laughing; laughing over serious matters . . . involuntarily . . . during anxiety" (Kent), and who, while seemingly resembling *Pulsatilla* or *Natrum muriaticum*, respectively, actually require the same remedy as their husbands.

In all spheres, in fact, *Lycopodium* courts inferiors and surrounds himself with them. Toward the competent he can be overly critical and even unjust, while inferiors bring out his magnanimity and allow him to play the role of savior. He loves to feel generous, understanding, forgiving, and tolerant toward erring or weaker mortals. Also, of course, inferiors are non-threatening. They will not challenge his insecurities and are unlikely to surprise him in some weakness or misstep (consciously or unconsciously *Lycopodium* is always protecting his aura of strength and invincibility). They offer him less competition and do not detract from his self-image. The dullness or incompetence of others permits him to shine the brighter.

When asked why he constantly made allowances for the incompetent persons around him, but none for the competent ones, a patient replied, "I realize that I can't bring my influence to bear on the former, so I don't bother to change them, while I can improve the latter, so I do criticize." This was an accurate assessment on one level, but it ignored the less praiseworthy motives—his dislike of competition and need to maintain a position of superiority vis-a-vis others.

Also, although shrewd and full of political savvy, *Lycopodium* is credulous. He can be deluded by appearances and exhibit surprisingly poor judgment of people. He is taken in by name-dropping, boasting, flattery, and self-promotion, and is impressed by "famous" personages per se. Conversely, he may overlook true worth in a modest individual. But his poor judgment may work ultimately to his own advantage: the person who is all "glitter" may be less than *Lycopodium* thinks he is but may still serve his immediate needs better than one who is true gold.

The type's oppression of those around him has yet another facet. Quite unconsciously he may encourage, even create, inferiority in others. His very competence and outward strength breed the opposite qualities in those who are close. After all, it is difficult to be around someone who is always self-contained, always in command, always gracious and charming in public, always self-assured, and always right. Others may be excused for giving up the struggle when confronted with so much viability.

For this reason, while he would seem to be a model parent or spouse—reliable, responsible, balanced, rarely a drunkard or a gambler—he sometimes exudes an indefinable oppressiveness that is especially hard to combat. Frequently one finds *Lycopodium* men married to chronically ailing women. Or a formerly capable and self-confident woman, upon marriage, becomes helpless and irresolute in the home, incapable of changing a fuse or keeping the household accounts. Even her care of the children or grocery shopping become inefficient when her husband is around, implying or showing her how he does them better. On a more serious level, the children may not live up to their potential and be uninspired and mediocre despite a fine education and all the "advantages." In contrast, the negative *Sepia*, erratic *Lachesis*, or neurotic *Natrum muriaticum* will raise productive, interesting, and happy children because they do not feel oppressed by the parental image.

Since much of this dialectic is subconscious, it is not only concealed from the average outsider but is usually unrecognized for the longest time by the principals involved. *Lycopodium* himself is certainly unaware of his influence, and the immediate family only vaguely senses that something is draining them of initiative. The psychologically overbearing individual can operate so imperceptibly, so like a soft blanket of moss, that the family members never suspect what is smothering them. The fiction of Henry James, whose elegant prose, infinitely subtle mind, and aloof disposition suggest a strong vein of *Lycopodium*, often explores the way in which one individual grows and flourishes through the willing or unconscious sacrifice of another.

On the overt or conscious level, this person who is so attentive as a colleague, so easy-going as a friend, so charming as an acquaintance, may be the harshest of dictators at home; a prominent characteristic is *Lycopodium*'s tendency to protect outsiders rather than his own. He has a quarrelsome side ("easily excited to vexation and anger": Hahnemann; "seeks disputes": Hering; and Allen has over 50 listings for his various types of "ill-humor, fretfulness, irritability,") that is often directed against his dependents and those who cannot or will not fight back. As one patient admitted shamefacedly, "The only person in the world I'm ever mean to is my wife." And if he cannot bully his wife, he will bully his children. This type needs their total obedience and unequivocal approval to reinforce his self-esteem and allay his underlying insecurity. Political animal that he is, *Lycopodium* perceives even family life in political terms. When he feels secure, he regards marriage and paternity as a balance of power and a ground for continuous delicate diplomatic negotiation. If his authority is not firmly established, he then resorts to a not-so-delicate jockeying for position.*

A *Lycopodium* patient being treated homoeopathically for severe renal colic, with blood and gravel in the urine, gave the impression of being attractive and good-natured in every way. Later, however, the physician learned that at home it was quite a different story. He was gracious and genial enough as long as he got his way and was obeyed implicitly, but he could be beside himself when opposed, expecting his family to exhibit their loyalty by accepting his views unquestioningly. He would tolerate no dissent on any issue, large or small. He insisted on deciding which members of the family were to do which chores and at which precise times, what his wife was to wear, and what food should be prepared. Any operation not performed to his precise specifications was made into an issue and an occasion for unpleasantness (*Nux vomica*). During treatment, however, as the urinary complaint cleared up, the patient's attitude toward his family began to change. He indulged in fewer political maneuvers and imposed his tastes less frequently. His wife gratefully told the physician that the family could now "breathe" around the father, whereas formerly she and the children had felt smothered. Yet the patient had not revealed this side of his character at all during the interview, and these traits were not used as indications for the remedy. This is merely a further illustration of how the constitutional remedy can act positively on all levels of being.

In connection with this case it should be noted that *Lycopodium* is capable of assigning moral dimensions even to artistic, culinary, and other tastes. If he dislikes fiction (which he often does), those who enjoy it will be made to feel guilty: "Why are you reading that frivolous book again?" he demands, "when you could be doing something helpful in the house—or at least reading something useful like the newspaper?" If his wife cuts her hair or dresses according to her own, not

---

* In Shakespeare's *Taming of the Shrew*, Petruccio exhibits a *Lycopodium*-like insistence on Katharina's unquestioning assent to whatever he says or wishes, as part of her wifely duties. If he says that the sun in the sky is the moon, she must agree that it is the moon. If he then reproaches her for her ignorance and insists it is the sun, she must accept the correction in perfect submissiveness. This, in exaggerated form, is the domineering *Lycopodium*'s subliminal expectation of his dependents' behavior in the home.

his, taste, she is being unfeminine, rebellious, and unnecessarily intransigent. If he likes beans and lentils (as is frequently the case—and of which he partakes with insufferable self-righteousness), those who do not are perceived as lacking some essential virtue.

To be sure, *Lycopodium*'s considerateness and charm *can* also be lavished on his family, and not directed only at outsiders. The surface of this individual will thus correspond to the underlying reality. But often enough these positive qualities are still mixed with traces of "imperiousness" (Hering) and a faint suggestion of superiority. These are simply bred into the constitutional type.

The overbearing manner reflects, in part, a deep, strong, conservative bent of mind: "Cannot bear any changes, aversion to undertaking anything new; aversion to appearing in any new role" (Kent). He is reluctant to change his job or residence, even if it means leaving a worse situation for a better one. He prefers to live where he has always resided, despite changes of fashion to wear clothes he has always worn, and continue to do what he has always done (in contrast to the restless *Tuberculinum* who is constantly seeking change). This quality is due primarily to caution—not, for example, to inertia, as is the case with *Calcarea*. He proceeds warily in most things. "What if things turn out to be worse than they appear?" he wonders. "At least here I know what to expect." Some have labelled this type "cowardly" (Kent) or "pusillanimous" (Hering), but, while these traits are also encountered, *Lycopodium* should rather be labelled cautious, conservative, circumspect, or wary.

Often the well-known symptom, "little things annoy" (Boericke), precisely describes his unreasonable irascibility at slight deviations from routine. In major upheavals *Lycopodium* can exhibit remarkable equanimity. He calmly accepts severe reversals. In a crisis he is magnificent: cool, supportive, reliable. It is the small changes that throw him completely off balance: "Hey, don't move that table! It was fine just where it was. I don't *care* if it gets more light in the new position." He is one of the few constitutional types to be actively upset by the disposal of an old dishrag, worn out and full of holes. *Sulphur* might hang onto the rag out of economy, but *Lycopodium*'s motive is different: although he, too, hates being wasteful, it is really his innate conservatism and tenacity that are disturbed by losing something to which he has grown accustomed. "I liked the old dishrag. I knew where the holes were and worked around them. I don't *want* a change of kitchen rag at this stage of my life. Why (turning to the culprit in irritation) did you throw it away? And why is everyone *always* working against me?"

All of which might appear to contradict our earlier assertions about *Lycopodium*'s viability and adaptability. This is part of his complexity. He is, indeed, adaptable on the intellectual or abstract planes; his psyche easily adjusts to changing ideas and circumstances in the world at large. But he is unyieldingly set in his ways and tenaciously conservative in all that concerns him personally (his habits, diet, health, family, etc.).

What further contributes to making him difficult to live with, for all his good qualities, is his cautious, often unduly apprehensive, attitude to money. He will practice needless economies ("parsimonious, avaricious": Hering) even if his earnings are adequate and secure, and at times (like *Arsenicum* and *Sepia*) he displays a miserly streak. After a long trip he will spend hours getting home from the station by cumbersome public transportation, arriving tired and irritated, rather than spend a few dollars on a taxi. Even when prosperous, he hates spending money on babysitters to give his wife some freedom. *Sulphur* and *Arsenicum* do the same, but *Lycopodium* is more apt to insist, or imply by a reproachful look, that this has nothing to do with spending money: it is the mother's *moral* duty to remain with her child at all times. He may eat poorly, not out of necessity, but because he does not like to spend money on food. He will refrain from buying fresh fruit or vegetables during the winter months, or forbid his wife to indulge in these for the family; and when living alone or cooking for himself, he will exist for months on grains or beans bought in bulk at wholesale prices. These last he will store away in the cellar where, with time, they become mildewed or infested with weevils. Then he will carefully and painstakingly salvage what he can of the contaminated food. He will spend hours doing some simple repair job (which should have taken minutes) with an old crooked saw, just to avoid buying a new one. Thus he is the man (seldom the woman) who is penny wise and pound foolish. A major difference between the money-conscious *Lycopodium* and his *Arsenicum* and *Sulphur* counterparts is that he does not enjoy *talking* about money as much as the latter. Also, he is usually less interested in acquiring material possessions.

We have been concentrating on the *Lycopodium* male (for the remedy is, constitutionally, predominantly a male one), but much of what has been stated can apply equally to the female. Although helpful and charming to outsiders, she too can be "dictatorial" (Kent) or a subtly suffocating influence on those around her. She, too, "cannot bear the least contradiction and at once gets beside herself from vexation" (Hahnemann). Thus, to be certain of his diagnosis the physician should look to the patient's family. If the members exhibit signs of oppression, or if the children are somehow not of the parents' caliber, or if the wife is chronically ill while the husband is strong and healthy, or if the husband appears repressed and unfulfilled for no tangible reason while the wife is serene, *Lycopodium* should be considered. With the remedy the homoeopath may be able to help not only the dominant member of the household but, indirectly, the others as well.

Detachment

Lycopodium needs to feel detached at almost all times and at almost any cost. Aloof from the turmoils of earth, he likes to float somewhere above struggling humanity, unruffled and unperturbed, regarding it from the lofty perspective of his detachment. He is interested, ready to advise and to help, but refuses to be emotionally involved. He realizes that his viability depends on some degree of detachment, and more than a modicum of emotional reserve.

To such an extent does he place a dignified distance between himself and small worldly concerns, that when a problem (personal, domestic, business, social, health) does arise, he will not meet it head-on. He may refuse even to admit its existence, rejecting whatever might disturb his detachment. He sticks his head in the sand, ignoring what he does not want to see and expecting the problem to go away.

One technique used to remain detached is humor. Wit is a notorious substitute for emotion, and resorting to humor is a classic way of preserving intellectual and emotional aloofness. Speaking of a *Lycopodium* friend or relation, patients will say, "He keeps me at a distance with his jocularity," or "He is pleasant enough but constantly maintains a joking aloofness that detracts from the significance of anything I say or do," or "He always makes a joke of an emotion or problem important to me, which dismisses it, and he then needn't confront it seriously." "Everything seems ludicrous to him" (Kent) because he doesn't really care.

He enjoys relating to people on an easy joking basis and often excels in light conversation and sophisticated small talk. Although Kent describes *Lycopodium* as desiring only familiar persons around him ("dreads the presence of new persons"), we also find that, like *Sulphur*, he enjoys large gatherings where strangers mix and merge, and where he can exchange witticisms with "important" people, or those potentially useful to his career, while the emotional demands remain negligible. This is quite different from *Natrum muriaticum*'s taste for small intimate gatherings, with close friends and family only, where everyone can engage in deep "meaningful" conversations.*

His humor can be described as "wry" or "dry," reflecting his innate sophistication, urbanity, and dispassionate intellect: examples from literature are the wry humor and caustic irony of Stendhal's *The Red and the Black* and *The Charterhouse of Parma*. At times he assumes the irritating tone of one who is detached from himself, knows and sees through himself, but does not expect others to do so. He is willing enough to make self-deprecatory remarks, but will not permit others to laugh at his expense. Highly conscious of power, and well aware that wit is power, he prefers to wield that weapon himself. At another's joke he will smile reluctantly, with the characteristic *Lycopodium* guarded or half smile, or will produce a repartee or counter-joke of his own and only *then* laugh.

"Sticks and stones may break my bones but names will never hurt me," is a well-known folk-saying, but, of course, names are what hurt the most—particularly when uttered in ridicule—and *Lycopodium* is careful to avoid becoming the target of another's humor. This is one reason for his caution and reserve, his conservatively understated manner. It may also explain why he is sometimes evasive and unwilling to answer questions directly or completely. This is due less to secretiveness than to a cautious reluctance to reveal anything about himself and his doings that may appear ridiculous.

On the other hand, he does not mind criticism of himself. In his detachment he is not easily offended. Pricks and even insults that would wound another roll off him like water off a duck—part and parcel of his

---

* Boenninghausen, interestingly, lists *Lycopodium* in the highest degree in the rubric "desires company," but does not specify whether of close ones or strangers.

apparent invulnerability. As long as criticism does not come from members of his immediate entourage and does not require him to change his life, as long as his surface is not seriously ruffled, he turns it away with a shrug or regards it as a bracing experience (*Sulphur*). He may even welcome it as a form of attention ("I don't mind what you say about me, as long as you spell my name right").

This all contributes to his aura of being good-natured and an easy person to deal with. Provided he is not seriously crossed and gets his own way overall, he often is just that. But a truly cooperative, easygoing, accommodating *Lycopodium* is a rarity.

He can be moody, alternately "merry, laughing at the simplest things" and "melancholy or low-spirited" (Hering). And the male especially has a temper, even though it is more controlled than *Sulphur*'s and erupts less frequently. Here again, the type lies somewhere between its partners in Kent's triad: the explosive, quick-to-anger *Sulphur* and the more even-tempered, hard-to-arouse *Calcarea*, and partakes of the natures of both. Being cooler and more self-possessed than *Sulphur*, *Lycopodium* is more likely to exhibit a "reserved ill humor" (Boenninghausen); if asked what is wrong, he will rarely speak out, much less complain, but his pained expression indicates that the question is unwelcome. Or he may temper his own or another's anger by resorting to wit, thereby defusing the emotion and heat of the situation. But when this slow-to-anger individual is finally roused, he can go off like a Roman Candle ("passionate anger": Hahnemann), displaying a surprising unreasonableness or vociferous defensiveness, even paranoia, and a nastiness stronger than *Sulphur*'s. His "maliciousness" (Hering), however, is usually limited to words alone. He is verbally nasty rather than physically violent. And the type is usually so well controlled that this side of his nature is not revealed to outsiders.

A pleasant bearing and good manners can be a form of detachment and substitutes for strong feelings. If a person assumes a proper look of concern, he need not become emotionally involved. In this sphere *Lycopodium* possesses consummate skill. Both socially and professionally he can listen attentively and intelligently to the problems of others without overextending himself emotionally or taking things too much to heart. His very reserve is reassuring; behind the self-contained and understated manner one senses that he could give more if he chose, whereas *Phosphorus* and *Natrum muriaticum* give all they have from the beginning, thereby exhausting their resources.

That *Lycopodium* remains ultimately detached, that his sincere interest lasts only as long as the other person is present, becomes apparent when, a few days later, he has completely forgotten what the other said. When the same conversation with the same person is repeated all over again, it is news to him. Although his memory might be jolted and he might think to himself, "Hmm — Fancy that! How interesting! It somehow rings a bell . . . Now, *where* did I hear this before?" he will still be genuinely surprised.

This instinctive placing of emotional distance between himself and others might explain why, when his memory begins to fail, the first things to go are people's names (*Sulphur*). Also (again like *Sulphur*), "He can properly speak about higher and even abstract things, but gets confused in everyday matters" (Hahnemann). He forgets conversations he has held not three days ago. A comparatively young and still intellectually vigorous individual will repeat himself in conversation like an old man. But unlike *Sulphur*, he does not repeat himself *verbatim*; *Lycopodium*'s conversational style retains some flexibility and diversity.

In his aloof detachment and lack of emotional expansiveness, *Lycopodium* resembles the moon that sheds light but gives no real warmth. This characteristic is especially felt in marriage where the individual often seems to go through the correct gestures of love and affection without the strong underlying feelings. Patients complain of the essential coolness of their *Lycopodium* mates, employing phrases like, "He pretends to care but doesn't really," "He's never there when I need him emotionally," "There's little substance in his fine words," or "He has no deep feeling for me — or for anybody it seems. I sometimes wonder if he knows what love is." This last is not necessarily an accurate analysis, but *Lycopodium*'s way of always holding something in reserve, of not giving himself entirely, understandably produces this impression.

One of O. Henry's working class vignettes, *A Harlem Tragedy*, humorously depicts a housewife's frustration at her husband's *Lycopodium* coolness. Two women are discussing their spouses, and one proudly displays her black eye and new blouse, both presents from her husband (the second following the first as a reconciliation gift). She then advises her friend to arouse her husband to anger so that, after being provoked, he too would respond with something exciting. The second girl goes home and, while at the washtub, berates her astonished and unsuspecting husband, calmly reading the newspaper, over her endless dreary household chores. She then lashes out at him with physical violence. Finally, she comes back, sobbing, to her friend. "What happened? Did he hit you back?" inquires the first girl eagerly. "Oh God," sobs the second, "he never touched me—he's—he's—washing the clothes."

Her husband recognized (or thought he recognized) the justice of the rebuke and reacted in a gracious, gentlemanly way, never suspecting that what she really wanted was some sympathy, some understanding, and above all some demonstration of passion.

The *Lycopodium* male, who thinks well of himself as a husband, is often genuinely surprised by his wife's dissatisfaction. "What has gotten into her? I am a good provider and a reasonable man, and I believe in marriage. What more does she want?" he asks. Indeed, he is often a steadying influence in a marriage. "Perhaps I am not all she desires, but I am still her anchor to windward," was one *Lycopodium* patient's answer to the complaints of his emotional and excitable spouse. He had a point. His very detachment and aloofness provided the ballast which prevented their marriage from capsizing.

On the negative side, however, he can be devoid of deep emotion, and this ultimate remoteness permits a man (or woman) coolly to desert his (or her) family ("flies from own children": Hahnemann) seemingly without a backward glance. In Kent's *Repertory* this *Lycopodium* characteristic is repertorized in the section, *Mind,* under the three rubrics, "Escape," "Forsakes," and "Indifference to her children." The nature appears not to assume guilt the way other constitutional types would do in similar circumstances. "What is done is done," he or she thinks. "I am now onto a new start and beginning a new life."

Possibly *Lycopodium* acts in this way because from the start there was no deep emotional involvement. For instance, upon marital separation, a man might maintain (much to his wife's hurt and surprise) that theirs was never a good marriage, that he never really loved her anyway. What he means is that, once the initial passion had subsided, he never was able to experience love on a profound level.

But the most common complaint of his spouse is, "Oh, he is a good enough husband, reliable, pleasant much of the time, or as long as I defer to him, and most would say I have no cause for dissatisfaction. But he seems to like everyone equally, myself included, and I would like to feel I am someone special to him." Indeed, *Lycopodium* does dislike making distinctions between people, instinctively regarding comparisons as "odious." Everyone has both virtues and defects and is therefore more or less on the same plane. He regards people collectively, in a dispassionate way, without seeking to single out certain ones for any particular liking or dislike. This is reminiscent of the stock situation where two children bring their drawings to their mother and ask her to decide which one is better; naturally she replies that they are both lovely, even if one is better than another. In his refusal to acknowledge distinctions, *Lycopodium* carries this considerate but somewhat patronizing attitude into the adult world.

Moreover, the male can be particularly indiscriminate in his admiration of women. If a member of the sex is merely pretty, he immediately decides that she is also good and intelligent; while if she injects a bit of flattery into her manner towards him, she invariably becomes brilliant. He harbors a vague respect for the weaker sex in general, often exhibiting an attractively protective manner. At the same time, he is convinced of the superiority of the male. *Lycopodium*'s gallant manner, in fact, often disguises an ineradicable sexual "chauvinism," a strong feeling that women have their allotted place in this world, which is essentially not to compete with men, as they do not have the necessary capacities. In family life the trait can be manifested in a glaring favoritism toward sons or, at least, greater deference to their wishes than to those of his daughters.

Perhaps, this attitude is why another common complaint of *Lycopodiums'* wives is that their partners do not "respect" them. Yet, it may be not so much a matter of his lack of respect, as his so obviously respecting himself, and his own sex, *more.*

The same can be true of *Lycopodium* women who instinctively play the same role as their male counterparts. Under a gracious manner toward men they harbor the deep-seated conviction that the male must be flattered, humored, and outwardly respected, but that women possess truer feelings and a more profound intuition and understanding.

Maybe the reason for *Lycopodium*'s "everyone is equal" attitude
is that, engrossed in his work and basically satisfied with himself, he
has little time or inclination for a profound interest in others *as individuals*, and particularly in the member of his family as distinct personalities in their own right. He loves them because they are his wife and
children but relates to them less for their own characters and merit than
for their relationship to himself. He takes for granted their love, care
and attention, and they, in turn, sense that he would love a different
set just as well.

Quite inadvertently, then, *Lycopodium*'s remoteness causes him
to neglect the individuality or specific needs of others, even those for
whom he has affection — which could suggest a lack of warmth or sensitivity. He may comment on his young son's fear of the dark, "When
I was Sam's age *I* never needed a light in the hall at night so why should
he need one? I consider his fear nonsense and an indulgence." Or, of
his daughter, "Why doesn't Nancy like her school? What's wrong with
the girl? If it was good enough for me, it should be good enough for
her. No, of course I won't consider letting her change schools."

In love outside marriage, the image of the moon recedes and yields
to *Lycopodium*'s more traditional love-image, corresponding to the remedy's origins. The moss spores, used in ancient times to make torches,
flare up brightly when ignited but die out rapidly. *Lycopodium*'s passions, similarly, can be urgent ("extraordinary sexual impulse": Hahnemann) but short-lived, flaring up only to subside quickly. His need for
detachment and emotional distance and his essentially cooler nature
can make it hard for him to sustain sexual passion for any length of
time. Thus, if after having been a responsible husband for a number
of years he begins to stray, it is because short-term affairs satisfy his
physical needs without any accompanying emotional demands.

Another factor here is that *Lycopodium*'s liking to charm, to impress and to be flattered, require more adulation than any one woman
can give him. The additional admiration he seeks, however, need not
necessarily come from a sexual relationship. Colleagues, students, followers, parishioners, patients or the public at large, can all help satisfy
his strong need for admiration.

The male exhibits a variety of sexual complaints, ranging from impo-
tence and mid-life sexual crises ("diminished sexual desire and power":
Hahnemann), through strong desire but inhibited performance (fears

of inadequacy may make it especially difficult for him to perform sexually with a woman he truly loves), to unsustained erections, premature ejaculation, or coldness of the genitals. In many ways *Lycopodium* is to the male sexual system what *Sepia* is to the female one. Both remedies cover a wide spectrum of functional and psychological disturbances.*

Lycopodium's detachment extends to relations other than marital and sexual: to relatives, colleagues and even friends. A sensitive portrayal of an adolescent's friendship with his *Lycopodium* classmate is found in John Knowles' *A Separate Peace*. The seventeen-year-old Phineas is portrayed in all the type's emotional equanimity and serene detachment as he quietly charms both teachers and fellow students.

The subliminal hostility he breeds in his best friend (the novel's protagonist), who is competing with him for eminence, arises from the complex mixture of emotions that *Lycopodium* not infrequently arouses in others. There is resentment of his natural talent and innate style, of his magnanimity and seeming detachment from petty feelings of rivalry, and of the relative effortlessness with which he succeeds at whatever he does while others have to strive and toil. There is resentment, too, of his calm self-assurance and the ease with which he relates to others while needing them less than they need him.

This is what makes *Lycopodium* appear psychologically invulnerable. He is not ungiving or without emotion: he can be moved by sentiment, as upon receiving a gift or "even to tears on being thanked" (Hering), and he himself feels gratitude. He is a good, dependable friend, and in dealing with him socially or professionally one senses consideration, thoughtfulness, often real kindness. But he sends out the subconscious signal: "Not too close, please, not too many emotional demands. I like you, but keep your distance." He does not allow others to penetrate the core of his reserve and thus remains ultimately inaccessible.

In fact, he baffles those trying to draw near. Though apparently inviting others to closeness, he maintains a frustrating distance they cannot bridge. He constantly eludes them by staying just beyond their reach. His sociable yet detached nature is symbolized in the key symp-

---

* Sometimes, in a marriage, the two types are like oil and water, that simply do not blend. Prescribing *Lycopodium* for the husband and *Sepia* for the wife has benefitted many such poor relationships.

tom described by Kent of wanting someone around, yet preferably *in the next room* and making minimal demands: "does not want to be talked to or to be forced to do anything, does not want to make any exertion." Indeed, *Lycopodium* cannot tolerate too much closeness, even of those he loves, and when his detachment is threatened, he becomes irritable, critical, sarcastic, caustic, or taciturn.

Not that he is without sincere affection, but his emotions are more likely to be channeled into intellectual commitments than personal ones. A *Lycopodium* patient admitted, for instance, that tears came to his eyes whenever he reread Lincoln's *Second Inaugural Address*. The emotions are there, but in a more remote area of the personality.

At times *Lycopodium* displays an arid imagination with respect to the feelings of others. Refusing to consider their true motives or desires, he is content to accept surface appearances, and may completely lack vision in personal relationships. Instead of attempting to understand or build on the overall structure that lies at the base of any deep relationship, he is always trying to "patch up" on a superficial level. Although he may possess an intuitive understanding of how to interact with people, he does not on the whole probe into the recesses of their minds. Others' feelings are their own concern, just as his are his own. He expects them to command their emotions just as he does his. Also, like many *Sulphurs*, he is not introspective or prone to soul-searching and self-analysis. If the physician suggests to him that he look into himself and examine what is transpiring in his heart, he does so willingly for about two minutes. Then he gets bored or, refusing to ruffle the calm surface, deftly changes the subject.

Lycopodium's need for detachment is fundamental to the careers he chooses and the roles he plays in them.

He works well within large institutional frameworks, not only because he is attracted to authority and power, but because by nature he is respectful of institutions as such. This is an important key to the nature. Both intellectually and instinctively he recognizes man's need for institutions to protect hard-won accomplishments and ideals. Unlike the innately anarchic *Lachesis* who senses the corruptibility of institutions and their tendency to destroy the very values they are created to preserve, *Lycopodium* recognizes them as the repositories of our highest civilized values.

Only extraordinary pressures can pitch this individual into the ranks of anarchists, revolutionaries, dissenters, protesters, or wild-eyed fanatics. He is a conservative who mistrusts radical changes. Even if he espouses unconventional ideas, he remains respectful of orthodox ones, profoundly sensing the importance of law and order. Rather than breaking with tradition and overturning the institutions, he will instinctively seek reform by working *within* the existing framework, improving administrative or legislative procedures or changing the establishment's laws in an orderly way (all of which enhances his aura of stability).

Furthermore, *Lycopodium* functions well within institutions because they provide channels through which feelings and impulses are directed in a controlled, contained and regulated manner. Through them he can serve others and yet remain, in large measure, detached.

Any institution *deintensifies* strong emotions and beneficial impulses so as to preserve them. The intensity and spontaneity of love are modified and deintensified by the institution of marriage, to help this precipitous and self-consuming emotion last longer. Religious institutions deintensify ecstasy and the difficult-to-sustain mystical experience into rites and services and convert burning faith into dogma. The sporadic intensity of artistic creativity and scholarly inspiration is rendered more systematic and long-lasting in educational institutions. Governmental institutions deintensify potentially anarchic personal freedom into regulations and order. Law deintensifies compassion into justice. This well suits *Lycopodium*. As in the sexual, so in the professional realm, his cooler nature renders him unwilling or unable to live in a state of continuous emotional fervor and involvement (in contrast to *Lachesis*). Institutions provide him with a respectable, dignified and sensible substitute for the heat and intensity of feeling that his nature eschews. At the same time, they supply a structure for *perpetuating* the values he so profoundly respects and whose necessity is so apparent to his conservative and practical instincts.

We noted earlier that *Lycopodium* functions well as diplomat or politician where his pragmatic instincts and somewhat sceptical manner stand him in good stead. Predictably, his mentality is also well suited for the law, a discipline which supplies his supple mind with scope for intellectual adventure while demanding a certain detachment. Lawyers and judges must excel in that which *Lycopodium* does instinctively: weighing, balancing, compromising, considering the interests of opposing groups and factions, or bending and reinterpreting facts to achieve viable solutions.

Our great Supreme Court Justice, Oliver Wendell Holmes, provides an excellent illustration of the constitutional type and mentality. First of all, he exhibited *Lycopodium*'s cleancut features that grew more dignified and handsome with age, the characteristic charming manner, subtle intellect and sophisticated style. On the other hand, even his closest friends (such as the James brothers) spoke of his essential coolness and insensitivity in personal relationships.

Lycopodium-like, Holmes enjoyed socializing and being lionized at the elegant home of Boston Brahmins and prominent Washingtonians, evincing there an almost tireless energy in sophisticated small talk, especially relishing his own repartee and witticisms. When asked by an admiring throng of Boston ladies what he thought of Emile Zola, whose risqué novels were then shocking Puritan New England, Holmes laconically replied, "Improving, but dull." Or, when at the age of eighty he was passed on the street by an attractive young woman, he sighed to his companion, "Oh to be seventy again!" These *bon mots* he would then relay to his unfailingly appreciative wife, who usually stayed at home, having neither the strength nor the desire to keep up his social pace.

Even in courtship and marriage Holmes was true to type. For twelve years he took for granted Fanny Dixwell's warm and unwavering friendship, giving no thought to her possible love for him. He admired her character and liked her as a very dear, old friend but kept her at a distance—dangling and waiting. When his unfeeling and aloof manner was finally called to his attention and his sense of fair play thus aroused, Holmes immediately set about correcting his remiss behavior by proposing to her and marrying her. The fifty-year marriage was by all accounts a happy one. There was little cause for friction: Fanny, childless and chronically ailing, allowed her own worth to be constantly overshadowed by her husband's and devoted her undivided attention to his wants and needs.

Holmes also exhibited the constitutional type's viability in his amazingly productive longevity as a Justice. He sat on the Supreme Court for almost thirty years, a major influence until the day he retired at the age of ninety-one! *Lycopodium*-like, finally, was the ultimate paradox of Holmes' life. His measured and aloof objectivity, judicial fair-mindedness, and intellectual balance prompted him to devote a large part of his long career to upholding the principles of American mass democracy of which he personally (an elitist by nature and upbringing) strongly disapproved.

In his combination of duty and dignity, sense of service and feeling for style (his book, *The Common Law*, is one of the finest examples of legal writing in the English language), blend of humanitarian concern with personal coolness and detachment, Holmes is a splendid representative of a largely *Lycopodium* nature.

In the ministry and other institutionalized spiritual paths *Lycopodium* is always willing to assume leadership and frequently achieves a position of eminence—as bishop, elder, guru. To function effectively, every institutionalized religion requires in its hierarchies these urbane, detached, socially-disposed and politically astute *Lycopodium* leaders. Thus he is not your lonely tub-thumper who goes out in all weathers to preach the Word of God from a soap box on busy street corners. This undignified posture he leaves to his *Natrum muriaticum* and *Sulphur* brethren. Nor is he generally a St. Augustine, ceaselessly wrestling with God and the Devil (*Lachesis, Sulphur*). *Lycopodium* does not have to wrestle for salvation. With God already solidly on his side, his conscience gives him few problems.

In daily practice he is straightforward and matter-of-fact about religion. He is either religious or non-religious, pure and simple. One patient proffered this typically dispassionate account: "I was brought up a Catholic, but when I was sixteen I began to have lustful thoughts. My religion taught that they were sinful, and, since it was impossible for me not to have lustful thoughts at that age, I gave up Catholicism. I have no quarrel with the Church or with religion per se, but it was simply easier to give up a religion which imposed difficult demands. Who knows, however? Someday when I am old and feeble, I may return to the faith of my fathers. We shall see."

If he is religious, he is serene and contained about it, accepting faith as a given of man's nature and with little doubt or soul-searching. With age, however, he sometimes develops a *Sulphur*-like inclination to religious melancholy "with doubts of his salvation" (Hering) and, in general, begins to manifest the more traditional *Lycopodium* symptoms: "despondency, satiety of life, seeking solitude" (Hahnemann, Hering). If he is lacking in natural piety, he simply has no interest at all in the spiritual sphere and cannot even understand that dimension in others.

Finally, and not surprisingly, *Lycopodium* ranks high in the medical profession, especially in the allopathic field. He innately commands all the attributes necessary for the practice of medicine: the correct deportment, the almost tangible exuding of self-confidence and capability, dignified concern and a cool collectedness in trying circumstances. His bedside manner and capacity to instill confidence in a patient cannot be surpassed. Then, too, his detachment serves him well in this profession, enabling him to tolerate with equanimity even those trying patients whom other physicians find so difficult. He instinctively knows how to ration his energies and preserve his resources against the emotional drain of demanding patients and those who refuse to help themselves intelligently. Thus, he is less prone than other conscientious types to burn himself out or become discouraged by the hard work of alleviating human suffering.

Self-Deception

Lycopodium's fourth prominent characteristic, *self-deception*, is the natural outgrowth of his self-esteem, viability and detachment. To preserve these three, the individual may resort to deceiving himself. Few types are so adept at blanking out undesirable realities and concealing from themselves what they do not want to admit ("None so blind as he who will not see!"). *Arsenicum* or *Nux vomica*, encountering a problem, say to themselves, "Here is a problem; now, how do I deal with it?" *Lycopodium* says, "Here is a problem; now, how do I *avoid* it?" It is thus less a matter of being unaware than of *refusing* to see that which is disagreeable or unacceptable. This attitude of willful blindness was symbolized in the behavior of Lord Horatio Nelson, who, while a captain during the Baltic Campaign, being signalled by the admiral's flagship not to engage the enemy, put the telescope to his blind eye and complacently declared, "I do not see the order." He proceeded into battle and fought on to victory.

From disregarding facts that interfere with his designs, *Lycopodium* goes on to forget what is fact and what is not. His poor memory, or more precisely his *convenient* memory, contributes to this, since he has a good memory for whatever reinforces his current policy but seems genuinely to forget whatever does not. This trait of accepting only as much reality as he can assimilate without threat to his detachment or his desires helps him remain serene and viable.

The defect of this virtue, however, is obvious. We mentioned earlier how *Lycopodium* patches up difficulties in relationships instead of confronting them on a deeper structural level; in the same way he is less willing than perhaps any other constitutional type to acknowledge unacceptable truths about his character, life-style, or attitude. He will agree to undergo family counseling or psychotherapy, only to withdraw just as he is beginning to reach some understanding not congenial to his self-image—some hitherto denied moral, emotional or intellectual inadequacy. "I do not require counseling. My wife may need it, but I don't. And I am not interested in discussing our problems any longer," he protests, refusing to delve deeper. In this respect he must be treated with extreme delicacy and tact, or he might not return for further treatment.

A patient will sometimes beseech the homoeopathic physician to help save his or her marriage, only to have the *Lycopodium* spouse deny, in real or feigned surprise, that any difficulty exists: "What problem? *I* have no problem. We never quarrel. We have a perfectly good marriage." Yet the wife has said that the husband has been impotent for months, chronically unfaithful, excessively remote, or constantly critical; or the husband, that the wife is dictatorial or subtly, but stultifyingly, overbearing in the household (the remedy may encourage reluctant or denying *Lycopodiums* to begin, or resume, counseling).

Lycopodium is unwilling to admit error, even when obviously in the wrong. Or the desire to aggrandize his self-esteem may be too strong for his veracity, and he will be compelled to exaggerate his exploits. Not content with being proficient in his own sphere, he refuses to acknowledge any limits to his capacities or listen to others' advice. Typical would be the intellectual who prides himself on his skill as an automobile mechanic: in actuality, whenever he sets out to prove this on the family car, it must later be taken to the garage for professional servicing. Curiously, in an attenuated version of that which Boenninghausen calls "fantastic illusions," he often takes more pride in these minor, and seriously defective, skills than in the ones where his true capacities are manifested. It is often difficult to distinguish between *Sulphur* and *Lycopodium* in the tendency to cover up or overcompensate for inadequacies. Possibly the latter is more discreet than the louder and more blatantly boastful *Sulphur,* but then, in seeking to impress others, he is more likely to deceive himself. This is especially true for males. *Lycopodium* women usually have too much dignity to magnify their accomplishments (like *Phosphorus* or *Lachesis*) or to boast about them overtly (like *Arsenicum*).

His self-deception emerges in yet another way. While he considers himself a model of level-headedness and moderation in all respects, he succeeds in this but imperfectly. In matters which affect him personally he can be as subjective and irrational ("arbitrary:" Hering) as anyone else. For instance, he may blindly defend someone he likes, even when the latter's misdemeanors or incompetence are clear to see. Indeed, his loyalty to those he chooses to support is often more commendable than his judgment.

A *Lycopodium* parent may defend the poor behavior of a favorite child in the most self-deceptive way (*Sulphur*). For example, the mother of a boy who had been asked to withdraw from four private schools and was now having problems in the public school, stated, "The trouble with this city is that there is *no* school that understands little boys. They just do not know how to deal with them." She would not even begin to consider that the problem might lie in her son. This woman was being treated preventively for a tendency to kidney stone formation: one stone had already been removed, and she was experiencing pains in the kidney area. Because she also had bloating after eating little as well as other *Lycopodium* digestive symptoms, this was prescribed in the 10M potency as her constitutional remedy, (alternating with an intercurrent course of *Berberis* 30x for the specific renal symptoms).* During the treatment the homoeopathic medicines once again demonstrated their beneficial "side-effects." As her health improved, so did her understanding. Inviting her hitherto unconsulted husband to lend a hand, she for the first time embarked upon a rational course of action to help her son. Yet, until this tendency to self-deception became manifest, the patient had appeared to be well balanced and eminently reasonable in every way.

This is characteristic of the type. The self-deception of *Phosphorus* or *Sulphur* is apparent to any student of human nature, but that of *Lycopodium* is concealed by an overlay of reserve and a balanced style, and emerges only in certain connections. Thus, despite some major

---

* When addressing the mental symptoms or administering a "constitutional" remedy, high potencies are generally employed; but lower potencies of a related remedy, or one directed to some specific physical symptom, can be given intercurrently. This method of using lower potencies more frequently, to supplement the occasional constitutional one, has been found to be effective in certain intractable cases or stubborn conditions. For an excellent discussion of the choice and use of potencies in homoeopathic prescribing, see Blackie, *The Patient, not the Cure*, pp. 97-101.

lacuna in his understanding, to the outsider *Lycopodium* may appear to be perfectly clearsighted and of exceptionally sound and fair judgment. He is most adept at portraying his thoughts and actions in the best possible light, regardless of his true motivations, and gives the impression of knowing what he is talking about even when he does not.

The following typical instance of *Lycopodium* self-deceptiveness occurred at a dinner party (social gatherings—where he tries to impress others—often reveal his true colors, and the physician can espy characteristics impossible to discern in the office where he is misled by *Lycopodium*'s front of rectitude and attractively understated manner). One of the guests was unassumingly explaining to an admiring group of listeners how, in an effort at spiritual self-refinement, he was undergoing various disciplinary exercises: the necessary daily meditation, giving up smoking altogether, and greatly moderating his intake of alcohol and meat. "For instance, I never eat any heavy meats, which tend to drag down the higher consciousness," he concluded.

The hostess, chancing to overhear this remark, exclaimed, "Oh, how unfortunate! Tonight I prepared an especially delicious roast beef. If I had only known, I would have instead . . . "

"Please," the *Lycopodium* hastened to assure her, "when dining out I eat *anything* that is served. The last thing I want is to inconvenience my hostess or impose my dietary restrictions on anyone else." This was said with such tact and feeling that everyone instinctively felt, "Now, that is *real* consideration. That is being a true gentleman!"

Well, when *Lycopodium* said he ate anything that was served, he meant it, for he had several helpings of the roast beef and swallowed them with obvious relish. One could only presume, after what he had said, that he was humbly sacrificing his spiritual development to put his hostess at ease. The only problem with this interpretation (as became apparent later) was that he repeated the same performance at other dinner-parties: the same talk of self-discipline and "heavy meats" and the same multiple helpings of pork, lamb or steak. Perhaps by "heavy meats" this *Lycopodium* meant elephant, giraffe, or hippopotamus!

Most surprising, however, was the reaction of his friends. Entertaining little doubt that he was as abstemious in fact as he professed, they continued to believe his words instead of his actions and to speak admiringly of his restrictive dietary habits. When reminded that he *did* eat heavy meats, even unto multiple helpings, they justified it as humility or politeness. So skillful, at times, is the charismatic *Lycopodium* at establishing and projecting an image, that the Emperor's lack of clothes is not noticed. This type of self-deception is more complicated than mere lying or hypocrisy. Because it satisfies some profound emotional need in him and supports his viability, *Lycopodium* genuinely believes that whatever brings him advantage *is* good and true, while everything disagreeable or distasteful must be wrong and untrue.

He often remains wedded to his self-deception for the simple reason that he does not *want* to change; and maybe there is no need to change. He is pleased with himself, successful by worldly standards, and wants to remain as he is: self-deceptive on certain subjects, to be sure, but an effective and viable member of society. After all, a pleasing self-deception can involve far less suffering and more ultimate productivity than the sometimes devastating self-knowledge of a *Lachesis* or *Natrum muriaticum. Lycopodium*'s indestructibility, in fact, reflects the unity of his nature that equips him perfectly for his task in life. As with the club moss itself little modification is needed for survival.

Sometimes, however, he displays a sincere desire to develop in understanding. This emerges particularly in the middle years, when his natural unity begins to break down. He then loses confidence in his own power and vigor, or sensing a discrepancy between the public image and the private person behind it, is consequently beset with doubts. "I feel that the rug I have been standing on so securely my whole life, has been pulled out from under me," "Apparently the foundation upon which I built my reputation was never solid," "The whole structure of my life has suddenly collapsed," "I don't know what happened, but suddenly my confidence is totally shattered," "Is my profession all there is to me?" "I wonder if I am a 'hollow' man—too concerned with the importance of appearances and lacking in emotional substance," are characteristic remarks. These patients can be helped with homoeopathic remedies, as the type possesses much good will. The hard part is getting him to *acknowledge* the deficiency. Once *Lycopodium* recognizes a weakness, he will conscientiously and intelligently set about rectifying it.

Lycopodium's self-deception should not be confused with, although it is complicated by, his specific understanding of "truth." He is the individual who would ask with Pontius Pilate, "What is Truth?" suggesting that the question has no answer. He is a sceptic and a relativist:

truth is a variable quantity, and today's truth is but tomorrow's error. It does not automatically follow, however, that he is cynical or self-serving. It is simply that he embraces the diplomat's, politician's or lawyer's understanding of truth. There can be, he feels, truth only for a given situation, for a given person, at a given moment. On controversial issues he can switch sides easily, playing the devil's advocate and directly contradicting the position he held last week, if only for the sake of intellectual balance. He feels instinctively that the truth does not lie on any one side, at any extreme, but somewhere in between and that progress and understanding are possible only by adhering to a middle course.

Thus, *Lycopodium* mistrusts extremes of any kind: intellectual, ideological, emotional, or those of taste or personality. He himself is low-key and collected, and he expects others to be the same. He is embarrassed by the eccentricities of *Calcarea*, irritated at the erratic behavior of *Lachesis*, annoyed at the unrestrained emotionalism of *Phosphorus*, and intolerant of the numerous peculiarities exhibited by *Natrum muriaticum*. He likes others to conduct themselves in a relatively conventional manner, both in public and private. Talleyrand voiced *Lycopodium*'s instinctive dislike of aberrant behavior when he instructed his colleagues before the diplomatic negotiations at the Congress of Vienna, "Surtout pas trop de zèle!" ("Above all, not too much zeal!").

Lycopodium also holds that truth must be flexible to remain viable. To be influential a man must adapt his idea of truth to the temper of the times. Everyone must engage in some untruth for the sake of his ultimate goal. Therefore, *Lycopodium* does not always try to tell the "objective truth." He prefers to tell people what they want to hear, what they are prepared to hear, or what he thinks they should hear; and to ask whether he is truthful is to ask the wrong question. He is, and he is not. He is frankly convinced that the ends justify the means. When challenged, he will openly admit to an elastic mentality, explaining that times and circumstances alter and that he is consequently forced to modify his opinions. Anyone in a position of authority acts on this principle to some extent and learns to respect it, but with *Lycopodium* the conviction is instinctive and is reflected in all his motives, actions and relationships, personal and professional.

And sometimes, what may seem like deceit is actually extreme circumspection or discretion. He is not untruthful, merely sparing with words, and giving out no more information than absolutely necessary.

The Patient

Last we come to a subject that must especially interest every homoeopathic physician: *Lycopodium*'s attitude toward, and behavior during, illness.*

As a rule he possesses "little confidence in physicians or their medicines" (Hering) and prefers to ignore physical infirmities. Illness offends his self-esteem and intrudes upon his detachment. He is irritated at weakness in himself, or even members of his family, and impatient with poor health. He may refuse to admit to any symptoms or ailments simply because he cannot be bothered. He cannot afford the time or the concern. He expects his body to serve him well, as it has always done in the past. Typically he thinks that he is above needing medical help and that a strong person should overcome sickness by willpower. He habitually uses such phrases as, "It's all in the mind . . . Forget about it and it will go away . . . I don't believe in doctors. I am perfectly healthy without them. . . . My own constitution will take care of the problem."

He is also the patient from whom it is difficult to elicit symptoms. Except for his main complaint he has none. He is the active young man who cannot remember when he was last ill but has chronic catarrh with persistent hawking up of mucus or a pain in the heel when walking. Or he is the energetic old man, looking and acting younger than his age but with an occasional bursitic pain in the right shoulder. Or he is the strong and sturdy child who for some reason cries before urinating, or is subject to right-sided septic and sore throats. Or she is the exceptionally healthy woman with varicose veins, particularly on the right leg, or a large cyst on the right ovary (the right-sidedness of most *Lycopodium* complaints or, alternatively, symptoms moving from the right side of the body to the left, is an important feature of this type—like the left-sidedness of *Sepia* or *Lachesis*). Nothing else, however, bothers *Lycopodium*—nothing at all! The individual is unaware of any modalities and is unresponsive when asked about aggravations or ameliorations, likes or dislikes. He eats all foods and drinks all beverages. He does not mind changes of weather or season and likes hot summers and cold winters equally. He is insensitive to mood changes in himself and others,

---

* Although the attitude described here is far more pronounced in males than in females, it exists in the latter also.

and few things anger or upset him (or so he says). The only modality of which he isaware is the (typically *Lycopodium*) late afternoon drop in energy: the 4-8 p.m. aggravation of symptoms, lowered vitality, or irresistible sleepiness. This is sometimes the sole physical clue the physician will elicit, apart from the patient's main complaint. Otherwise, like the moss from which the remedy derives, little in the external environment perturbs this individual.

Consequently, he may feel superior to the ordinary rules of life. Indeed, he can ignore basic dietary and health precautions and still remain fit and well. An example was the elderly *Lycopodium* bachelor who, for reasons of frugality, existed for nearly two decades on prepackaged cookie mixes and Kool Aid but only called his physician once every few years for an infrequent case of influenza, being otherwise in very good health. Alternately, *Lycopodium* may strain his constitution too far and suddenly break down physically or psychologically in middle age. He may lose his sexual or intellectual vigor relatively early ("cannot read what he has written; makes mistakes in writing; leaves out words, letters, or syllables; vanishing of thoughts or cannot grasp a thought; inability to think of the right word or uses wrong words for correct ideas—says plums when he means pears, memory weakened,": Hahnemann, Hering), or, while seemingly in "perfect health" and without any warning, may die of a heart attack, a massive stroke, or another sudden and overwhelming condition. The cause may be a miasmatic flaw—a congenital weakness that emerges with age, but often he depletes the capital of his strong constitution by living off it heedlessly.

Sulphur, especially in the male, can manifest a similar paucity of symptoms, which may be genuine or may reflect an inability to observe himself. These two hardy types sometimes seem scarcely to know the meaning of illness, or even pain, going through life without ever suffering from a headache. One *Lycopodium* patient in his seventies asserted that he had experienced pain only once in his life—when shot in the arm during World War II. However, this very characteristic of symptomlessness, once it is established, can serve as a guide to the remedy.

A man in his mid-forties sought homoeopathic help for a curious numbness or paresis of the lower half of the body. It had started a year earlier in the right big toe, moved up the legs past the groin, and was now at the waist. He could move his limbs, but walking was an effort, as he had to concentrate on every step. Moreover, his sexual performance was now affected. He was prescribed *Phosphorus*, then *Conium*, because of the ascending pattern of symptoms, but without effect. Other symptoms were sought in vain. The numbness was not aggravated by walking, sitting, or lying down; neither in the morning nor the evening. It was not ameliorated by heat or cold, by strong pressure or gentle rubbing. And he had no other complaints. "Otherwise I feel just fine," he insisted. This was the clue, and a dose of *Lycopodium* in high potency caused the numbness to recede down the body to the right big toe whence it had originated. Another dose three months later removed the sensation from the toe, and that was the end of the case.

There is an amusing variant of the "no symptoms" *Lycopodium*. The office visit begins with the patient announcing that he is a perfectly healthy man.

"Why are you here then?" is the obvious retort.

"Because of my wife. She told me to come."

"Well, you are fortunate in your constitution" (the patient inclines his head in modest acknowledgment of the indisputable fact). "Let's see, however, if we can detect some symptoms or weakness . . . "

"But I have no symptoms. I tell you, I am *perfectly* healthy."

"I agree. You may not have any *symptoms*, but everyone has at least some physical *peculiarities* that are an integral part of his constitutional economy. Let me just try to pinpoint a few of these. . . . "

Under such soothing treatment *Lycopodium* relaxes and begins, on cross-questioning, to admit that "Yes, in fact I have been subject to athlete's foot for years, but that is because I got it in the army. I never had it before." Also, he has a regular winter cough, "but it is never bad—not debilitating or anything like that. And it is probably because I once had pneumonia as a child." He does have flatulence beginning an hour after meals, "but that I inherited from my father who has it worse than I do." Although his wife claims that he is grumpy and low-spirited in the mornings, "it is perfectly normal in view of the fact that I wake up around 4:00 a.m. and find it difficult to get back to sleep." Or he may occasionally experience a low-grade pain in the small of the back or between the shoulder blades. "Yet it is nothing important, not even regular, so I wouldn't call it a real symptom."

The interview proceeds in this manner, with an alibi or justification for every symptom, the patient all the while convincing himself

that somehow his symptoms are not his own and that he is not ultimately responsible for any weakness of his constitution.

Whence comes this unawareness and denial of symptoms? Why
does *Lycopodium* need to remain reassured of his flawless constitution
and physical invincibility? Some fear of illness is certainly involved, but
such factors as his threatened dignity and self-esteem or desire for emotional detachment also play a role.

Anyone who has dealt with a *Lycopodium* during illness knows
what an uncooperative patient he can be ("headstrong and haughty
when sick": Boericke). He forgets to take the medicine when directed
and fails to report new symptoms or even to give an account of his
progress generally. "Don't keep asking me how I feel all the time, doctor. It's *your* business to know that. After all, *you're* the physician!"
And if pressed for symptoms, he becomes cranky: "You know I never
notice these things. I am not interested in my symptoms."

"Well, begin to notice. Get interested," urges the physician.

"It's too late in life to start now. *You* notice," is the cavalier reply.

Even when he finally accepts homoeopathic aid, he may resolutely
refuse to make the smallest concession to help the remedies along. One
patient suffered from chronic insomnia in the early morning hours. For
this and other symptoms, he was given a dose of *Lycopodium* and told
to stay off coffee. He slept much better for a week, but then he resumed
drinking coffee, his insomnia returned, and he asked for more medicine.
It was suggested that he should again give up coffee rather than take
another constitutional remedy, and to this he retorted, "What nonsense!
You should give me medicine that permits me to drink coffee at night
and *still* sleep; otherwise, what is the use of your remedies? I could
give up coffee on my own, if I wanted to. I don't need a doctor for that!"

"Still, you must give us time, and if it is ruining your health, perhaps . . . "

"Coffee is worth the price. I *refuse* to give it up!" was the adamant
reply.

This constitutional type even equates physical weakness with moral
deficiency. He feels that the person who lives "right" should not fall
ill. "Look at me," he instinctively thinks when hearing of others' illnesses, "I live right and am perfectly healthy. If others were more like
me, they too would be in good health." All this can be unspoken, even

subconscious, but the "I am healthy because I lead a virtuous life" conceit is a form of self-righteousness peculiar to *Lycopodium*.

There comes a time, however, when he can no longer close his eyes to the unpleasant realities of his physical or mental condition, when he must relinquish this ostrich-like attitude. The apprehensiveness and underlying insecurity described in the books now emerge. Once his veneer of physical invincibility begins to crack, *Lycopodium* can panic and escalate his illness into a crisis.

He will now exacerbate any small illness into a life-threatening condition. If a sore appears in his mouth, it must be an early stage of oral cancer; if he has a respiratory complaint, it must be the sympathetic cough of organic heart disease; stiffness in the neck with mild headache must be "chronic meningitis" (as one patient put it); flu-related dizziness and nausea must be congestive heart failure. Much of his panic reflects his view of illness as a "crisis" requiring (as he thinks) drastic curative measures.*

This tendency to exaggerate his illness, once it occurs, has other roots in the *Lycopodium* psychology. He dislikes being subjected to the indignity of small ailments, such as the "common" cold, which place him on the same ignominious plane as other suffering mortals. He wants an ailment worthy of his self-respect. He knows that even individuals of unquestioned rectitude, like Job, are occasionally subject to devastating afflictions.

Subconsciously then, and at other times quite consciously, in his impatience to be restored *immediately* to normalcy and good health, he will opt for removal of an organ ("Let's get it out and over with, once and for all!") or some other form of energetic intervention rather than interest himself in preventive measures or in the slower process of repair and gradual strengthening of the body. Constitutional treatment with *Lycopodium* may change the patient's attitude despite himself, but prior to such a conversion he will create a no-win situation for the homoeo-

---

* Parenthetically, the *Lycopodium* patient (except those in the medical field or who have had long experience with illness) can be remarkably ignorant of anatomy and physiology. Unlike the medically informed *Arsenicum*, *Natrum muriaticum*, or *Sulphur*, *Lycopodium* usually has no conception where the liver is (he points to the stomach), or the stomach (he points to the abdomen), or even where the kidneys are (which he thinks are located near the bladder).

pathic physician. If the cure is slow, he insists that the remedies are not working and balks at continuing treatment; if the cure with homoeopathy is swift, he decides that he did not really need medicine after all, that his own strong constitution took care of the problem. If the duration of cure lies somewhere in between, he wishes fervently that the remedies would "make up their minds one way or another, and either *work* or *not work!*"*

In view of his general mistrust of medicine this is not surprising, but other factors are also involved. Homoeopathy, like few other medical disciplines, requires the patient to relinquish his detachment, become aware of his physical and emotional life, and do his share of noting and reporting symptoms. Whereas *Arsenicum* delights in working hand in hand with the physician, and, in his authoritarianism, even tries to take over the case himself, *Lycopodium*'s authoritarianism operates in reverse. He resents the painstaking involvement by the patient that homoeopathy demands. He does not in the least desire a peer relationship with his physician and is prepared to defer entirely to his expertise. He is paying good money for the physician's specialized knowledge and expects him to make all the decisions—just as, were the physician to come to him for legal or other professional advice, he would assume full responsibility and not expect the client to interfere. Not for him is today's do-it-yourself medical philosophy, with everyone dabbling in healing in a sort of holistic stew.

Finally, given his conservatism, the unorthodoxy of homoeopathy makes him nervous. "What do you want me to go to a homoeopath

---

* This personal mistrust of medicine is curiously revealed in the *Lycopodium* homoeopathic physician himself. He deeply respects the remedies per se. He knows the value of regular constitutionals and prescribes them with good results to his patients. But he cannot spare a thought in that direction for himself. He puts off taking a remedy until later, until tomorrow. . . . He then betrays his subliminal reluctance by conveniently forgetting. One such physician, notorious for ignoring his own health, was asked why he would not even permit a fellow physician to prescribe. "Remedies are for the weak and feebleminded," he replied, "and there are plenty of those around. A strong person like myself does not need constitutionals." This answer was a characteristically *Lycopodium* jocular evasion of a serious question, with the flippantly arrogant reply containing more than a grain of his true feelings.

for?'' he asks his wife testily. "Why shouldn't I continue to patronize my regular doctor?—And what *is* a homoeopath, anyway?" (this last, after it has been explained to him a dozen times). As with the moss which takes several years to germinate spores and a decade and a half to achieve full development, *Lycopodium* takes a long time to accept a really new idea. He is obdurate, "defiant" (Hering) and impermeable to suggestions; the most obvious facts do not penetrate. Eventually, however, the slow-changing individual does come round, in his own good time. And, once ready to accept a new idea, he becomes just as unyielding the new way.

The unforgettable behavior of a *Lycopodium* patient, nursed with homoeopathic remedies through a serious illness, serves as an appropriate case with which to recapitulate some salient points of this personality type. On contracting a pain near the liver he hastened to a specialist and returned full of self-importance. "The doctor of internal medicine says that I have bladder stones and that the *entire* gall-bladder will have to come out—the sooner, the better. And possibly the pancreas too—because it's obviously in bad shape." His manner showed clearly that the very idea of such radical measures impressed him tremendously and that he considered them befitting a strong man visited with a strong disease.

He arranged an operation, but meanwhile an infection supervened, and the surgeon was wary of proceeding with a weakened and feverish patient. At this point the wife decided to turn to homoeopathy for assistance, and the patient (despite never quite trusting "those little white pills") received the classic *Chelidonium* 200X for the acute symptoms, together with tincture of *Chelidonium*, *Chionanthus*, and *Hydrastis* to be taken in water at regular intervals.

After twenty-four hours the temperature had subsided, and the discomfort was lessened—although the patient himself insisted that the medicine was "not working." However, to a *Lycopodium* this often means that he is not *completely* cured.

"Give it another day before we change the prescription," was the physician's suggestion.

"Why? Homoeopathy may work with others but it doesn't work for me" (another typical *Lycopodium* comment). "Shouldn't I go back to my regular doctor again? And how long must I continue taking these disgusting drops? They taste just terrible!'' (meaning: mildly bitter).

The next day the pain and signs of infection had virtually disappeared, and the patient declared triumphantly to the attending homoeopath: "Now I am ready to have the gall-bladder taken out.''

"But why remove it if you are getting well?''

"It's got to be operated on sometime. You're not suggesting that I go through another such attack again, are you? Anyway, one thing I refuse is to take any more of that *foul* tincture.''

His *Lycopodium* nature was just itching to have the operation, so he would not have to worry or ever think about his gall-bladder any more. With the aid of his devoted wife that crisis was somehow weathered, and he made a good recovery. But if there had been the mildest relapse, he could not have been kept from the surgeon's knife.

After an uneventful convalescence he commented to the physician: "I am grateful for your work, but I hate the side-effects of your remedies.''

"What side-effects are you talking about?'' was the astonished query.

"Your medicines have altered my character and forced me to change my life-style long before I was prepared to do so. When I'm tired, they make me want to rest—whereas I used to be able to keep going without sleep. When I'm hungry, I have to eat, instead of relying on a quick drink as formerly. I love coffee and was able to drink ten cups a day; now one is enough. I used to assert myself in the home; but now, unless I watch out, I find myself—a self-respecting man—complying with my wife and daughters like a regular lamb. What have you done to my formerly strong constitution and character?''

The homoeopathic remedies are triple-pronged, affecting the patient's past, present, and future. *Lycopodium* can reach back to the time before the patient lost his vigor and self-confidence and help him recapture it; it can encourage him to confront and overcome present insecurities and inadequacies, substantiating what is hollow in his facade of strength and competence; finally, acting for the future, the remedy can prevent an individual's fine intellect and mental capacities from deteriorating with age. In such ways does potentized club moss enable the *Lycopodium* patient's appearance of heightened vigor, intellectual strength, confidence, and serenity to become, or to remain, a reality.

Sepia

THE remedy *Sepia* shares important characteristics with several other polychrests—*Phosphorus, Pulsatilla, Sulphur, Lachesis Arsenicum*, and especially *Natrum muriaticum*, with which it is frequently compared. This does not prevent it, however, from being a major constitutional remedy in its own right, with a personality distinctly its own.

Sepia is made from the fresh ink of the cuttlefish—an independent creature which swims alone rather than in a group and lives in the crevices of rocks in the cool depths of the sea. When in danger it sends out clouds of ink to cover its escape, and when securing its prey it ejects the ink for camouflage. Thus the brownish-black liquid serves both defensive and aggressive purposes.

The remedy is predominantly female. The classic picture is the woman seeking emancipation from her traditionally passive and too limited role as wife and mother in the home. Homoeopathic *Sepia*, however, comes in different guises. For a better understanding, it must be divided into three distinct faces: the worn-out overworked housewife or emotionally withdrawn woman; the contented career woman; and finally, the dissatisfied complainer.

The Overworked Housewife

Margaret Tyler gives a graphic vignette of the first face, describing a tired housewife with her sallow, bloated complexion and free perspiration, who can stand neither stuffy rooms nor cold air, who suffers from constant backache or headache, is constipated, and has an overall "dragged-down" feeling. So worn out is she with the cares of home and children that she only wants to lie down and rest; her very eyelids

droop from weakness (*Gelsemium, Causticum*). In her run-down condition she feels stupid, dull, forgetful; and when overwrought she feels
she must hold tightly to something to keep from screaming. At times,
driven to an extreme of irritability, she lashes out at her children and
especially her husband. From this picture arises the image of the rebellious dissatisfied woman who wants to leave her husband and children
("aversion to members of family": Kent) and "get away from it all."
Or she has simply become "indifferent to her loved ones" (Hering).
But *Sepia* is more complex than that, and the terms "aversion" or "indifference" must be qualified.

In certain cases, *Sepia* can indeed be found lacking in maternal instinct, as evidenced by the remedy's success in animals who refuse to
nurse or care for their young (and may actually attack their offspring:
Tyler), but she is not intrinsically devoid of emotion. Feelings run strong
and deep in this type. She loves her husband and children dearly but
is too exhausted to feel *anything* but the need to get through the day's
work and survive to the next. She simply has no physical or emotional
energy left for love.

All manifestations of love—marital, parental, filial, and even close
friendship—are a drain on her reserves of energy and an obstacle to
her need for a certain amount of privacy and independence ("company
aggravates, amelioration when alone": Kent). The cuttlefish, after all,
is a solitary animal. *Sepia*'s immediate family, being the greatest emotional drain, is naturally the greatest threat. She may see her children
in direct conflict with her need for self-expression, and so she fights
the emotional bonds that stifle the growth of her individuality. Where
another woman would see them as enhancing her mental development,
she feels them to be a hindrance.

Sepia experiences love not as excitement or enjoyment (*Phosphorus*), not as a blessing as natural and necessary as the sun (*Pulsatilla*), not as a rare and beautiful gift or unattainable ideal (*Natrum muriaticum*), nor as a human's inherent due which can almost be taken for
granted (*Sulphur, Lycopodium*), but rather as a responsibility—or even
a burden. She thinks of love somewhat as follows: "These people love
me. They expect something of me. I must live up to their expectations
and not disappoint them. I've got to do well as wife, mother, sister,
or daughter." Yet how does one express love toward, for example, one's
children? *Phosphorus* and *Pulsatilla* easily pour out affection and ca-

resses; *Natrum muriaticum* provides instruction, instinctively assuming the role of teacher; *Calcarea* indulges her children and enjoys them in an effortless empathy; *Arsenicum* enjoys taking command and organizing her charges' lives. For *Sepia*, however, love has no easy outlet, no natural form. Kent has an interesting phrase in this connection, "Love does not go forth into affection." Love is not absent, but the manifestation of love is benumbed and cannot be expressed.

So she falls back on *duty*. Even when at the end of her resources, her sense of duty keeps her going until gradually she begins to resent her incarceration and struggles against the ties that bind her. In her wretchedness she projects gloom, just as the cuttlefish ejects its cloud of ink. No one can spread darkness around herself like a discontented *Sepia*. Then she begins to think of leaving home, to escape from the burdens of imposed love.

Actually to *do* so—to forsake her home and family—a woman must usually possess *Lycopodium* in her nature. For *Lycopodium* does not feel guilt, regret or self-condemnation as other types do. The more purely *Sepia* woman might want to get away but is restrained by a sense of duty and guilt. So she stays on to complain, nag, and perhaps to fall ill from the strain.

Furthermore, she is proud, as well as dutiful, and in the best sense of the word. Though needing independence and possibly desiring a career for emotional fulfilment, she will still put much care into a task uncongenial to her nature. She tries hard to do things the "right" way. But the right way is so difficult for *Sepia*! She is like a puppy raised among kittens who tries to climb trees and spring onto tables, not realizing that she is a dog and not a cat. The housewife's pathology arises from the sheer physical stress of an uncongenial role.

Whitmont, adapting Jungian psychology to the homoeopathic method, interprets this aspect of the *Sepia* psyche as rooted in a conflict with the other sex within her. Every individual is composed of both male and female genes. The conscious personality has the attributes of the dominant sex, while the unconscious bears marks of the opposite sex and performs a complementary balancing function. In the healthy individual these two forces (the Yin and the Yang) work together harmoniously, but in the *Sepia* woman an imbalance occurs. Failing to find a healthy or satisfactory outlet, the unconscious male in her begins to surface in a way she can neither understand nor control, while her suppressed femininity (which takes on a dark character by virtue of its suppression) retaliates in the form of certain aggressive characteristics and neurasthenic conditions. On the physical plane this struggle manifests itself, not surprisingly, in malfunctioning of the female reproductive organs.

Thus *Sepia* should be considered for sexual and menstrual complaints of all kinds, including frigidity and the disturbances of menopause; it should also be considered for disorders of pregnancy, such as tendency to abort and morning sickness, as well as for severe postpartum depression (''baby-blues'') and other ailments while in childbed or nursing. The remedy is further effective in uterine displacements and disorders such as prolapse, ''bearing-down'' sensations, fibroids, and violent stitches upwards from the vagina. Hering has six pages of frequently-encountered ''female'' symptoms. Perhaps most dramatic of all is its power to counteract female sterility. There have been many ''*Sepia* babies'' whose existence the mother attributes to this homoeopathic remedy. *Calcarea* and *Natrum muriaticum* are the other two frequently effective remedies, and *Natrum carbonicum* sometimes works when these classic remedies fail (Kent).

Even when not lacking in maternal instinct, *Sepia* does not take readily to motherhood. It is too binding, too psychologically draining, and too physically exhausting for her constitution, which often exhibits a picture of low thyroid, low blood pressure, or adrenalin deficiency.* Hence the mental symptom, ''indifference to those loved best'' is doubtless the result, rather than the underlying cause, of her problems.

This distinction is important, since it explains why, contrary to expectation, *Sepia* frequently makes a good, even an excellent mother. The woman whose outlook on life is soured or dreary and whose personality is tiresome will still raise independent, contented, creative children who, reacting healthily to their mother, are charming, attractive and a pleasure to be around. This is partly because she is not overly protective, sentimental or self-imposing. She is often matter-of-fact and stands no nonsense. She does not oppress her children (as does *Lycopodium*) or attempt to mold them according to some preconceived image (*Arsen-*

---

* The whole picture of adrenalin disturbances as related to the physiological and psychopathological action of *Sepia* has been discussed by Whitmont and Gutman.

icum). It is hard enough for her to live with one *Sepia* (herself), let alone encourage her offspring along similar lines. She respects the child's personality and lets him be himself, yet without overindulgence.

She can be unsociable and "averse to company" (Hering). She does not want to go out, largely because of the physical effort which sociability demands (as one patient said, "I don't even have the strength to comb my hair before going out, to raise my fork to eat or to pull the muscles of my mouth into a smile"), and she is too fatigued to delight in music, museums, nature, or even her friends. Uninterested in what others are saying, reluctant to contribute anything herself, too tired to follow the conversation ("concentration is difficult": Kent), she may answer in monosyllables: "she feels stupid . . . with difficult flow of ideas" (Hahnemann); "incapable of mental exertion" (Boenninghausen); "language comes very slowly, has to drag out the words to express ideas; forgets the chief points" (Hering). All of the foregoing contribute to the general picture of "indifference."

Yet, once she *does* make the supreme effort and attends a social gathering, once the adrenalin is stimulated to flow, counteracting her sluggish and "ptotic" state, she comes alive, is good company, and enjoys herself thoroughly.* In fact she may become "very excitable when in company" (Boenninghausen). Amelioration of physical and mental symptoms from strenuous (as against mild) exertion is a guiding symptom (Boger). Otherwise, she only wants to crawl into her lair and be *left alone*, not touched, approached or bothered, just allowed to sleep: "avoids the sight of people" (Kent); "wishes to be by herself and lie with closed eyes" (Hahnemann). For many of her symptoms are markedly better from sleep, even a short nap (*Phosphorus*). Unlike *Lachesis*, whose symptoms are worse from sleep, or *Natrum muriaticum* who needs a long, deep sleep to feel better, *Sepia* can lie down feeling hopeless and depressed and wake up a short time later with the gloom temporarily dispelled.

In her unsociability she may at times resemble *Natrum muriati-*

* * *

* *Sepia*'s weary, "dragged-down" emotional state finds its physical counterpart in ptosis: the "dragging" or "bearing-down" sensation or prolapse of any part of the body, but in *Sepia* particularly of the uterus.

cum's loner mentality; also, like *Natrum muriaticum*, she may be "worse in company yet dreads to be alone" (Kent). But her loneliness proceeds from a different source. *Natrum muriaticum* needs the love she appears to be pushing away and suffers from its absence. *Sepia*, however, is truly seeking to escape from close emotional ties and the obligations they impose, and can be content without them.

In certain cases her emotional unresponsiveness takes the form of what Tyler calls a "stony" or "frozen" indifference. This emotional apathy may develop from some profound sorrow or disappointment in a reserved individual who cannot allow herself to feel because she cannot afford it. A case in point was a 26-year-old woman with amenorrhoea who, three years earlier, had suffered severely from an unfortunate love (in *Sepia*, as in *Natrum muriaticum* and *Ignatia*, profound grief can lead to cessation of menses). Since that time she had been cold and unresponsive with her family and friends and toward the world in general. She had seemingly withdrawn into some chilly arctic region where she was determined to remain remote and uncommunicative. No one was able to reach her in any way. She was polite and dutiful, but completely indifferent: "the death of a near relative or some happy occurrence leave her equally unaffected; no trace of her former love for friends, or even for her own child" (Hering).

For an older person, buffeted by fate, the attainment of such mental serenity may be desirable, even at the cost of some lack of emotional response. But in a young woman on the brink of life such aloofness from the richness and variety of emotional experience is sad. The patient consequently received a dose of *Sepia* 50M.

Initially there was no dramatic change. *Sepia* can be a slow starter. Yet on a visit two months later she was a different person—not carefree or even happy, but more caring and responsive, and her menses had resumed. No further remedy was prescribed, since the single dose had obviously reached some deep level of her emotional disharmony and was beginning to heal it. Instead, the remedy was allowed to continue dispelling her "stilled" (Kent) or suppressed emotions, as she blossomed into a warm, lovely and now happy human being.

According to Pierre Schmidt, Hubbard and other authorities, *Sepia* (like *Sulphur*) can be prescribed with benefit for patients who are unable to respond to other indicated homoeopathic remedies, just as they cannot respond emotionally to life.

In addition to being an independent constitutional type, the remedy can be indicated during a *temporary stage* in a woman's life. It has proved invaluable for adjustment to the increased sexual demands of marriage; when a woman is trying to resolve the conflict between home and career; for the one who has "never been the same" since childbirth, an abortion, or a miscarriage; during the change of life, etc. Upon receiving *Sepia* these women often revert to their basic *Phosphorus*, *Calcarea*, or *Pulsatilla* selves. Thus the physician should recognize the episodic as well as the chronic state of the *Sepia* psyche.

Altogether, the first face of *Sepia* is characterized less by absence of emotions than by the attempt to escape them. Either she needs independence or seeks a self-imposed emotional detachment after having been injured in her feelings—contrasting with *Lycopodium*'s ingrained or inherent detachment. In particular, love is sensed by the housewife as a confinement and burden, even as she tries to counteract these feelings with duty.

The Career Woman

Sepia seeks to emancipate herself from the *burden of love* by moving into a world comparatively devoid of personal emotions, into a profession. This brings up the second face of the remedy, the woman who has an enjoyable career or is doing some interesting work concurrently with her housewifely duties. Because she is intellectually occupied and in her proper element, she comes to the physician for a specific physical complaint rather than for the overall tiredness and mental depression of the housewife: for menstrual and uterine disorders, and urinary complaints, such as urgency, or loss of control when laughing or coughing (*Causticum*); for anemia, backache (especially in the sacrum), or headaches; for arthritic pains; for hair falling out in bunches or early graying; for constipation or skin complaints. *Sepia* is a remedy of choice in various eczemas, adult acne (*Natrum muriaticum*), seborrhea, brownish or yellowish markings on, or discoloration of, the face, and skin troubles beginning in the middle years, such as small flesh-colored or brown warts appearing on the neck or in the axillae (armpits), skin turning blotchy, a sallow complexion with brown rings around the eyes or mouth, liver spots on the face and hands, and a host of digestive complaints reminiscent of *Sulphur*—all of which symptoms are thoroughly repertorized in the homoeopathic literature. One guiding symptom is a "longing for vinegar, acids, and pickles" (Boericke) as if to stimulate the weak or sluggish digestion, and the common craving for sour pickles during pregnancy is a *Sepia* indication.

This intellectually and emotionally fulfilled woman is usually between 25 and 55, with a strong will and penetrating mind, whose lifestyle exhibits a striving for self-realization. The remedy is frequently encountered in feminist champions of women's rights. Whatever her field of professional endeavor, she is efficient, well-organized, and intelligent. Her clear intellect thus contrasts with the better-known symptoms: "mind is dulled, thinking is a great exertion, thoughts flow slowly, words come slowly," etc. Often her clothes tend to blacks, browns (the cuttlefish's ink) and dark reds. Her dress and appearance may be "arty," but it is a stylish rather than a Bohemian artiness. In the creative arts, she often takes up drawing and painting, and of the performing arts she prefers dance. A keynote of the remedy is the modality "better from dancing" (H.C. Allen). Even headaches abate as soon as the woman starts to dance. In fact, dancing is often a passion with her, possibly because she feels free and unconstrained. The action sublimates, at least temporarily, all surfacing of the emotions which she finds so burdensome and which she has been trying to suppress. There was doubtless much *Sepia* in the genius of Isadora Duncan and Martha Graham, with their search for new ways for the body to express its inner emotions through dance.

These women claim to be better from any "violent motion" (Boenninghausen) or activity: jogging, tennis, soccer, swimming in cold water (Boericke; although they do not like cold air), anything bracing and vigorous, in preference to a quiet game of croquet, strolling in the park, or weeding the garden ("I *need* to feel that I've used my body vigorously"; "When I take exercise, I like something that is going to knock me out!"). Like the cuttlefish whose limbs or tentacles are always in motion, dancing in the water, they are more comfortable from moving about and worse from any fixed or "locked" position, such as kneeling in church, standing for any length of time, bending over to do the wash (hence *Sepia* is known as the "washerwoman's remedy"), or even sitting. Often when sitting they must cross their legs to relieve the sensation of pressure and "bearing down . . . into the vagina" (Hering). This may be why they are prone to travel sickness, and their symptoms (such as headaches or constipation) are aggravated by sedentary travel. Long periods of immobility exacerbate their poor circulation and intrinsic *stasis* (Farrington's term).* Perhaps for the same reason, i.e., amelioration from stimulation, they are "cheered by thunder and lightning" (Kent—*Sepia* is the only remedy listed under this rubric).

This *Sepia* type can be spirited, creative and attractive, but even when socially outgoing she may still lack the warm sympathy of *Phosphorus*, the natural sweetness of *Pulsatilla*, the strong humanitarian dimension of *Natrum muriaticum*, or the generous self-sacrifice of certain *Lachesis* individuals. As long as she is predominantly *Sepia* and without the benefit of homoeopathic remedies, she may appear deficient in feminine receptivity and the finer shades of emotional responsiveness. Possibly during the process of her social and psychological emancipation she has acquired a certain insensitivity.* *

Being clever, objective, and generally right, she feels quite free to tell others their mistakes and point out their shortcomings. For example, at a homoeopathic course, after one teacher's somewhat long-winded presentation, a student came up and asked him, "Have you ever taken *Sulphur?*" A bit nonplussed, he replied, "Yes, I have taken *Sulphur* in the past. Why?" "Strange," she said, shaking her head, "it doesn't seem to have worked for you." And, turning to her fellow students, "I simply can't understand it; it didn't seem to have worked on him at all. I wonder why?" She was entirely accurate in her judgment, the teacher was raggedly dressed as well as ponderously exhaustive in his delivery. Yet it took a *Sepia* to point it out to him in such "delicate" terms.

Thus she possesses a certain directness or matter-of-factness of speech and conduct (*Natrum muriaticum*). A guest might thank her hostess at the end of a dinner party in the following manner: "Many thanks for a nice evening. It was lovely seeing you and your husband again, even though this party was not as good as the one I came to last year. Your friends are not as interesting as they used to be." This is

---

* "Stasis" is defined as "a stoppage of the normal flow of liquids in any organ or vessel of the body; a slackening of the blood current as in passive congestion; impaired motion of the intestines with the retention of feces" (Webster).

** However, *Sepia* does possess psychic or mediumistic sensitivity. One imagines the swarthy gypsy fortune-teller as a*Phosphorus/Sepia* type.

not the way most people would thank a hostess, but she might be correct; the dinner party might not have been one of the best; and the accuracy of her remarks might make such frankness acceptable even if not necessarily desirable.

Also, at times this *Sepia* harbors a too outspoken "I am right" attitude (*Arsenicum*; the *Lycopodium* woman disguises it better). Indeed, she may be competent, clear in her observations, and possessed of an astute, if at times limited, judgment of people and circumstances. But others do not always want to be reminded that she is right. Men, especially, would far rather she were less often correct in her remarks; they would prefer her a little more ignorant and softer.

Even in friendship she may be too outspoken, her unsentimental approach verging on hardness. She greets an old friend with a hearty, "My, you *have* put on weight!" or "What are you doing with yourself these days, Ellie? Still nothing, as usual? Just hanging around wasting your time?" Or, a woman beginning to get along with her new stepchildren and genuinely enjoying their company, will let them embrace her but then append bluntly, "Oh my dears, I didn't think I would *ever* want to kiss you!" Honest, to be sure, but there are more subtle ways of communicating these feelings.

Still and all, while the forthright *Sepia*'s comments can make one feel uncomfortable, in a curious way she is not usually offensive, being candid and blunt rather than malicious. It is hard to take umbrage at facts that cannot be disputed, especially when delivered in the dispassionate, objective tones of a weather forecaster announcing that today's temperature is 74 degrees with a twenty percent chance of rain.

In all these instances we are speaking of *Sepia*'s insensitivity to others. With respect to herself she is sensitive enough, and in all meanings of the word. Not only is she physically hypersensitive to odors, noises, light—all of which can make her irritable and aggressive—but she also is extremely touchy and easily offended by criticism. Her "hardness" or "coldness" can be merely the outer shell of an extremely vulnerable (*Natrum muriaticum, Calcarea carbonica*), dependent (*Pulsatilla*), and helpless (*Phosphorus*) individual. Moreover, she understands her own nature well: her judgment of herself is as forthright and objective as her judgment of others. In the consulting room she is straightforward and not self-deceptive, aware of her weaknesses as well as her strengths (significantly, this remedy is *not* listed in Kent under the rubric "want of self-confidence"). And, on closer acquaintance, her commendable qualities become apparent: fairness, candor (*Sepia* is rarely hypocritical), sense of responsibility, trustworthiness, and, perhaps most important, integrity. You know where she stands on important issues.

If married and childless, this woman might say, "I am quite certain about not wanting to have children. My maternal instinct is not highly developed. I am perfectly content with my husband." And she is. For *Sepia* is not by nature promiscuous; she does not seek new thrills in love but leans toward long-lasting sexual relationships. If married to the right man which she frequently is, being discriminating and choosing well, she will remain loyal and sexually satisfied for life.

Or, if unmarried and asked if she misses it, she might reply, "No, I miss a good, strong ongoing relationship with a man, but I don't want marriage. I don't want to be tied down. I choose to remain single." And there are other variations on this basic theme: "When I was married, I felt it my duty to clean up after my husband and prepare his meals; after that I couldn't get down to my painting, so I always felt worse when he was at home and resented having to take care of him. I am happier now in a freer relationship," or "I get irritated at my husband's hanging around me too much. I love him, but I need my own space to operate in, and he curtails it."

Thus she is not necessarily antipathetic to sexual relations per se, as the traditional picture of *Sepia* suggests. This picture probably arose because, until recently, sex for women was associated with marriage, housework, and childbirth. Nor is she outwardly unfeminine and lacking in sex appeal. She can be quite the contrary, with her frequently lithe, graceful, trim figure. Sometimes, especially when combined with *Arsenicum*, she is the "dark, proud beauty," a woman of strong and dominant character who radiates competence and is highly attractive to the other sex. Such a woman often has a quiet, unassuming and obliging husband.* But, to do her justice, in return for her husband's devo-

---

* P.G. Wodehouse repeatedly relies on the classic set-up for comedy, in which compliant, gentle, weak, yielding *Pulsatilla* heroes are strangely and inexorably attracted to these strong-minded, clever *Sepias* who immediately begin to push them around, undertaking to reform them or "improve their minds" through serious reading. In one story, the valet Jeeves, attempting to console his mild and empty-headed master, Bertie Wooster, over the rupture of his engagement

tion, she will be a most supportive wife. Interesting herself in his work, helping him with good advice and her clear intellect, she is often an admirable partner for her unaggressive mate.

The remedy, however, also befits women who display masculine tendencies in both looks (narrow pelvis, tendency to a moustache) and manner; or who display sexual indifference, complete loss of sexual desire, "aversion to husband" (Kent), or, in the extreme, "dread of men" (Hahnemann). There can also be post-coital irritability ("discouraged," "anxiety after coition": Kent) and/or aggravation of symptoms. This does not mean that she necessarily prefers the same sex, although homosexuality does exist in the *Sepia* picture, as it does to some degree in all of the polychrests discussed in this book; she simply has little sexual interest or energy (at other times, although the desire is present, the flesh is weak, and the pain on sexual intercourse is "intolerable" [Hering]). This picture is found in the woman who cannot decide whether or not to marry for fear of being subjected to increased sexual demands. She is content to spend time occasionally with the man she loves, but no more than that: "I'm not so sure . . . Frequent sexual relations throw me off balance . . . Maybe marriage is not for me . . . " The remedy may help resolve her ambivalence, either way.

The second face of *Sepia* can be proudly independent. She has always managed on her own and wants to continue doing so. Scarlett O'Hara in *Gone With the Wind*, with her passion for dancing, her pride in independence, her sharp business mind, and her constant striving for self-expression, exhibits much of this face. Characteristic, too, are her admirable loyalty and responsibility toward her family—a long and heavy burden on her; her own type of honesty about herself; and her directness, combined with insensitivity toward others. Her other side, with its drive and at time unscrupulous determination, is more *Arsenicum*.

Sepia's pride can take the form of a lofty reserve. She is frequently a private person ("quiet, introspective": Hering), keeping her feelings to herself and discouraging any intrusion. Not easy to get to know or to understand, she may appear withdrawn and unresponsive. Indeed,

to a *Sepia/Arsenicum* woman, says, "I think you would have found her educational methods a little trying, Sir . . . It was her intention to start you almost immediately upon Nietzsche. You would not enjoy Nietzsche, Sir. He is fundamentally unsound."

she does not lightly reveal her emotions, being often of a retiring and introverted disposition. This may be due partly to an artist's visual, i.e., non-verbal, way of responding to the world and to her problems, but, in any case, she is (once again) seeking escape from her emotions rather than deficient in them. When she lets down her defenses and allows her troubles to pour out, a softer and warmer facet often emerges. During the office consultation she will weep freely when telling her symptoms, and, like *Pulsatilla* but contrary to *Natrum muriaticum*, she benefits from the release of pent-up emotions ("weeping ameliorates symptoms": Kent).

She also possesses a just pride, stemming from her sense of duty and the fitness of things. In any collective venture, for instance, she might at first feel imposed upon. Even the most dutiful *Sepia* does not feel instinctively, but must learn, that for a communal enterprise to succeed, everyone must do *more* than his or her allotted share. Once she understands this her innate pride compels her to discharge her duty scrupulously ("I'm as good as anyone else"). Then she is most easy to cooperate with in a direct businesslike way.* In general, her manner is more often at fault than her heart. For she is basically considerate and has good will. She will herself offer assistance to those in need, less enthusiastically than *Phosphorus* perhaps but more reliably.

---

* Few situations more clearly bring out an individual's true nature than a long-standing arrangement for driving children to and from school. No one is easier to cooperate with than the "benevolent" *Sulphur* who spontaneously offers to do more than her share, is ready to bail others out in an emergency, and who can be relied on completely, while no one is more difficult than the lazy selfish *Sulphur* who will exploit a situation for all it is worth. *Lycopodium* can always be counted on for full cooperation because, with her sense of what is correct and her natural reliability, she will do her share graciously and without fuss but will not, as a rule, exert herself to do extra. *Natrum muriaticum*, on the other hand, will do more than her share out of fear of not doing enough and unwillingness to be oppressed by feelings of indebtedness. At some point, however, she begins to resent it bitterly and self-righteously, and wants to back out and throw up the whole cooperative arrangement. *Calcarea* is reliable and helpful, but with a tendency to run late, having been detained by flustering over some minor crisis at home. *Phosphorus*, as might be expected, will spontaneously offer to take overtime; in intent and words she is most

The Complainer

The third face of *Sepia*, the dissatisfied complainer, is actually the negative image of the conscientious housewife (typical here is the originally quiet, compliant, often artistic woman who, with an unsatisfactory or too stressful marriage, turns bossy and nagging), the contented independent career woman, or the emotionally remote one. Because she is frequently encountered in the physician's office, however, she will be treated as a separate type.

The traditional words used to describe her are: "critical, vexed at every trifle, scolding, fault-finding, bemoaning, lamenting, discontented with everything, easily offended, peevish and disposed to quarrel, great irritability from slightest cause, disagreeable, constant ill humor," etc. (Hahnemann, Hering, Kent, and others). All of these are accurate and easy enough to spot, as her straightforwardness readily reveals her negativity; in fact, it bristles from her entire being. She concentrates on the dark side of things ("all her troubles present themselves in a sad light to her, so that she is despondent": Hahnemann), is convinced that she is being badly used and that others do not like her. Or, lacking emotional generosity herself, she attributes the worst motives to what people say and do. In the physician's office she may be reluctant to admit to improvement under treatment, and sometimes she talks as if barring from her sphere of vision even the possibility of cure, as in the following characteristic dialogue:

"Oh, the pain in my back is no better. Not better at all! I don't know why I even bother to come here. We're not getting anywhere really."

"But remember, your period now comes once a month instead of every three weeks, and there are fewer accompanying headaches."

---

generous, but when the time for action comes, she not only wriggles out of the extra driving but even out of her share. When others take over for her, she may forget to repay the favor. *Pulsatilla*, desiring to cooperate, will usually do beautifully and, if she begins to slip in her share, allowing others to take over, will respond appropriately if this is pointed out to her. *Arsenicum* will religiously carry out her part of the bargain and, given the chance, will organize and conduct the whole car pool, deciding for everyone who is to do what. Strong on equity and intellectually realizing the advantage of full participation and cooperation, she is completely reliable even though outraged (like *Natrum muriaticum*) at anyone who does not pull her load.

"That is true [with moaning reluctance] but, oh! I know that you will never be able to cure my back."

"Give us time and we will."

"I don't know. We still have to see if my periods remain regular. I haven't been really well since I was ten years old, and no improvement has ever lasted . . . " and so on.

Thus an *undisguised* negativity distinguishes this *Sepia* from other types, whether due to an inability to conceal her nature, a need to feel rejected, excessive candor, or simply a complete lack of interest in producing a good impression.

Occasionally, though, her negativity is disguised. A highly attractive, cheerful, responsive, young woman who had been manifesting the remedy's physical symptoms since childhood was being treated for life-long constipation. Yet the mental picture did not fit. Only toward the end of the interview, when the physician finally thought of asking her what she disliked in herself, what she would change, she said, "I am always undermining the love of anyone close to me. I did this with my parents and now I am doing it with my boyfriend who started talking about marriage. Instead of being loving, I keep complaining to him that he doesn't really love me or that if he knew me better he wouldn't. I don't know why I put myself down in this way. I've nagged away at him so much that now he has dropped all thought of marriage. I know I have this tendency to ruin close relationships, not only romantic ones—although with acquaintances and not-so-close friends I am as happy and sparkling as the day is long." *There* was our *Sepia*!

This type may think she has a raw deal in life and that fate has treated her worse than others. A futile "envy" (this symptom should be raised to a higher degree in the Kent *Repertory*) frequently lies at the root of her discontent. She abstractly envies others their good fortune or success: the rich their money, celebrities their fame, women in politics their power, and artists their genius. A memorable example of such envy was the dancer being treated for sciatic pains who complained, "Why is it that when Isadora Duncan performed her dancing to symphonic music, the public considered it beautiful and innovative, but when I perform my modern dances to the sounds of humpback whales singing [whines, groans, eerie screetches, and whistles]—something *really* innovative—the critics call it grotesque?" (Why indeed!)

More concretely, she may envy one friend her job, another her nicer home, a third her more interesting husband, a fourth her apparent lack of problems. She even envies her own husband's satisfaction at his work. She feels that he is growing and *his* mind is expanding while she, tied to the home, is contracting and her mind deteriorating, with no sense of fulfillment in life.

Her envy is altogether different from the well-known *Lachesis* jealousy, which is an obsessive and passionate possessiveness of some loved one or of some all-engrossing activity or idea. *Sepia* covets that for which she herself has no aptitude, or to which she has no legitimate claim. She chronically worries that others have something she lacks and is inordinately fond of regarding the pastures on the other side of the fence as greener than her own. When a housewife, she wants independence and a career; or if working part-time, she bitterly resents her housework, ranking her job above her family life. But when the children grow older, or she separates from her husband and is free to pursue her career, suddenly her priorities alter; she will conceive an overwhelming aversion to her work and, in a classic negation of everything she had previously striven for, will want her husband, children or home-life back again.

She can be, moreover, the patient with whom nothing seems to go right, who becomes brooding and withdrawn ("sad, dejected": Hahnemann), and who, in her misery, is unable to react or to feel. There is no joy in her life, and, if there were, she would be incapable of appreciating it. She is nauseated by the very smell of food—one of life's basic pleasures—sometimes just by *thinking* of her favorite dish. And she is tired and drained by eating instead of being energized. She emanates utter dreariness. Nothing in her social or professional life interests her or gives her happiness. She finds people dull or stupid: "aversion for social intercourse amounting to contempt" (Hering). She sits in the physician's office looking and feeling empty, with no ambition, no drive, no emotional life ("great indifference toward everything; no proper sense of life . . . [feels] as if did not care what happened": Allen), at times secretly wishing that something—anything—would happen to relieve her apathy and ennui: "I can't seem to get what I want from life. Is this all there is to it? Do I even have a *right* to a meaningful life? Why can't I experience happiness, as others do? I wish I knew what a normally happy life is! This emptiness inside me is frightening," are among the more common laments of the *Sepia* suffering from long-standing misery or indifference. Women in this state may experience unaccountable bouts of sadness with involuntary crying, weeping "without apparent cause" (Hahnemann), or suddenly become irrational, unreasonable, and uncontrolled, in a state of hysteria reminiscent of *Ignatia*.

All these feelings, as well as her sadness, depression, and numerous anxieties, have a prominent time modality; like *Pulsatilla*, they are aggravated in the morning and/or evening.

Another prominent *Sepia* modality is the left-handedness of many complaints (*Lachesis*, *Phosphorus*). In the occult sciences the left side has traditionally been regarded as pertaining to the emotions, the irrational, and the unconscious, while the right side represents the intellect, rationality, and consciousness. Thus her predominantly left-sided symptoms in yet another way suggest an imbalance of the emotional, rather than the intellectual, sphere.

This face of *Sepia* has two ways of reacting when in a really black mood. Just as the cuttlefish's ink serves as a screen behind which to hide, the woman retires into a dark moodiness and deliberately cuts herself off from others. Despite being urged to talk and communicate her feelings, she maintains a cold silence. She will refuse to answer the door or the telephone because she does not want anyone to offer sympathy or interfere with her misery, and because any "conversation aggravates" (Kent). She feels truly indifferent to others at the moment and wants to be left alone, while *Natrum muriaticum*, who will do the same, is perversely rejecting what her nature actually craves.

On the other hand, just as the cuttlefish's ink also serves as a weapon of attack, *Sepia* may become loudly dissatisfied, highly irritable, "quarrelsome" and "impatient" (Kent), especially with her mate, and at times "inclined to be vehement" (Hering). She is then spiteful in her verbal thrusts, lashing out at those nearest in sporadic fits of aggressiveness while taking a perverse pride in her sharp tongue (*Arsenicum*, *Lachesis*). At such times everyone around her must walk on eggs for fear of provoking an aggressive outburst—an ejection of that black cloud of ink. There is in this person much "suppressed anger . . . about former vexations and past events" (Kent) that is just waiting to erupt; also, "violent ebullitions of passion, with trembling (particularly of the hands), can be brought on by a mere trifle" (Allen).

Whitmont reconciles this duality of behavior under stress by referring to the physiology and anatomy of the cuttlefish. To paraphrase:

the cuttlefish is a mollusc (a soft gelatinous body encased in a calcareous shell), but of all the molluscs it is the most highly developed for action, since the half of the body with the tentacles is permanently outside the shell. Thus, one part of *Sepia* (the feminine) is passive, withdrawn and unmoving, enclosed and cut off from the world by a protective hardness. This is the part which, under stress, retires into indifference; the other part is not only free and active but moves rapidly through the water and shoots out its tentacles with swift accuracy to catch its prey. This attacking mode, concludes Whitmont, is her aggressive (masculine) form of reacting under stress.

However, the cuttlefish is not a truly aggressive animal, and *Sepia*, faced with real opposition or a threat, is apt suddenly to collapse and become spineless. This gentler, yielding, irresolute side of the nature should not be disregarded. Like *Pulsatilla*, she can be incapable of making decisions and full of tears and self-pity, even seeking consolation. In this respect she differs from the threatened *Lachesis* who, snake-like, becomes more rigid and ready to attack what menaces her.

The negative *Sepia* can even be quite uncivil to, or high-handedly spurn, those proffering help. She does not want to be beholden to any-one and is resentful at needing help or being ill. Occasionally also she *wants* to play the martyr and resists any attempt to deprive her of that role. She is the woman who sits the friendly neighbor or relative down at the kitchen table and pours out all her moanings and lamentations, tirelessly "relating her grievances" (Kent). She must prove to others, as well as to herself, that life is not fair to her, and she vents her martyr-dom by complaining. Such for example is old Mrs. Gummidge in *David Copperfield*, who is always groaning that she feels "more than others do," a damp raw day, a smoking fire in the chimney, or the burnt pota-toes at dinner; and who exploits her long-standing bereavement to ceaselessly lament, "I'm a lone, lorn creetur and everythink goes con-trairy with me." *Sepia* is listed in the Kent *Repertory* under the rubric, "complaining," in the first degree; in our opinion it should be elevated to the third degree.

Each remedy possesses its own way of being negative in the home. *Pulsatilla* becomes whiny, *Arsenicum* scolding and aggressively asser-tive, *Lachesis* erratically violent, *Phosphorus* unreasonably demanding, *Sulphur* rude and surly, and *Natrum muriaticum* self-righteously argu-mentative. But *Sepia* nags and bemoans her fate, is "never happy unless annoying someone" (Kent).

Another aspect of her discontent is her extreme intolerance of contradiction. If crossed or criticized, she flies into a passion of justification (*Natrum muriaticum*) or becomes nasty (*Lycopodium*). This may be why marriage can bring out her negative traits. The marital state entails a certain amount of conceding or deferring to one's partner, and she "permits no opposition to her opinions" (Kent). In an argument with her husband, for example, she flares up shouting in anger and begins to tremble; and then, to be sure to have the last word, she storms out of the room slamming the door behind her. Although she might later admit to herself that she was wrong, her pride makes it near-impossible for her to apologize (like *Natrum muriaticum* and in contrast to *Pulsatilla*).

Like *Arsenicum* and *Lycopodium* she can actually become "miserly" (Hering)—the housewife, for instance, displaying a reluctance to buy food for her family. Even when there is no financial need, she may pride herself on how *little* money she spends on groceries. To ascribe this to a subconscious dislike of family would be too facile, since this trait is found even in a woman who genuinely loves her husband and children. It is rather the trapped and mentally starved housewife's substitute for an intellectual challenge; once *Sepia* gets out of the house and puts her mind to more interesting challenges, she stops thinking so much of economy (although she will never become a spendthrift). Her miserliness arises also from a subliminal "fear of poverty" (Kent), of being left without shelter, food ("fear of starvation": Hering), or clothing. It is as though she has gone through these deprivations in some past incarnation and can never lose her fear of them, whatever her financial status. In Kent's *Repertory*, under the rubric, "Delusion: thinks [s]he is poor," *Sepia* is the highest remedy listed.

Sometimes she manifests a low-grade chronic selfishness, whose constant refrain is an insistence on her own needs: "I want . . . I need . . . Why don't I have . . . " The characteristic can take an acute form where she requests more and more of others ("greedy": Hering), until no one wants to help her any longer.* She then complains that life is against

---

* At such times she is reminiscent of the fisherman's wife in the fairy tale, *The Fisherman and the Sea*: A poor fisherman one day caught in his net a little goldfish who spoke to him in a human voice, "Please,

her, that people are not doing enough for her, that they avoid her. Perhaps they do, but in all probability she has brought this state upon herself. "Character is fate" said the Greeks, and the truth of this axiom is seldom exhibited more clearly than in the negative *Sepia*.

The various constitutional types have their typical ways of breaking, or not breaking, relationships. Briefly, *Pulsatilla* will make any concession to prevent a rupture, while *Lycopodium* employs wit for conciliatory purposes: like *Pulsatilla*, he may make the first gestures of reconciliation, but without the latter's accommodating sweetness. *Phosphorus*, we recall, dislikes hostile feelings and will try to avoid a falling out, yet occasionally finds herself in the midst of discord arising from some confusion or misunderstanding in the relationship. With *Lachesis* something has changed in *her*; there is no confusion, just a sudden reversal of the original feeling of friendship; in both types, however, the rupture can be repaired. *Sulphur* is quick to quarrel but equally quick to forgive and make up; after the initial explosion she forgets what it was

---

kind Sir, let me go, and in return I shall grant you any wish you may ask of me. For I am a magic fish. Just call for me, and I shall come to you." So the kind fisherman let him go and, returning to the mud hut where his wife was sitting in front of a broken cooking pot, told her about the goldfish. "What a fool you are" she scolded him, "you should have asked for a new cooking pot; can't you see that ours is broken? Go back at once and ask the fish for one." So the old man obeyed, and the goldfish came at his call, promised to fulfill his request, and disappeared into the bright blue sea.

On returning home, the fisherman found his wife sitting beside a brand-new pot. But after a time, she again showed signs of discontent, "Why did you only ask for a pot?" she complained, "when we also need a new hut. Go back to the goldfish and ask him for one." So the fisherman again went back to the sea, which was now less blue and shiny, and called for the fish . . . And the same events were repeated several times until his wife was living like a queen in a palace.

However, she was still dissatisfied and demanded to rule over the sea as well as the land, and that the little fish be made to serve her personally. The poor browbeaten fisherman trudged back to the now angry, dark, and seething sea and called the goldfish who, on hearing the wife's latest request, said nothing but, with a flick of his tail, disappeared into the deep. The fisherman then returned to find his wife sitting by the original mud hut with a broken pot in front of her.

all about, and thus there is no real falling out. *Arsenicum*'s judgmental attitude leads her to sever relations with others who are not performing up to her standards or who venture to rebuke her; while willing enough to criticize others, she does not appreciate being criticized herself. *Natrum muriaticum* will put up with much abuse to avoid a rupture but then suddenly cuts off relationships out of hurt feelings (sometimes justified, sometimes not), disappointment in others, a sense of guilt or of insufficient approval; to repair the rupture is always difficult and sometimes impossible. *Calcarea* is not easily provoked but, if offended, will withdraw to nurse the wound, although not with *Natrum muriaticum*'s morbid resentment and seldom with her finality. *Sepia*'s third face does not have to break with others, as others break with her. But her first two faces are restrained, considerate, and often dignified in relationships; out of principle they will not permit themselves to quarrel (*Lycopodium*).

Many of *Sepia*'s negative characteristics, can be markedly changed by the remedy. After a dose in high potency, she becomes a more satisfied and agreeable person. The woman who used to regret what she lacked is now grateful for what she has. An originally complaining patient will return saying, "Yes, my life is still dull, but at least my children are intelligent, and I am thankful for that" or "I graduated from Radcliffe *magna cum laude* which has had to serve as training for washing dishes, cleaning the house, and changing diapers, but my husband is a good man, and I am fortunate in that respect" or "Life, after all, does not *owe* me more than I've got, and I realize it's up to me to make the best of that." Even the complaining tone of voice, the nasal twang or drawl which so often reflects *Sepia*'s discontent (also *Staphysagria*'s: Boger), becomes modified.

Still others volunteer that they have become conscious of the fruitlessness of envy: "You can always find *someone* who has what you don't have." And some patients apologize handsomely for their previous demeanor: "I really was quite convinced you would not be able to help me, and that I was wasting my time and money here. So I want to apologize if I showed it in my behavior." Thus, homoeopathic *Sepia* performs the dual function of lessening some of the patient's inherent negative tendencies and making her more conscious of others, so that she can at least keep them under control.

A middle-aged European woman came to the clinic with a complicated picture of dysmenorrhea, headaches, arthritis, burning pain in the stomach after eating, and other symptoms. She made an unfavorable impression, with her irritation at the physician running a little late and displeasure at the (to her) unfamiliar manner in which the homoeopathic interview was conducted ("The homoeopaths in Europe do not spend their time asking me to describe my favorite meal; they stick to the more strictly pathological symptoms"). She was also without a good word to say for America ("a country too big, where the inhabitants are making what seems like a concerted effort to eradicate its natural beauties"), or about Americans ("who are always looking for quick easy solutions to everything"). So, without further ado *Sepia* was prescribed in high potency, and she was requested to return in six weeks.

In less than half that time she called in to say that her last period had been easier and her headaches were improved, but that the joint pains in her arms and fingers were worse than ever, and she was developing a painful abscess around one fingernail. What should she do? "Nothing," she was told, "but soak your finger in *Calendula*, and let us know how you are coming along." Two days later she phoned in to report that the arthritic pain had lessened, but that the finger was even more infected and painful. Thereupon it was suggested that she come to to the office immediately.

It was one of those hectic days, with several emergency calls and acute cases coming in, and out-of-town patients hurrying to catch flights, so that it was a good while before the physician got around to this woman, (prescribing *Myristica sebifera* 200x, that wonderful "specific" for felons and paronychiae). Yet she never complained at the delay and, when he finally got to her, was all understanding. No one could have behaved more graciously under the circumstances. Obviously the *Sepia* had already taken effect and by way of the paronychia was expelling not only her physical ills but her disagreeable personality as well.

This is possibly why, to use one of Hubbard's graphic phrases, "The second dose of *Sepia* is *always* a mistake!," and why in chronic conditions many months should go by before it is repeated. If the physical symptoms persist, as they sometimes do, it serves better to go on to other medicines. The remedy, like the individual, seems unable to respond well to too many demands. And also, when *Sepia* is well chosen, the attitude is so altered that another dose is not needed. The remedy dispels the dreariness and discontent and brings about a more buoyant, positive frame of mind; it can liberate a woman from oppressive gloom, for which there is frequently no tangible reason, into the bracing sunshine.

The Male

Although this remedy is indicated far less frequently in males than in females, it was actually discovered by Hahnemann in a male patient: a painter displaying unusual symptoms whom Hahnemann observed constantly licking the tip of his brush while painting in sepia ink (i.e., "proving" the remedy).

The physical symptoms most frequently encountered in males requiring *Sepia* are: tension headaches, nausea from the smell of food (*Arsenicum*), chronic sinus and nasal catarrhs, rheumatism or arthritis in the legs, a rundown, allergic constitution, and severe constipation with or without urging (like *Natrum muriaticum*, *Sepia* often retains anger or resentment via the stool), occasionally with the sensation of a ball-shaped object in, or a knifelike pain shooting up, the rectum. His sexual energy is low (he is reluctant or too tired to make the necessary effort), or he may entertain an "aversion to the opposite sex" (Kent); and sometimes, for whatever reason, he presents a picture of deliberate and longstanding suppression of the sexual urge.

The male mental symptoms are at times a curious corollary of the female ones. In both the traditional sexual roles are reversed, reflecting once again the *Sepia* "greener pastures" syndrome—and, on a more profound level, reflecting the phenomenon of what Jung called the "anima" (the woman in a man).*

The woman seeks to emancipate herself from the passive, receptive female role, the world of home and emotions, into a life of action. The male, conversely, wants to disengage from the active world of politics and business and lead a quieter, more contemplative life. The formerly energetic, hard-working man, now middle-aged, is "indolent" (Hahnemann), discontented with his job, and tired or worn out emotionally. He wants only to stay at home and spend time at some low-keyed occupation or hobby, or simply to be left alone ("indifferent to everything, insensible and apathetic": Hahnemann).

The male can also be irritable ("he becomes angry with every trifle": Allen), with what is traditionally regarded as a Welshman's type of dourness or "moroseness" (Hahnemann). He may display little interest

---

* This thesis, applied to *Sepia*, is discussed in detail by Whitmont.

in—at times actual hostility toward—his wife and children ("aversion to members of family": Kent). He is too tired for any occupation ("no disposition to work": Hahnemann), and "it is even an exertion to think" (Allen); or, like *Natrum muriaticum* he "dwells on his past troubles . . . and is occupied with sad memories" (Hahnemann). Yet he, too, is better from strenuous activity: chopping wood, spading the garden, brisk five-mile walks. In fact, he needs a powerful stimulus to get going or to feel any emotion. He worries about the future (in a whiny tone) and about his mind being dull ("dullness of comprehension; inability to collect or express his thoughts": Allen). *Sepias* of both sexes have various "confusion of mind" symptoms: "after eating, after coition, from mental exertion, when spoken to, when walking, during hot weather, before menses" (Kent). He may be slow-acting and forgetful from over-stress ("inattentive and distracted": Hahnemann), but, like the female, the male seldom gives the impression of stupidity. *Sepia* does not, as a rule, make overtly stupid moves or say foolish things. Above all, he does not harbor a higher than warranted idea of his own capacities. The nature is capable of judging dispassionately and does not suffer from a groundless, overwhelming ego (*Phosphorus, Sulphur*).

Little more can be said of the male *Sepia* than has been said already of the female, but the following is an instance where the remedy was prescribed solely from the mental symptoms. A patient was lamenting her intellectual husband's recently changed behavior. "He has always had a first-rate mind, but recently, instead of being interested in anything significant, all he talks about is the household budget and the high price of groceries; also, he complains if there is a bit of unused food left lying in the refrigerator. When he comes home from work, even as he turns the key in the lock, he can smell something aging in the refrigerator and goes straight for the culprit. Or he nags if I use the wrong kitchen utensils to cook with. He just hangs around me being picky and petty over everything. I wish you could do something for him."

The physician asked for more symptoms. "I don't know of any. He is disgustingly healthy, and even if he had other symptoms he wouldn't talk about them. And he won't come to this clinic because he dislikes doctors" (*Sepia* is not as eager to visit doctors as *Arsenicum, Pulsatilla,* and some other types—although Kent does list the medicine in the second degree under "anxiety about health). But if you give me a remedy I will see to it that he takes it."

She did, however, recall one incident illustrating her husband's blunt behavior. At a lecture they had attended the husband approached the speaker and asked, "Are you *sure* you are the same person whose picture is on the back of your books? I would never have recognized you! You've certainly aged since that photograph—and where is your hair?" (indeed, the picture had been taken twelve years previously).

Had he been a *Natrum muriaticum*, who has a tendency to put his foot in his mouth, he might have blundered into making such a remark but then, sensing its gaucheness, would immediately have tried to right it: "I *am* sorry. I mean *of course* the picture is still like you— yes, now I see that you haven't really changed at all . . . " compounding the awkwardness of the situation by his apologies. But this man made the statement half matter-of-factly, half in jest, leaving the speaker with no choice but to laugh and forget it. On this scanty, but sufficient, evidence the physician prescribed *Sepia* 1M.

At the next visit the patient stated that immediately after taking the remedy her husband developed severe knee pains which lasted a week or two (he had had occasional stabs of pain there in the past, possibly the first signs of an incipient arthritis which was now being dispelled by the remedy). Meanwhile, his upset over leftovers on the back shelves of the refrigerator had diminished; he no longer talked about the price of groceries and was back again to his caustic but intellectual self.

The Child

While *Sepia* is primarily an adult remedy, it should not be neglected in children—both girls *and* boys. Physically, these children manifest constipation, eczemas and other skin eruptions, ringworm, inability to tolerate milk (from which they get constipation or stuffy noses), chronic loss of appetite, a propensity to catch cold at every change of weather, or enuresis (especially early in the night, so that if caught and taken to the bathroom before 10 p.m., the child will stay dry till morning).

But, here again, negativity is most often the key to the remedy. *Sepia* children can be disgruntled, critical of their parents, teachers, and friends, interested in neither work nor play, scolding, uncooperative, and naggingly discontented. Once they become active, however, on the playing field or at a party, and get all the "bile and vinegar" out of their systems through exercise, they play as happily as other children. Generally they are serious and reserved rather than fun-loving, and do not socialize easily with other children. Feeling too tired to go out and play, the child is nevertheless hypersensitive and highly "excitable" (Borland) and, of course, finds energy to complain. Lucy van Pelt of the *Peanuts* cartoon strip is a regular little *Sepia*. She is clever, chronically dissatisfied, takes pride in her bad temper and in annoying or psychologically bullying others, and even enjoys feeling martyred.*

In his rejection of affection, the child's behavior sometimes suggests that he feels even the love of his parents to be a burden. But the remedy is also important for the child brought up in an orphanage or "home," or whose parents are divorced or travel frequently, leaving him behind with sitters or relatives, i.e., for the youngster who, consciously or unconsciously, feels neglected (*Natrum muriaticum*).

Yet, in children as in adults, just one dose of *Sepia* can cause such an alteration of character as to bring to mind the anecdote about the difference between a pessimist and an optimist:

Two little boys were sent to clean out a stable full of manure. The pessimist grudgingly worked for a while, then stopped, complaining: "What's the point of all this? We'll never be able to finish this job. There's still so much left to do, and the work is so boring!" But the optimist, shovelling away harder than ever, replied, "With all this manure around, somewhere in this pile there has *got* to be a pony!"

---

* Typical here is the scene in which Lucy, standing by the window with her brother watching the rain splashing against the panes, complains that it *always* rains on Sundays, as if deliberately to ruin her play day. Linus intercedes, "It doesn't always rain on Sundays. Last week we had a good day . . . " At which point Lucy turns on him with a black look and a threatening fist, and he quickly amends his tone. "You're right, it *always* rains on Sundays. You are a very unlucky person." And Lucy is mollified.

Sulphur

THIS chapter discusses what is probably the most useful and widely employed of all constitutional remedies—*Sulphur*. For even as elemental sulphur is generously diffused throughout the earth's crust beneath the surface vegetation, so a *Sulphur* layer lies beneath the surface of all the varied constitutional types, serving as the homoeopathic common denominator of mankind.

Versatility

Hahnemann from the first recognized *Sulphur*'s special significance to homoeopathy when he established it as the leading anti-psoric remedy in his theory of chronic diseases.* Since he regarded Psora as the causal miasm at the root of most chronic conditions, a large propor-

---

* After nearly two decades of practice Hahnemann observed that many of his patients with acute diseases responded to the similar remedy only temporarily and then suffered relapses. This led him to conclude that underlying these acute diseases were a number of chronic "miasms" or diseases which had to be removed before the supervening acute disease could be cured. In 1828 he published his *Chronic Diseases* which hypothesized the existence of three basic chronic diseases: Psora, Syphilis, and Sycosis (gonorrhoea). They assume the most versatile forms (Hahnemann wrote two large volumes of their symptoms) and were to be cured by *Sulphur, Mercurius,* and *Thuja (Arbor vitae),* respectively. Of Psora Hahnemann wrote: "Psora is that most ancient, most universal, most destructive, and yet most misapprehended chronic miasmatic disease which for many thousands of years has disfigured and tortured mankind, and which during the last centuries has become the mother of all the thousands of incredibly various (acute

tion of patients—even those of a different constitutional type—will manifest the *Sulphur* diathesis at some point in their treatment.

There are thus definite *stages in illness* that call for this medicine. Because of its well-attested power to bring latent symptoms to the surface ("where there is paucity of symptoms to prescribe on": Hahnemann) and to cleanse the system of the effects of previous allopathic drugging, *Sulphur* is often the first remedy used in a severe chronic case. But it is many-faceted and equally efficacious in the middle of a course of treatment when other remedies fail. It has a unique capacity to elicit a response and prod stagnant cases into progress: "When carefully selected remedies fail to act, *Sulphur* arouses the reactive powers of the organism" (Hering/Boericke). If it will not resolve the case by itself, it will enable the patient to respond to the previously ineffectual simillimum.

The deep-delving remedy is also invaluable in complaints tending to relapse ("seems to get almost well, when disease returns": Hering) or for ailments continually recurring even under homoeopathic treatment. And, finally, *Sulphur* frequently plays an Omega as well as an Alpha role in acute and chronic ailments. In childhood ailments and such protracted diseases of adults as pneumonia, heart conditions, rheumatoid arthritis, influenza, and mononucleosis, it terminates the illness or hastens convalescence and cure.

In certain stages of life it often benefits constitutional types other than its own. In infancy and early childhood it clears up diaper, food, and heat rashes, cradlecaps, eczemas, and digestive problems. It is also most effective in the pimply and difficult adolescent years. Later it is indicated in the midlife crisis of men and the menopausal period of women. Although other "female" remedies (*Lachesis, Sepia, Pulsatilla*) might be better known for the hot flashes and other symptoms of these years, *Sulphur* is also needed—especially to counteract the onset of growths, both malignant and benign (H.C. Allen). Finally, the remedy has proved invaluable in many infirmities of old age.

Sulphur is so powerful that it may usurp the role of other remedies, as shown by the following example. A man of thirty came to homoeop-

---

and) chronic (non-venereal) diseases, by which the whole civilized human race on the inhabited globe is being more and more afflicted" (*Chronic Diseases*, I, 9).

athy for treatment of an embarrassing complaint. Three years earlier he had lost his normal voice after a severe and prolonged bout of influenza, and since that time sounded like a woman. Although he had been to a number of ear, nose, and throat specialists and speech therapists, he had not yet succeeded in getting back his former male voice. The physical symptoms pointed to several lesser remedies, among them *Spongia*, and *Rumex crispus*, but the mentals were pure *Pulsatilla*. Everything was there: the plaintive tone, the emotional behaviour, and the dependent manner. However, since he had taken a long course of antibiotics for his influenza, the physician started the case with a dose of *Sulphur* to counteract any residual allopathic drug effects and to act as a "reconnoitering agent" until other remedies could be investigated. As it happened, no other remedy was ever needed, since the one dose of *Sulphur* took care of the entire case. At the subsequent visit the patient was once again talking in his normal masculine voice.

Another typical case was an older man with a heart condition whose symptoms perfectly fitted the picture of *Tarentula hispania* (anguish; extreme restlessness; a need to walk about, although he was worse from motion; a sensation "as if the heart were wrung or twisted" [Boericke]). But he lived out in the country, and there was no way of getting this unusual remedy to him quickly. Because he also wanted the windows open and occasionally experienced a rush of blood to the head, as a stopgap measure he was advised to take the *Sulphur* he had on hand. By evening, however, his case had been so steadied by this medicine that a change in prescription was not justified. It is a cardinal rule of homoeopathic practice not to change horses in midstream; if a remedy, even if seemingly second-best, is doing the job, the physician should stay with it until its action is exhausted. *Sulphur* was repeated shortly thereafter, and the patient remained in good health.

What type of individual requires *Sulphur* when it is operating within its own legitimate and well-defined sphere and not stealing the show from its lesser brethren? It is not easy to describe a remedy whose action is so polyvalent. What is more, it is extremely rich in those polarities, variants, oppositions, and "shadow sides" which are the hallmark of the polychrests. Yet its personality has very definite features which in this analysis will be classified under the following headings: 1) *Sulphur*'s selfish and materialistic side together with its polar opposite: generosity and anti-materialism; 2) *Sulphur*'s physical and emotional erup-

tiveness and heat, with all its ramifications; and 3) *Sulphur*'s intellectual slant of mind together with its antitheses: pseudo- and anti-intellec-
tualism.

Selfishness, Materialism, Generosity

Selfishness is a prominent feature (Kent), but the remedy hardly
holds a monopoly on this universal human trait. Each constitutional
type has its own variety of selfishness. *Phosphorus* is convinced that
the whole world revolves around himself; *Sepia* asks for more and more;
Silica shirks responsibility; *Pulsatilla* constantly demands to be petted
and protected; *Natrum muriaticum* insists on doing everything his own
way; *Arsenicum*, like *Nux vomica*, is calculating and unrelenting in his
own behalf; *Calcarea* and *Lycopodium* tenaciously refuse to yield an
inch despite another's needs; and *Lachesis*, when his feelings are aroused,
becomes oblivious to the desires of others, or even their existence.

An extreme form of *Sulphur*'s selfishness is encountered in the blatant egoist ("egotism": Hering), most particularly in the churlish male
whose insensitivity permits no consideration for others. He strongly
approves of people helping each other in life, provided this is not expected of him. Completely engrossed in his own world, he will not
put himself out for anyone, grumbles or becomes "peevish" (Hahnemann) if asked to do even the smallest favor; yet he expects others to
look after his comforts. Kent offers a graphic illustration of this trait:
"Everything that he contemplates is for the benefit of himself . . . There
is absence of gratitude . . . He will sit around and do nothing, and let
his wife take in the washing and work her fingers off taking care of him;
he thinks that is all she is good for . . . A state of refinement seems to
have gone out of [him]."

The belief that toil is good for a woman is a subliminal if not overt
tenet of many *Sulphur* males. He is the man who comes home to a wife
laden with household cares and small children and ask her roughly,
"Why didn't you rake up the leaves as I asked you to? What do you
mean you didn't have time? What *have* you been doing all day?" He
is convinced that nothing is difficult, fatiguing, or important to anyone
but himself.

Nor is this true only in the home. Generally "indifferent to the welfare of others" (Kent), the selfish *Sulphur* is reluctant to give a minute
of his time or an ounce of his energy to some communal enterprise

and, even if a concerned partner, barely does his share of the work. He does not have to cooperate or express his gratitude because everything is owed him. Others should feel privileged to help him out.

Sometimes the *Sulphur* child's aggressive unwillingness to cooperate, attributed to selfishness, is actually generated more by an extreme independence and resentment of outside interference. "I want to do it my own way!" he insists. "By myself, by myself!" he cries angrily, pushing away help as he struggles to tie his shoe laces or attempts some other difficult task. He is convinced from an early age that he knows best and demands to be left alone to try. *Calcarea* children can also be independent but are less pugnacious about it.

Sulphur can also be materialistic. This is manifested in a love of money and/or possessions as well as in the attitude: "What's mine is mine, and what's yours is negotiable." The quality emerges at an early age: the child can be quite ferocious in snatching away toys from others while protecting his own tenaciously. "It's mine! . . . Don't touch! . . . I want *your* ball! . . ." are among the first phrases of the *Sulphur* child. The remedy was once successfully prescribed for this reason to an eighteen-month old boy with a complicated respiratory-tract infection: while sitting on his mother's knees he tugged at her earrings and shouted "Mine . . . mine" with an angry and determined expression on his face.

At times, however, the reverse is encountered. Instead of grabbing, babies will insistently thrust a toy or rattle into another's hand. A six-month old *Sulphur* girl was brought in for treatment of an amazingly thick cradle-cap: a layer about 1/8 inch thick that could be peeled off in slabs. During the interview, she tried with amusingly insistent grunts to force her teething ring on the physician and would not rest until he had accepted it. An older child will approach whomever he has taken a fancy to and generously hand over his book or stuffed animal in the same assertive manner.

As *Sulphur* grows older, he begins to *collect* things: rocks, shells, stamps, matchboxes, locks and keys, or baseball cards. He even collects broken toys fished out of trashcans — whatever catches his fancy, regardless of worth. He is by instinct a pack rat, hoarding whatever he can lay his hands on. The young girl will collect numerous dolls or tiny animals and china objects which she crowds onto her shelves where she can see them all. She will spend hours sorting and rearranging these pretty things, while the boy is more likely to shove his collection into a drawer or leave it in a pile on the floor.

The child is "extremely pleased with his possessions" (Borland). He is proud of them, talks of them, displays them. He is not even envious of a rival's possessions, although he would always like to add to his own. However cluttered and messy his room, he knows exactly where everything is and cannot bear having anything moved or removed. He must be able, at any moment, to lay his hands on some particular object and dislikes anything to be out of sight or reach. The pockets of a younger *Sulphur* boy will be stuffed with his favorite objects, while the older boy squirrels away the household stationery supplies in his desk drawer, so that other family members always know where to find the best pens and erasers, the scotch tape or staples.

The same quality is found in the adult. His desk is easily recognized by the papers heaped up or scattered around, so that it would appear impossible to find anything. Yet he can in a moment locate the smallest memorandum and is distraught if his wife or secretary suggests putting things in order; in fact, he regards clutter and messy surroundings as "comfort." Alternately, while he may possess a theoretical desire for neatness, and is upset by ambient dirt and mess, he will not bestir himself or lift a finger to clean up. Both at home and in the office he wants others to pick up after him and is enraged when they do not (in either type, following a prescription of *Sulphur*, the patient may return saying, "I don't know what happened, but after I took the remedy, I felt inspired to clean up my desk and pick up my room"). At times the apparent neatness of *Sulphur*'s abode is purely superficial, and disorder reigns beneath the surface order. If a closet door is opened, all the contents—hastily pushed out of sight—will come tumbling out. His desk drawers are rat's nests, with thread, string, paper clips, and paper entangled in an undecipherable bundle (*Arsenicum*'s closets and drawers are as impeccable as the room's outward appearance).

In his strong attachment to each item he may be unwilling to share his possessions and will hang on for dear life if urged to do so. He resents even lending impersonal and easily replaceable objects, such as a pair of scissors, is nervous when they are not on his desk, and remains so until they are returned. This need for tactile contact with his possessions, keeping them on his person or within reaching distance, is a particular *Sulphur* characteristic.

A vivid illustration was the eczematous three-year-old who walked into the physician's office with five—not one, but five—"pacifiers" (rubber nipples) in his possession: one in his mouth, one tightly clenched in each fist, and the remaining two dangling from each arm where he could see them. If any of the five disappeared, he would fly into a passion. This situation called for *Sulphur*. Soon after receiving a course of the remedy his eczema started to resolve, and before long he came to his parents and said, "I think, in fact, I'm getting too old for my pacifiers. I'm going to give them *all* away to Santa Claus. Do you think he will come in the summer [it was July] to get them?" However, being *Sulphur*, he requested an electric train in exchange for his well-chewed pacifiers.

During his boyhood stage *Sulphur* loves swapping his goods and seldom emerges the loser in these transactions. Here again, however, the reverse is encountered in the child who will happily trade a good camera or brand new BB gun for an irresistible sack of worthless old toys and feel proud about it.

He hates to part with any object, even the most useless. A thirteen-year-old girl, ordered to discard some of the books and toys she had outgrown, wailed piteously, "How do you expect me to get rid of them when I can't even bear to throw away my fourth-grade math and spelling tests?" The adult remains constitutionally unable to throw things out. The woman cannot dispose of her grandmother's illegible letters, her children's outgrown shoes, or a long outmoded lamp. The man cannot clear the clutter out of the cellar: remnants of rugs, pieces of linoleum, parts of machinery, and even stacks of newspapers. Each of these objects *Sulphur* finds impossible to discard because, "Who knows?—some day it might come in handy."

The child may have an "astonishing money sense" (Borland). A four-year-old will accost an adult with the perceptive remark: "That's an expensive coat you're wearing." The boy has a sharp eye for bargains and insists that his parents shop accordingly: "Why do you buy your film at the drug store when it's much cheaper at the supermarket?" Predictably, these price-conscious boys are reluctant to lend money, even to their parents or friends who they know will repay them in due course.

This intrinsic sense of value can be manifested in more subtle ways. The father of one ten-year-old had been invited to give the graduation address at a state teachers' college. Upon hearing of this honor, the children responded with enthusiasm and praise—all except the youngest boy, who was silent. When the father sought his reaction, the boy laconically replied, "A state teachers' college is all very well, but Harvard would have been better."

As he grows older, *Sulphur* becomes more discriminating in his collecting but retains the same tenacious grip on his possessions. The intellectual child now insists on *owning* his books. He is no longer content to borrow them from the library and will appropriate those he likes from the household shelves. He wants his books there, on his own shelf. The youngster who likes music wants his own stereo and keeps all his favorite records in his room. The adult continues to amass books and records. His impressive collection may include several editions (or recordings) of any single literary (or musical) work.

Later the financially successful person needs to satisfy his collector's instincts on an even grander scale and starts acquiring *objets d'art*. The museum-like decor of his home is rivaled only by that of an *Arsenicum*, but *Sulphur*'s rooms will be crowded with objects, while the *Arsenicum* connoisseur is more select. Both types share a specific form of materialism, wanting to *own* whatever they appreciate. If it were possible, some *Sulphur* or *Arsenicum* would by now have purchased Versailles or the Taj Mahal.

In polar opposition to the above, however, *Sulphur* is also the child who spends his weekly allowance treating his friends to candy and comic books, generously giving away his belongings to all and sundry; or the day before examinations he will lend his textbooks and class notes to a friend, philosophically accepting the possibility that he himself will get poorer grades. A girl will give her scarf to someone who admires it, saying that she does not need it herself. Nor will she later resent giving it away, as might *Phosphorus* or *Natrum muriaticum* after a similar gesture. Thus the extremes of selfishness and generosity are strangely encountered in this remedy.

At times he is too generous for his own or another's good. A brother will perform the household chores of a younger sibling in addition to his own. Or, walking home from school, he will regularly carry the other's books and coat. He fails to understand that such behavior is not healthy for himself or the sibling but will reply that he is free and has the time: "I don't mind. Johnny is tired, why *shouldn't* I do it?" while Johnny magnanimously allows his brother to do his share of the work. In such cases each would probably benefit from a dose of *Sulphur*.

The adult can behave in the same mistakenly generous manner.

He willingly supports brothers-in-law and other family members who are loafers and hangers-on, repeatedly bailing them out financially and otherwise, at times to the detriment of their own characters.

Some *Sulphurs*, moreover, demonstrate a complete lack of interest in material things or financial matters. They can be almost simple-minded in this respect, overlapping with *Calcarea* in the sense of being not quite "with it" in practical matters. They are not "slow" like *Calcarea*, but their heads are so far in the clouds, they are so engrossed in thought, that the "real life" around them passes by unobserved.

Total indifference to possessions may reflect a conscious ascetic determination to dispense with chattels for the sake of spiritual or intellectual development (*Natrum muriaticum*); or it might simply represent the type's natural predisposition: a reluctance to be burdened with worldly goods. Like Thoreau or Rousseau he seeks to return to the simplicity of nature and is content to own the barest minimum for survival. He will live in dingy surroundings, refusing to own anything of value. The small boy who owns nothing but an old ball and a battered bicycle, yet is so satisfied that he cannot think of a birthday or Christmas present, is usually *Sulphur*; on the other hand, the boy who presents his parents with a foot-long list of what he wants and *needs* for Christmas is also *Sulphur*.

He may also profess lack of interest in goods and chattels, while the reality is the precise opposite. The one who most loudly proclaims his anti-materialism is often the most strongly attracted to money and possessions, supporting the truth of the contention that underlying any strong denial is its exact opposite.*

Even the *Sulphur* who seeks possessions and enjoys owning them may exhibit a truly anti-materialist streak in his attitude toward clothes "indifferent to personal appearance" (Kent). The adolescent or young adult likes to dress in an ill-fitting sweatshirt, torn sneakers and jeans

---

* One of the *Doonesbury* cartoons portrays the scruffy and unshaven *Sulphur*-looking Mark Slackmeyer, who in clothes and behavior is rebelling against his upwardly-mobile middle-class family. He is addressed by his mother: "Mark, dear, I was wondering what you think of material possessions?" He responds self-righteously, "Surely you must know, Mother, that Marx, Christ, Gandhi, and I are all in agreement that material possessions are the curse of mankind." "I am glad to hear you say that," she replies brightly to her appalled son, "I just backed over your motorcycle."

(practical, durable jeans are essentially *Sulphur*—hence their universal popularity), due less to an intrinsic lack of aesthetic sense than to his need to *hang on* to his belongings. By dint of being long with him and much worn, his clothes have become a part of himself, and how can anyone throw out a part of himself?

For the same reason the adult *Sulphur*'s preferred outfit might be a twenty-year-old tweed jacket with well-worn elbows or poorly applied patches, and a pair of creased and ill-fitting trousers seemingly acquired from Goodwill Industries. He likes to feel comfortable in these old favorites, these true and trusted friends (*Natrum muriaticum*). "Without a wife to attend to him he would wear [a shirt] until it fell off in rags" (Kent).

Here too, however, the opposite is found. He can be highly clothes-conscious, dressing nattily and expensively and seeking to impress his peers. Yet even when well-dressed, some detail will remain shabby: the shoes are worn at the heels or scuffed at the toes; the collar is crumpled or the tie awry. Most typically, the socks are mismatched. Despite all the expense and attention to sartorial elegance, some one feature will be overlooked ("can appear very smart but always something wrong": Blackie), and the overall impression is still that of *Sulphur*.

Attachment to his old ragged clothes introduces another facet of this type's pride of possession, described in the homoeopathic texts as: "fancies himself rich" (Boenninghausen), "thinks himself in possession of beautiful things; even rags seem beautiful" (Hering). He extravagantly admires whatever belongs to him and sees virtue where no virtue lies. This feeling goes beyond the child's preference for a worn baseball card or broken tin soldier, or the adult's particular attachment to some ragged shirt. It is exhibited, for instance, in the parent who takes pride in the child of little intrinsic merit. Of his scheming, grabbing son, he will boast, "He will make a fine businessman some day"; of a lying, cheating daughter he will venture, with real admiration in his voice, "She is so clever—much cleverer than our other children. She is certain to succeed in life." Of this same daughter the *Sulphur* mother will say, "She has real flair! Other girls are dull by comparison."

Pride in one's children is a universal trait, to be sure, but this characteristic is quite different. Other constitutional types may overlook their children's defects and exaggerate their attributes, but are more objective in their judgment. *Arsenicum* is critical, even though boastful; *Sepia* is dispassionate and without illusions, as are usually *Natrum muriaticum* and *Nux vomica*; *Pulsatilla* is gentle and forgiving, but sees clearly; *Calcarea* may indulge poor behavior but will not defend it. None will condone a child's selfish or unattractive traits. But *Sulphur* (also *Lycopodium*) can hardly see a defect in his possessions and instinctively thinks: "If it's mine, it must be admirable." At times he may even vaunt his own clever, but not very commendable, conduct, boasting of actions which others would prefer to conceal.

Sulphur's aptitude for business is another manifestation of his innate feel for the practical and material. He often exhibits sound financial sense, whether running a small grocery store or managing a large corporation. Some are more interested in economics and finance as such than in accumulating personal wealth; others appear to have as their sole life's goal the wresting of a fortune from compliant or defiant opportunity. Money to them is the measure of success, and they judge another's capacities and talents by how much money he earns. This individual is usually systematic and careful with his wealth. He does not overextend his purse or squander his fortune on wild schemes or risky investments (as might *Lachesis* or *Phosphorus*) but hangs onto it for the sense of pride and power it gives him. Later he enjoys donating it to large, prestigious institutions or establishing his own charitable foundation. He thus satisfies his generous as well as acquisitive instincts, and succeeds in serving God and Mammon both.

Some are tight-fisted, disliking to lend money or to spend it on others (*Arsenicum*). The husband complicates his family's life by insisting on unnecessary petty economies (*Lycopodium*). He sets the home thermostat uncomfortably low and refuses to buy a kettle with a whistle that works or a new lampshade that better suits the decor. He loves economy for its own sake, although each individual has his own particular quirk. One drives his large car several additional miles to buy gas a few cents cheaper than at a nearby station. This is not a fantastic deal in view of the time involved and the wear on the car, but it is the kind of economy *Sulphur* cannot resist. A successful writer types his manuscripts on the reverse sides of letters, bills, and other scraps of paper which most people throw away; he even becomes agitated when his family does not follow suit. After a dose of the remedy, however, these parsimonious tendencies abate and family harmony is restored. The patient may allow his family a warmer house or the extravagance of clean stationery, while continuing to use scrap paper himself. The homoeopath repeatedly finds how by "unblocking" one member with a constitutional remedy, the dynamism of the whole family is affected for the better.

Such behavior exemplifies *Sulphur*'s dislike of waste. He enjoys nothing more than making dinner out of "leftovers" or salvaging a "perfectly good" piece of wire from a dismantled dishwasher to repair the electrical system of his car. He is also irresistibly attracted to "bargains." If he can buy a cantaloupe or avocado at a reduced price on his way home from work, this makes his day. Never mind that it is overripe and therefore worth only half the price; he derives satisfaction from the very principle of the thing.

He may carry his bargain hunting to such an extreme as to be left with the need to give away part of what he has bought, but he loves this too. For generosity coexists with his love of economy. He unstintingly feeds and boards friends and relatives for days at a time but cannot resist saving a few cents on a half-rotten avocado.

The wealthy individual characteristically spends his money ostentatiously—on expensive cars, stereos, oversized mansions and other status symbols—or in other ways displaying a *nouveau riche* mentality. One patient described himself as "heavily into conspicuous consumption." Whether well off or not, he is fascinated by the *price* of things and by how much others earn, and this constitutes the principal theme of many of the non-intellectual *Sulphur*'s conversations (also *Arsenicum*). Sometimes, indeed he cannot stop talking of money! Anyone who is fond of pronouncing with special relish and unusual frequency the phrases, "millions of dollars . . . billions of barrels . . . thousands of shares . . . " is certain to have *Sulphur* somewhere in the picture. Yet this same affluent individual will talk just as happily about the high price of string beans or soda water.

In concluding this section a quite different side of *Sulphur*'s fascination with the material should be mentioned: his love of working with his hands and with the earth. Boys are often fascinated by gadgets, mechanical or electrical. They love to tinker with motors, tape-recorders, radios, pocket calculators, and bicycles. They take them apart and put them together for hours at a time, often revealing from an early age a sound understanding of their functioning. At any age the type not only enjoys, but actually needs, to work with tools—in carpentry, building, plumbing, mechanical repairs, and the like. Any inventor will have a strong *Sulphur* streak — whether a genius like Thomas Edison or an unknown tinkerer in his cellar, plugging away for years on a solar-powered can opener or noiseless blender ("when he gets an idea in his mind he is unable to get rid of it. He follows and follows it until finally accidentally he drops into something, and many times that is how things are invented": Kent, *Lectures on Homoeopathic Materia Medica*, Sulphur).

Likewise, the tenacious small farmer who ekes out a bare existence from the soil, the hired laborer who enjoys manual work in the garden or yard, the prosperous planter with his newest technological improvements and expensive machinery, as well as the desk-bound businessman who happily relaxes in his vegetable patch — are all following their *Sulphur* inclinations.

A banker in his late fifties sought homoeopathic help for an enlarged prostate; the symptoms were urinary dribbling, and uncomfortable pressure when sitting. Several possible remedies were being considered when the physician asked about his hobbies. "I *love* my vegetable garden with its turnips and squashes," he replied. "There is nothing in the world I like better than getting my hands *dirty* in the soil." That remark decided the physician on *Sulphur*, and, even though other medical consultants had recommended removing the prostate, or at least trimming it, several doses of this prescription in high potency (interspersed with occasional prescriptions of *Sabal serrulata* — a prostate specific — in low potency) made the operation unnecessary.

The Heated and Eruptive Personality

Having touched upon the wide range of materialistic characteristics which *Sulphur* embodies, we move now to his "heat." In former times sulphur was called "brimstone," from the Middle English words for "burning stone." The element has long been used for such purposes as the manufacture of matches, gunpowder, etc., and this yields the type's characteristics of heat, burning, eruptiveness, and flare-up.

On the physical level, as the classic texts relate, he is usually warm-blooded, uncomfortable in the heat, and with a tendency to perspire freely — all over the body and especially on the face. He has warm hands, often with red or sweaty palms, and red ears which may or may not protrude from the head. If the face is not red, it easily flushes scarlet with heat, exertion, or annoyance. The orifices of the mucous membranes—lips, ear canals, anus, nostrils—may be bright red, even if the rest of the skin is pale; and his skin breaks out into red, hot, itching eruptions of various kinds: eczemas, rashes, pimples, or boils (many of the patient's deeper-seated complaints are manifested on the skin). When a patient complains of burning pain in any part of the body, *Sulphur* is one of the first remedies that comes to mind (also *Phosphorus* and *Arsenicum*). A major guiding symptom, for example, is burning of the soles of the feet at night, to such an extent that the patient keeps them outside the bedcovers. Even young children "kick clothes off at night" (Hering) or unzip their pajama suits to expose their burning feet. The patient may exhibit areas of *disturbed* heat, such as warm hands but cold feet (or vice-versa); warm body but cool hands; warm head but cold body, and so on. An uneven distribution of body temperatures points strongly to this remedy (also to *Lachesis*).

Although sensitivity to cold should not preclude a prescription of *Sulphur*, as a rule this remedy likes the feel of cold air, so that even in winter he sleeps with the windows open. In cold weather he will don only a sweater and trousers, ignoring hat, gloves and jacket. Parents must constantly struggle with these children over the wearing of overcoats. They wriggle and resist, arguing that they do not need one, and define a sweater as "something a child has to wear when his mother is cold." Aggravation from a heated room, warm weather, a warm bed, heavy clothing, or a warm bath (better from a cold shower) are other modalities pointing to the remedy.

He may suffer from "aggravation in the spring" (Kent—in whose *Repertory* the modality should be raised to the third degree). When the weather turns warmer, a host of symptoms will emerge (*Lachesis*) or the patient will feel low in energy (*Natrum muriaticum*). Just as all of nature throws off the old and takes on new life, so his constitution seems to undergo a "spring cleaning" (elemental sulphur, of course, is a powerful cleansing agent—hence the use of sulphur baths, soaps and drinking waters). His tendency to hang tenaciously onto old and useless objects has already been discussed; in the same way this type may resist relinquishing his old self until the coming of spring forces a constitutional upheaval that presages physical and mental change and growth.

In children this "heated" or eruptive nature can be seen clearly in both the physical and mental spheres. The infant is active, restless, and colicky, at times "intolerably passionate and hard to quiet" (Hahne-mann). He is always hungry, exhausting his mother with continual greedy nursing, and continually on the go, fussing against whatever holds him back or holds him still. He may lie awake crying at night, wanting to be fed and amused, then sleep most of the day (*Psorinum*).* One of these night-time babies, a five-month-old boy, was brought to a homoeopathic physician for a severe case of diaper rash. The skin on his buttocks and groin was not only raw, raised, bright red and shiny-tight like a balloon, but also cracked and so inflamed that the heat could be felt a foot away. How the baby could stand it was a mystery, but he was a tough little fellow (as *Sulphur* often is) with a demanding but basically sanguine disposition. He received three doses of the remedy in high potency at twelve-hour intervals. Not only did the rash begin to subside immediately, disappearing completely in a few days, but his inner clock was also changed. Thereafter, he began to sleep at night and do his playing and eating during the day. Numerous *Sulphur* babies have been encouraged by this remedy to keep more sociable and civi-lized hours.

A similar picture is found in older persons. The adult who "takes short naps" (Hering) during the day is often *Sulphur*. He can drop off to sleep in an instant, anywhere, anytime, in any position, however much commotion is around him. Conversely, at night he can hardly get to sleep "on account of great flow of thoughts" (Hering), or, once asleep, "wakes frequently or becomes wide awake suddenly" (Boericke); he also wakes at 3, 4, or 5 a.m. and sometimes cannot fall asleep again (Hahnemann lists more than 50 symptoms relating to "sleep"). Some-times the type gets a second wind later in the evening, this being the time he loves to talk or socialize. Students claim they cannot start study-ing before 9:00 p.m. (*Lachesis*). "Irresistible drowsiness during the day, wakefulness at night" (Hering) summarizes it.

At night the young boy will leave his bed innumerable times on various pretexts to postpone the dreaded moment of going to sleep. He cannot slow down, cannot bear to be left out of anything, and refuses to end the day. In girls *Pulsatilla* is more likely to get up at night, from

---

* This is in contrast to the *Lycopodium* baby who "cries all day and sleeps all night" (H.C. Allen). The *Calcarea* baby's physical symptoms may resemble *Sulphur*'s, but he is usually more chilly and placid.

dislike of remaining alone in her dark room, coming timidly downstairs to seek companionship.

Sulphur hates being washed ("dread of being washed in children": Hering), dressed, put to bed, or seated at the table.* Youngsters may have to be tied to their chairs (literally) to keep them sitting through a meal. Later in school they cannot sit quietly at their desks but squirm around or constantly jump up. The boy practicing the piano will get up half a dozen times in half an hour, going to the bathroom, getting a drink, stretching, or for whatever other excuse he can conjure up. Sitting still, and especially *standing* still, are intolerable. Even in the adult, standing is a "most disagreeable" (Hering) position, aggravating a number of symptoms.

As the boy grows older, noise-making and movement continue to be intrinsic to his nature: slamming doors, banging things, tumbling downstairs, loud shouting, fidgeting about, and making noise for its own sake. Adults are constantly telling him, "Keep quiet! Be still! Sit down!" or "Stop it—whatever you're doing, stop it!" But *Sulphur* needs to be active. He loves to be outside playing ball, riding his bicycle, and engaging in various strenuous activities. He is not only energetic but also inherently creative, initiating projects and seldom allowing himself to be bored.

Some boys must be always talking. If they have nothing particular to say, they will babble or talk nonsense in order to fill the unendurable silence or attract attention. Often they are quiet only when listening to music. Even here, however, the music must be stimulating, and the youngster plays it at a volume which deafens others but bothers him not at all. He may later join a school band or orchestra, or an informal jazz or rock band, as he enjoys making music in a group—the louder the better. He also likes his books, movies, and television programs to be full of excitement, fast action, and lively stimulation. The lyrical, poetic or introspective modes are not for him.

The disposition can be fiery and pugnacious. When angry, these boys sometimes resemble little bullocks: their eyes get red and small, their faces darken, and they act as if "seeing red." They are not necessarily obnoxious—just obstreperous and constantly asserting them-

---

* Although the following picture is found more frequently in boys, naturally it applies also to girls.

selves. In fact, they may be remarkably uncomplaining, possessing the positive, buoyant outlook of those two charming *Sulphur* immortals, Tom Sawyer and Dennis the Menace. They emanate heat, but, like fire, also radiate cheerfulness. When the rowdiness level reaches that of the terrorizing youngster in O. Henry's *The Ransom of Red Chief* (where the boy's kidnappers are willing to pay his father a premium to take him back), it is time to administer *Sulphur*. It helps to cool them down — at least to the point where the family's eardrums and nervous systems can be preserved.

The maturing lively boy may turn his creative energies to trouble-making, with a most disruptive influence on the class. Not that he is scheming or underhanded; he is usually open and straightforward, "up front" even in his negative behavior. He disrupts by overtly bullying others, causing commotion, or displaying the persistent aggressiveness of the show-off. This may be one reason why young boys are notoriously more difficult to teach than girls; any group of the former will necessarily include several *Sulphurs* who are energetically determined to be noticed. Continually striving for effect, he brags loudly or tells obvious lies about imaginary feats. He might steal money, pen-knives, or mechanical pencils from his classmates' desks or lockers or from stores in order to boast about these "macho" accomplishments to his peers.

In contrast, the boy who is the social core of the class is also frequently a *Sulphur*. He is still making waves, still asserting himself, but in a constructive way, by manifesting his leadership qualities. He energetically organizes group activities, plans class entertainments, and works hard to carry them through, generously ensuring that there is fun and participation for all. The benevolent *Sulphur* leader does not discriminate among the members of his group. Although he may have preferences, he keeps them to himself. In his all-inclusiveness and high sociability he is anxious primarily to further the group's welfare.

Given the heat-emitting and commotion-causing qualities of this remedy, it is hardly surprising that *Sulphur* is the "ace of spades" of homoeopathic adolescent remedies.

Formerly an early riser, the adolescent now wants to sleep late in the morning; he lies in bed a long time before getting up, then arises grumpy, quarrelsome, or totally uncommunicative. *Sulphur*'s time modality contains a characteristic polarity. Some are slow to wake up, feeling groggy, heavy, and irritable in the morning and wishing they could sleep until noon. Others, like *Arsenicum*, leap out of bed in the morning, "lively" (Kent), fully alert and "prepared to meet the day with a glad cry." Age is usually a factor: the early risers are children and the elderly, while the adolescent or young adult is the late sleeper.

Although he used to love breakfast, he now wants nothing in the morning but makes up for it by nonstop snacking throughout the day or eating late into the night. The student inevitably comes home from school ravenous and parched and is always making sandwiches for himself or nibbling on cookies and other sweet carbohydrates for quick energy. He craves ice cream and *ice cold* carbonated drinks (*Phosphorus*). He drinks quickly, in large gulps, as if to cool down his overheated mind and body.

Sulphur at every age displays much thirst, draining glass after glass of cold liquids (*Arsenicum*, also constantly thirsty, drinks in sips). The child endlessly demands milk (even though it might disagree with him) or fruit juice; the adolescent guzzles sodas and milk between and during meals; the adult male drinks cold water or beer all day. Some can down several highballs before a meal, followed by large quantities of wine at the meal itself.

He often has a strong head for alcohol and, when inebriated, gives little indication of it except for increased gregariousness and a tendency to talk louder. On the other hand, *Sulphur* is a principal remedy for alcoholism (together with *Nux vomica* and *Lachesis*).

Although he prefers his drinks cold, *Sulphur* likes his food "hot," i.e., spicy, peppery, highly seasoned. His palate is sophisticated, with a liking for exotic or unusual dishes. Some might consider it a jaded palate that can be stimulated only by strong flavors, in contrast to the bland preferences of *Calcarea*. A strong interest in good food, fine wines, and the culinary arts is frequently found in men and women with *Sulphur* in their natures. Their dishes show inventiveness and love of experimentation. Even young children display the instincts of gourmet cooks, enlivening their food with spices and serving dishes in unusual combinations.

Whether young or old, fat or thin, strong or weak, the individual can consume enormous amounts of food. These are the appetites usually termed "bottomless pits." When asked about food preferences, he will reply that he likes everything ("I am onmivorous," is characteristic), although the child will most often say "Pizza!" and then add the classic *Sulphur* aversions: liver and broccoli (or lima beans, brussels-sprouts, and spinach). But, in a true reflection of the remedy's polarity, it has also cured cases of complete loss of appetite (as when suffering from depression).

His table manners may exhibit utter disregard for appearances. He eats greedily, even with his fingers, or thoughtlessly helps himself to the lion's share of a dish, leaving the remains to be divided among several others. One new patient, seeking help for arthritic pains and a persistent bronchial cough that woke him at night, apparently feeling very much at home in the physician's office, helped himself without being asked from a bowl of ripe peaches left by a previous patient; with the juice running down his chin and shirtfront, he described his symptoms in a loud voice and with much laughter while munching on the peach. This excessive informality, compensated for, however, by his expansive good humor, immediately indicated *Sulphur*, and several doses over a six-month period allayed his physical problems—although the medicine did little for his bad manners.

The other side of *Sulphur* is a feeling of sluggishness and fatigue, with sleepiness after meals, due to the impaired digestion underlying many of his problems. He may have difficulty assimilating food ("defective assimilation": Hering) and a tendency to stomach acidity, resulting in heartburn, empty or sour eructations, contractive pains, ulcers, etc.* The commonly encountered 11:00 a.m. aggravation, in which the individual experiences lightheadedness, a marked energy drop, and an "empty, all-gone feeling" (Hering) is *Sulphur*. In more extreme cases, there may be accompanying dizziness, headache, sweating, and uncontrolled irritability, suggesting that a hypoglycemic drop in blood sugar could be responsible for the remedy's "worse-before-meals" (Boger), "weakness and hunger an hour before mealtimes" (Kent) modality.

---

* Hahnemann lists over 300 symptoms for the digestive system, some of the most frequent being: "headache after a meal, with pressure in eyes . . . above the eyes, and nausea; during or after a meal perspiration in the face; immediately after a meal pressure in stomach; after eating but little, abdomen feels full, with oppressive breathing; after dinner much fatigue; regurgitation of the food an hour after eating it," and so on for nine pages (*Chronic Diseases*, Volume II).

The adolescent may look unwashed and unkempt, with pimply skin, waxy ears and dirty finger-nails. Some have a constitutional antipathy to soap or are unwilling to take the time and trouble to bathe ("averse to washing": Hering). They may consequently give off a dismaying odor of "garlic" or "spoiled eggs" (Kent), but seem unaware of themselves, or at least unperturbed by it. Others, on the contrary, have an offensive odor *despite* washing (*Psorinum*), and these may be extremely sensitive to their own odor ("disgust to the point of nausea about any effluvia arising from his own body": Hering). Naturally, all these symptoms are found in the adult as well.

The boy's nails are likely to be bitten to the quick (*Natrum muriaticum*), or he will constantly pick at them as well as at his nose, pimples, scalp, or skin. At this stage his very hair may change in texture and become unmanageable: wiry or kinky or growing every which way, as if reflecting the rebellious nature of its owner. Often the adolescent develops a typically *Sulphur* lankiness and stoop: "does not walk erect; stoops or bends over forward walking or sitting" (Hering).

This adolescent makes his presence felt in the home far more than most other types. Either he fidgets constantly or lies slumped on sofas or draped over chairs, right in the center of things. Certainly, growing so fast and changing so much, he feels weak and tired, but even this is manifested in a restless, heated form. When a teenage *Sulphur* enters a room, if only to collapse in a chair, it suddenly becomes too hot and too small.

The mental heat of the *Sulphur* adolescent is familiar to parents and teachers. At his best, he is the classic intellectual live wire: alert, imaginative, sceptical, with a talent for mimicry, eager to ask questions, point out pertinent exceptions to what an adult says, and engage in verbal combat. His sprightliness, intellectual curiosity, and engaging brightness add much to class discussions. But teachers still wish he would exhibit more diligence and care in his schoolwork. He has plenty of raw talent but fails to approach the level of performance of which he is so eminently capable (the antithesis of *Arsenicum*). Both at home and in school his innate resistance to authority leads him to devise ways of *avoiding* school (or house) work, and he will expend more energy on this than it would have taken simply to do the job. Yet, when he does choose to interest himself in anything, which is rarely that which is asked or expected of him, he displays surprising application and meticulous care. And once getting to his homework, he finishes it off in an hour, where another would take several. In contrast to the circuitous and amorphous ways of *Calcarea*, there is directness and focus in *Sulphur*'s approach to an intellectual or other challenge. He goes straight to the heart of things, his powers of concentration are excellent, albeit short-lived, and all the while he retains a buoyant attitude. Instead of complaining when overwhelmed with schoolwork or other obligations, he will take a positive view, "All this is good for me. At least I don't get bored, and there is nothing worse than being bored. Also, it keeps me out of trouble—always an important consideration!" In general, his restless intellectual and physical energies require much stimulation; he is easily bored and so deliberately seeks out new challenges.

At worst the adolescent is irritable, *uncooperative*, critical, and dissatisfied ("censorious": Kent), even when others are trying to please him. Loudly and aggressively he proclaims his universal discontents: unfair teachers, non-understanding parents, too much responsibility, too little recognition. He loafs around the house, seeking quarrels everywhere, refusing to do his chores, and pulling a disappearing act when most needed. If pressed to do his share of work, he spends so much time arguing disagreeably that it is easier to do it for him ("I *like* being argumentative and aggressive," he freely admits).

All in all, the *Sulphur* adolescent is probably most responsible for the institution of boarding schools. While *Calcarea phosphorica* and *Natrum muriaticum* seek to escape from adults (the *Phosphorus* adolescent, we recall, continues to share his life with his family), it is the adults who seek to escape from *Sulphur*. The remedy, however, can temper all this. It has repeatedly eased those stressful and disruptive adolescent years, rendering them interesting, constructive and happy for both child and parent.

A dramatic example of the powers of *Sulphur* was seen in the treatment of a thirteen-year-old boy with La Tourette's Syndrome—multiple dyskenesia—of five years' standing. Despite strong doses of central nervous system depressants he was manifesting over 100 different kinds of tics, grimaces, and grunts which had compelled his withdrawal from school. But underlying this dazzling variety of choreic symptoms (suggesting a number of possible remedies) was the boy's obviously *Sulphur* character and personality. He was rude and sulky with his parents, reluctant to answer the physician's questions, irritable, and curt. Extracting information about symptoms was an uphill battle. And he seemed totally insensitive to the trauma his asocial behavior was causing his parents. For these reasons *Sulphur* 50M seemed indicated and was prescribed. The case was long and complex, and from time to time he needed the more specifically choreic remedies such as *Mygale* and *Agaricus*. But repeated prescriptions of *Sulphur* kept the case moving forward. Judging when to repeat the remedy was facilitated by the fact that his attitude changed for the better whenever he received a dose, while his mood and behavior deteriorated as its effects wore off. Under homoeopathic treatment he was able to return to school and lead a normal adolescent life, almost entirely free of tics and other choreic symptoms.

In the adolescent girl the *Sulphur* picture is somewhat modified. She is cleaner and neater than the boy and less prone to feeling misunderstood and discontented. Her room, however, is equally untidy, looking as though a hurricane had passed through, leaving wreckage and devastation in its wake. The floor is littered with clothes, both clean and dirty, commixed and intermingled with books, papers, and other debris that she seems quite unable to pick up ("I like organization, but not in my room. If I were to pick it up, I couldn't find anything anymore. Anyway, it would take me at least three weeks to do so!"). While adolescence is a notoriously untidy period, that of *Sulphur* is especially so. Many young patients have declared that they *love* the "chaos" in their rooms and in their lives, finding it exciting and stimulating (*Arsenicum*, in contrast, cannot tolerate disorder even during these years).

A hallmark of the *Sulphur* girl, or an indication of any adolescent's need for this remedy, is a comprehensive and overflowing collection of cosmetics and shampoos; and a dead giveaway is her treatment of the toothpaste in the bathroom. She *always* leaves the cap off the tube with the paste oozing out all over the sink! This inability to replace the cap on the toothpaste tube is an almost universal trait of adolescent *Sulphur* girls. Their parents all complain of "oozing toothpaste."

The teenage girl requiring *Sulphur* begins to emit more mental heat than before, becoming argumentative, egocentric, and impatient. As with the boy, her presence in a room makes the atmosphere oppressive. But it may be due to her loud voice, raucous laughter, and uncontrolled vivacity more than to disagreeable behavior. She is easier to deal with than her male counterpart, perhaps because she is usually less purely

Sulphur, and her behavior is modified by some other constitutional picture. It is generally the *Natrum muriaticum* girl who has the hardest time during adolescence.

After the adolescent years, the heat of the personality is moderated somewhat, although the adult may remain feisty and assertive. *Sulphur* is recognized in the chaotic yet effective executive or professional person overflowing with plans and projects and chronically surrounded by clutter and commotion. In fact, he seems to operate best in a profusion of mixed sensory stimuli. The child does his homework surrounded by family or while watching a television show; he constantly interrupts his studies to strum on a guitar or make forays into the kitchen. The adult likes his office to be a beehive of activity; if working at home, he does not object to loud music in the background, continual interruptions by his children, or by telephone calls (in contrast to *Nux vomica* and *Natrum muriaticum*). And he will jump up from his desk to momentarily repair the toaster or change the spark plugs in his car. To work productively he does not need long stretches of uninterrupted time. Continual and varied assaults on his senses only stimulate his creativity.

The onset of middle age generates a resumption or increase of the emotional heat. The male, especially, grows more critical and belligerent: "the mood is quarrelsome and contentious about everything" (Hahnemann). In the home he is unreasonably irritated over minutiae (*Lycopodium*, *Nux vomica*) and prone to raise his voice when things do not go his way. He can be bullying and abrasive with colleagues and subordinates, blustering and bombastic with friends and acquaintances. Yet the remedy in high potency can defuse this "high explosive," changing the patient from an egocentric, overbearing despot into a reasonable, if still aggressive, human being. *Sulphur* has an open-hearted, good-natured side which the remedy often accentuates and brings out. While the type's potential flammability still remains, the remedy imposes a layer of control which would otherwise be lacking. Moreover, the *Sulphur* type pleases the physician by reacting to the remedy with rapidity, in contrast to the adult *Calcarea* or *Lycopodium* who are slower and more difficult to change.

This brings up the topic of the *Sulphur temper*. At any stage of life he erupts easily. The temper outbursts are strong but not lasting. "Quick to anger, quick to subside," was Hering's way of putting it — like a volcano which blows its top and spews its sulphur but is then quiet again. Minutes after his outburst he has already forgotten it.

A patient once stated that, when her *Sulphur* future husband proposed, she had hesitated on the grounds of his explosive temper. "Don't worry about that, my dear," he assured her. "Vesuvius is quiet most of the time." And this proved to be an accurate self-characterization.

Sulphur is argumentative, finding in verbal battles an outlet for his pugnacity. He is not particular about the topic and often enjoys argument for its own sake (like the Irishman in the joke who, seeing two men pummeling each other in a bar, inquired: "Is this a private fight, or can anyone join in?"). He is thus ready to jump with both feet into any dispute, unlike *Arsenicum, Natrum muriaticum, Nux vomica* or *Lachesis*, who equally enjoy a heated debate but are more selective about the subject-matter.

He loves to fire off that first shot at Fort Sumter, and will frequently provoke fights, but rarely feels distressed or resentful afterwards (as does *Natrum muriaticum*). And those caught in a dispute with him should also forego resentment, not only because it is difficult to best him in an argument but also because he himself bears no hard feelings — once the internal pressure has been relieved and the steam has escaped ("excitable mood; easily irritated but quickly penitent": Hering). In fact, he looks forward to the next one and remembers with pleasure the more exciting discussions and arguments of his life. A young boy's best friend will be a fellow-*Sulphur* with whom he quarrels and makes up interminably, at times even engaging in exhilarating physical fights. Teenage "best friends" will engage in interminable arguments over the relative strengths and weaknesses of their favorite athletes or whether photography is a major or only a minor art form; while older students will stay up nights disputing whether Freud or Jung have had a greater impact on world thinking or heatedly debating which is the greater — a perfected lyric or an unfinished symphony. To *Sulphur* argument is a form of basic communication or interpersonal relationship, as well as a mental stimulus.

Possibly he gets over his quarrels easily because they remain largely intellectual. While he may become momentarily emotional, his feelings are seldom deeply affected. His love of contention — as both mental exercise and exchange of ideas—overcomes any wound. Anyway, he can extract the maximum intellectual exercise from any topic, just as *Phosphorus* can extract the maximum fun from a situation, *Lycopodium* the maximum prestige—and *Natrum muriaticum* the maximum hurt.

This fundamentally intellectual, rather than emotional, approach to life renders *Sulphur* resilient in setbacks and reversals, in contrast, for example, to *Calcarea*. When an undertaking falls through, he wastes no time on regrets but immediately immerses himself in another. The same is true for romantic or other emotional attachments. His feelings are ardent, but if he suffers a loss or rejection, he easily turns somewhere else, thinking "There are as good fish in the sea as ever came out of it."

Another facet of his heated personality is a strong *need for personal recognition* and to be at the center of things. Like Teddy Roosevelt, he insists on being "the bride at every wedding and the corpse at every funeral." He enjoys boasting loudly and at length of his future plans, his complex projects, and his varied achievements. The *Sulphur* homoeopath, for example, can be recognized by his way of saying, "*I* cured his pain instantaneously . . . " "*I* was able to stop the hemorrhage after ten minutes . . . "—instead of "*Arnica* cured . . . *Belladonna* stopped the bleeding . . . "

He may also exaggerate. Believing with P.T. Barnum that "the naked truth, poor thing, is a downright impropriety and must be dressed up like a pretty woman," he can be carried away and aggrandize his accomplishments. He will claim to be in superb physical condition when he actually only runs an occasional lap with much panting and sweating. He will boast of giving up smoking when it has been for a very short period of time; by resuming it and dropping it over and over again he repeatedly gets credit for a strong will. Or he brags of all the important people he knows, when he might just have exchanged a few formalities with them (like *Lycopodium*, he is readily impressed by famous personnages). He vaunts his correct political or financial predictions—which may be only hindsight. Or he builds a reputation on what he is *intending* to do, without necessarily following through.

Usually he thinks highly of himself, but, not surprisingly, the opposite is also encountered. Borland avers that *Sulphur* may not be as hale, hearty, and self-confident as he appears but resents having his bluff called and, adamantly refusing to listen to good advice, sticks stubbornly to an erroneous decision rather than admit a mistake (*Lycopodium*). His eruptiveness is seen in his impatience. He does not suffer delays or fools gladly. He cannot tolerate physical impediments to his projects ("cannot get quickly enough what he wants": Hahnemann) and is impatient with those who are slow to understand his meaning or to appreciate his innovative ideas. In dealing with others he can be blunt and at times hard-hitting, expecting them to be equally energetic and productive. Generating big ideas, he then needs others to carry them out, and surrounds himself with people who are willing to work fourteen hours a day at the menial, monotonous or ignoble tasks (the drudgery) to implement his magnificent plans—while he is already onto a new idea, devising ways of setting others to work on *this* one, and has little patience for repeating or explaining, as is often needful when leading others. As Whitmont puts it, "The *Sulphur* personality, acting as a catalyst, always feels he must keep things and people on the move; he must always take the initiative, lest things become stagnant." Thus his strong ego can be intimidating, making others feel insecure, slow, and dependent. This is encountered in father-son, husband-wife, teacher-student, master-disciple relationships, and the like, where the dominant member of the pair is *Sulphur*. Nor is he content to remain the power behind the throne, as are, at times, *Natrum muriaticum* and even *Arsenicum*. He likes to be firmly and visibly *on* the throne, his reign obvious to all.

When not balanced by one of the more sensitive constitutional types, he can have a very thick, even "rhinoceros"-like, hide. He treads heavily on the sensibilities of others, sometimes quite inadvertently, at other times rather unconcernedly. He is often unaware of what people think of him, partly because (in contrast to *Lycopodium*'s constant awareness of his image and *Natrum muriaticum*'s unending search for approbation) he does not care. Even when shrewd about others, he can be remarkably dense about himself and among the least introspective of homoeopathic types. He is the energetic man of action and big ideas, pleased with himself and incurious about critical self-analysis.

In concluding this section, a few words are in order on the "benevolent" *Sulphur* (the polar opposite of the heatedly aggressive individual described above). Sometimes this remedy is appropriate for patients who yield *no* negative mental symptoms or characteristics: the well-disposed serene man without emotional hang-ups or chips on his shoulder, the jolly, cheerful woman who is well-inclined toward the whole world ("uncommon cheerfulness; lively and good-humored disposition" Allen).

For instance, the type can be exceptionally hospitable. The very act of throwing a party, bringing disparate and incongruous personalities together into a harmonious and successful whole, gives him immense satisfaction. This overflowing benevolence may sometimes appear unmanageable and too indiscriminate. Like an enthusiastic but inexperienced cook, he insistently combines the most incompatible ingredients (persons) into a common pot (social ventures), sanguine that a delicious dish will result (a good time will be had by all). Although the odds may seem heavily against him, his concoctions often succeed, seasoned as they are with his own abundant good spirits. Thus the irrepressible bon vivant, the Falstaff who is determined to experience and enjoy life on all cylinders and to pull others along in his wake, is frequently a *Sulphur*.

Not only does this buoyant, optimistic individual from time to time lose himself in pleasant daydreams ("reveries": Boenninghausen) of grandeur, greatness, happiness, and fulfillment, these same themes recur during sleep. His dreams are "happy" (Hering), marked by action, adventure, color, and imagined accomplishments. He flies through the air, observes exciting battles, travels to unknown places, and finds himself in such funny situations that he laughs in his sleep (*Lycopodium*) and sometimes wakes up singing (Hering). He is what Boger calls a "hopeful dreamer" who realizes many of his wishes in his sleep. Patients, in fact, sometimes complain that the cure effected by a *Sulphur* prescription has also deprived them of their formerly engrossing dreams. Terrifying, anxiety-laden, and vexing dreams are, certainly, also found strongly in the constitutional picture, but these are common to other types as well and are thus less useful to the physician than the adventurous and exciting ones.

Sulphur, too, is the spontaneously generous man or woman whom everyone instinctively approaches for help: money for refugees, room and board over a prolonged period for some lost soul, or the expenditure of time and energy on some charitable cause. Other constitutional types, to be sure, contain individuals who are equally kind, but *Sulphur*'s irrepressibly sanguine outlook, healthy geniality, cheerfulness, and robust kindness (reminiscent of the Cheeryble brothers in Dickens' *Nicholas Nickleby*) make him a strikingly benevolent figure.

A middle-aged businessman emanating a *Pulsatilla*-like sweetness came to homoeopathy for a number of long-standing complaints. His digestive system had been woefully impaired by long sojourns in the Orient. His pancreas, gall-bladder, and liver were also affected, and he suffered as well from the allopathic medications prescribed for these various complaints. He had burning, itching hemorrhoids, hypertension, and various heart symptoms (periodic palpitations, intermittent missed beats, and episodic angina). Everything was aggravated by the stress of his high-powered job and his tendency to eat, drink, and smoke to excess. His history revealed a traumatic childhood: the loss of both parents before the age of six and subsequent experience of being passed from relative to relative and from school to school. His physical picture and medical history suggested several remedies, among them *Sulphur*, but the physician could find no negative mental symptoms to guide him to the correct remedy—only a serene and benevolent attitude toward mankind. There were no childhood resentments (*Natrum muriaticum*), no criticism or intolerance of anyone (*Nux vomica, Arsenicum*). He was entirely content with his family, considering that he had the best possible wife and children; even his secretary and housekeeper were the best possible. His house was full of *objets d'art* collected in the Orient, and his generosity brought him an equal number of friends. This was the epitome of the "benevolent *Sulphur*," and the remedy, given systematically in ascending potencies, predictably relieved most of his symptoms and kept him in reasonably good health for an extended period.

Intellectualism and Creativity

Sulphur's third prominent aspect is intellectualism. Whether blue-collared worker or high-level executive, artist or physician, he displays a scholarly or philosophical slant of mind. He loves theorizing, rationalizing, weaving abstract or hypothetical systems, and the storage and retrieval of practical or statistical data. Such occupations as the study of the Talmud—the unending interpretation and elaboration of the Torah—are typical of *Sulphur* (although the finer splitting of hairs involved in Talmudic studies appeals also to the *Arsenicum* mind). He cultivates his mind and intellect with the same assiduous energy another *Sulphur* will direct to a business operation or piece of landed property.

This intellectual bent can be seen in the curious inquiring minds of young children, especially boys. At an early age they begin to read newspapers, magazines, and such improving works as encyclopedias, dictionaries, military histories, and, especially, the *Guinness Book of World Records*. Even in fiction their taste will incline toward the historical or scientific; they like their fiction full of facts. Sometimes they possess an "amazing aptitude for languages" (Borland) and are fascinated by them. When an adult patient knows (or claims to know) four or five languages well, *Sulphur* is invariably strong in the picture. On some level all such intellectual acquisitions can be seen as extensions of the *Sulphur* "collector's" instinct. He amasses facts and information, acquires knowledge and stores words, both native and foreign, much as he collects objects—voraciously and indiscriminately.

He may possess a prodigious memory. Once some bit of information lodges there, it stays and accumulates interest as surely and safely as money in a bank, to be brought out whenever some expenditure is needed. If a lecturer makes an error in quoting a literary or historical reference, it is a *Sulphur* who will catch it and correct the speaker (also *Arsenicum*). A *Sulphur* homoeopath will often have an exceptional memory for materia medica, even the beginner remembering the differences among the various *Kali* (potassium) and *Natrum* (sodium) salts and reciting whole rubrics from Kent's *Repertory*. As a conversationalist he has a vast store of quotations from poets classical and popular, ancient and modern, one for every occasion.

A boy of five or six can rattle off scores and league standings of the various football or baseball teams as well as the statistics of individual players. Skeptical comments about the accuracy of his information are received with composure and a precise indicaton of the source. Nor does he add, "So, there!" as *Sulphur* is not prone to gloat. He simply announces the fact. But the sheer demonstration of his phenomenal memory conveys an implicit challenge, "Dispute that if you can!" Clever young Linus van Pelt in the *Peanuts* comic strip is a typical *Sulphur*, freely reciting esoteric passages from the Scriptures or bringing forth profound observations in the most matter-of-fact way. On the other hand, whether adult or child, the type can be intellectually aggressive and overbearing—a Mr. Know-It-All who consistently expresses his views in an annoying "without fear of contradiction" tone.

It is thus ironic that *Sulphur* should be a principal remedy for weak or failing memory: increased forgetfulness, recurring absent-mindedness, a *Calcarea*-like loss of concentration. The remedy immediately comes to mind for patients who forget the names of familiar streets, friends, family members, and the like ("startling forgetfulness, especially as to proper names": Hahnemann). "You, you, Tom, I mean Tim—whatever your name is . . . " he will say to his son-in-law, Ted, who has been in the family for fifteen years (*Lycopodium*). And he cannot for the life of him recall who came to dinner last night ("So forgetful that even the most recent events are only obscurely recalled": Hahnemann). At the same time, he remembers complex mathematical formulae, little-known dates in history, and obscure literary references. Such *Sulphur* strengths and weaknesses of memory could reflect the individual's natural inclination toward the abstract, factual, and scholarly, rather than the purely personal.

An elderly *Sulphur* homoeopathic physician of the writer's acquaintance, who was beginning to forget the names and faces of even his best and oldest friends, could still discourse at length about complicated cases he had treated many years ago: "Oh, yes, that woman who got *Sepia* 10M for her keratoconus [a rare eye disease], followed by two doses of *Tuberculinum* 1M and a dose of *Sulphur* 200x—how *is* she doing?"

The classic image of *Sulphur* is the "ragged philosopher" (Hering): the unkempt, scraggly bearded, scruffily dressed, absent-minded professor, his mind lost in great thoughts—to the exclusion of everything and everyone else. He lives in his own world of ideas and abstractions where learning and books are more important than human relations and emotions.

Studying in a library, he will lose all sense of time and come home hours late for dinner. If preparing his own meal, he will start reading a book and forget to turn off the gas under the burning pot. He may be virtually incapable of survival on his own. He is impractical and inept with his hands, especially in the finer motor movements (*Natrum muriaticum*). Far from being the manually dexterous and mechanically adept type discussed earlier, he is unable to drive a car successfully or even to use a typewriter, while opening a can of soup, untying a knotted piece of string, pouring liquid from one bottle into another, let alone fixing a slipped bicycle chain, are all traumatic experiences.

This unworldly individual of philosophic bent, to whom scholarship and intellectual pursuits are as natural as breathing ("disposed for literary work": Allen), appears quite different from the materialistic

Sulphur aggressively defending his own interests. But the opposition is more apparent than real. Both types are *accumulators*: one accumulates knowledge, scholarship, and theories, i.e., spiritual or intellectual goods, while the other accumulates money, land, possessions, i.e., worldly or material goods. Some manage to accumulate both.

The professorial *Sulphur* can be identified by his manner of reasoning. He provides a philosophical underpinning for every opinion and will offer a whole theology in support of some simple action. He is well informed on any subject but expostulates on it in a too exhaustive fashion; or, sparked off by some random observation or comment, he amplifies these into philosophic monologues.

The individual who sometimes appears brilliant, sometimes merely tedious, is probably a *Sulphur* (who is a bit of both). He knows so much — yet, despite the valuable and mind-enrichening information pouring out, his *impersonal* style of presentation makes the listening difficult. He himself, of course, is unaware of producing on the listener an impression like that of Gladstone on Queen Victoria, who remarked irritably in a rare flash of wit: "He always addresses me as if I were a public meeting." Indeed, when patients of other constitutional types start expressing themselves pedantically, ponderously, or long-windedly, it may well indicate that the time for *Sulphur* is at hand.

His writing style is exemplified by the scholarly and monumental work whose every page is studded with informative data, every sentence documented by a lengthy footnote (which is often the "meat" [concrete rendition] of his abstract or theoretical treatese), and every phrase weighty with significance — the type of important and influential book that every educated person feels he must at least hold in his hand once in his life (examples of which are given below). While the usual fate of these highly specialized volumes is to be placed in a position of prominence on the bookshelf with a silent promise to read them at some later date, *Sulphur* scholars have provided much of mankind's intellectual dynamism over the centuries.

The poorly organized lecturer with enormous information at his disposal is often *Sulphur*. The extremely disorganized one will write his ideas on scraps of paper or the backs of envelopes which fall out of his folder or notebook, or which he fishes out of his pockets as he lectures ("Ah, yes, another point to remember . . . "). He knows his material well but overwhelms his listeners, failing to realize that these masses of information so fascinating to him, may be less interesting to others (except, perhaps, to a fellow-*Sulphur*). Every college student has experienced such a professor and wondered why he was ever hired, let alone tenured, to be thus inflicted on unfortunate students year after year.

But there is a reason. He must be respected for the legitimate scholar that he is, even when not the most inspiring lecturer. Those who can remain attentive in class will always learn from him. His weakness is the need to communicate *everything* he knows, and his thoroughness may give the impression of pomposity. Listeners soon become glassy-eyed waiting for him to end.

This is not the only constitutional type who loves overmuch the sound of his own voice. *Lachesis* is a worthy competitor, and everyone loves to discourse on subjects which interest him. It is the styles that are distinctive. At a gathering *Sulphur* can be espied holding forth in the midst of a crowd of listeners. The man who, after recounting his world travels in typical *Sulphur* "enumerating" or "quantitative" style (Imagine,! only last week I was dining in Paris at the *Tour d'Argent*, where the meal cost me . . . then I took a two-mile walk round the Louvre and saw at least 500 paintings . . . And the week-end I spent in Rome, where I visited most of the monuments and ruins from the second century B.C. to the fifth century A.D. . . . And only *three* days ago I was in Istanbul, where I toured the famous Porphyrogenitus Palace—the finest specimen of Byzantine civil architecture left in the city . . ." and so on), points to his head, appending, "My most interesting journeys however, have always taken place right up here," and then proceeds to launch into his latest theories on various subjects—is hardly a caricature of this type.

Even in everyday conversation *Sulphur* tends constantly to theorize and occasionally to pontificate, with mere mundane topics taking on grand dimensions. He expresses himself with as much eloquence on the merits and drawbacks of ballpoint versus fountain pens as on the difference between Positivism and Structuralism in contemporary philosophy. Some converse without the least give and take. Their conversational egocentrism is illustrated by the anecdote of two men talking: when the first has finished a long monologue, he turns to his companion and says, "Enough of me. Let's talk about you. Tell me, what do you think of my new book?''

As early as adolescence he begins to exhibit conversational insensitivity. At meals and other family gatherings the boy assertively talks only about what interests *him*: the difference between his own cassette recorder and his friend's more expensive one or the problems with his motorcycle carburetor. He drones on and on, playing the pedagogue, knowledgeably but insistently instructing others in the mechanics of tape-recorders or motorcycle engines.

As is to be expected, however, *Sulphur* is also found in the opposite extreme: the adolescent from whom not a single extra word can be extracted. He answers questions in monosyllables or with grunts of assent or denial, behaving as if every utterance costs him a dollar. Possibly he feels a subliminal dread that by talking he might give something away for nothing.

Sulphur's penchant for monopolizing conversation is often seen in a reluctance even to listen to others. If he cannot deliver monologues or remain at the center of the discussion, he will doze off while others are talking. Then, waking with a start, he will announce, ''Well, I guess it's time to go home,'' rise and leave. Once he has had his say, there is no further reason to remain.

When he does try to take an interest in others, he may ply them rather ponderously with questions. Sometimes he enters the gleaned information in a little notebook, kept for the particular purpose of storing knowledge for future use. He has little talent for small talk and is not socially adroit; in contrast to *Lycopodium*, his attempts at gallantry or light conversation are often laborious. At a cocktail party an obviously *Sulphur* man was addressing a large handsome woman, ''I always admire the way you move, my dear,'' he said, ''like a swan gliding on the water.'' He paused. She beamed. And he added, ''Considering your weight, close to 200 pounds, I estimate, it's surprising how gracefully you walk.'' Then he moved off, convinced that he had just delivered a welcome and gracious compliment.

Sulphur is not renowned for quick wit or repartee, in contrast to *Arsenicum, Lachesis* or *Nux vomica*. That does not mean, however, that he is not interesting. If he can overcome the tendency to harangue his audience, he can be a fascinating conversationalist, even while domineering. His restlessly creative and ever-questing mind is inventive and, original, bursting with insights, generating theories about the knowable and the unknowable, like a volcano erupting in all directions.

In the physician's office this patient recounts his symptoms in a comprehensive and knowledgeable manner, attempting to provide what he calls (and which is indeed) a "complete and methodical report" of his case. One patient with a frayed and bulging briefcase (often the hallmark of a *Sulphur* who cannot get himself to dispose of, or leave behind, any of his papers) came seeking relief for long-standing digestive problems: he suffered from dullness and lethargy after meals, which was better when moving about; he had hard, knotty or burning stools, alternating with diarrhea, and burning itching hemorrhoids. The characteristic physical symptoms and the dog-eared briefcase amply indicated his need for *Sulphur*, but, as if unwilling to leave any room for doubt, he proceeded to corroborate them with mental symptoms. In a measured monotone and using learned language, he entered into an exhaustive treatise on the nature of his problem. "I suspect, as does my internist, an enzyme deficiency. When feeling poorly—No, let me rephrase that—at my worst, I feel that the gastric juices, due to a moderately severe endocrine imbalance, are not performing their proper functions . . . The doctors are all in agreement that the necessary chemical changes are not taking place. We are possibly speaking here of an inborn error of metabolism, of which modern medical science has yet to establish the curability . . . " and so on (*Sulphur* patients love to employ solemn scientific phrases).

Usually what he says is medically informed and scientifically accurate, but after a while the physician's attention starts to wander. Little enjoyment is afforded by a *Sulphur* expounding a futile hypothetical diagnosis of his liver, kidneys or enzymes; his delivery simply does not grip the listener's attention (also, of course, most of what he says is irrelevant for homoeopathic prescribing). Whatever the cause of his alleged deficiency, whatever the imbalance of his endocrine system, whatever chemical changes are, or are not, taking place in his stomach due to his metabolic dysfunction, after two minutes of such a discourse the physician immediately recognizes the *Sulphur* picture—and *that*, after all, is what counts!

Therefore, whenever the physician feels like crying out to a patient, "Stop telling me so much about things I don't want to know!" Or, "Spare me, I beg you, these learned explanations!" he should consider prescribing *Sulphur*.

Often the patient will return changed and sounding less like a medical textbook, allowing the physician to ask his questions in his own way and exhibiting more finesse in his conversation. Repeatedly homoeopaths have remarked after such a patient's second visit, "I never would have believed it! When he recounted his symptoms the last time, it sounded like the weekly train schedule between Washington and New York—there was no life, just facts. Now, what he says actually carries emotion and human interest!" In general, *Sulphur*'s conversation can be lacking in the human dimension, indicating overdevelopment of the intellect at the expense of the emotions.*

Arsenicum, given the opportunity, will also present his case at length, giving a blow-by-blow account of its history and nature with as much scientific detail as *Sulphur*. In their manner of talking about health and disease these two remedies often overlap, especially in the male. Both love to describe in detail all they have read about their particular ailment (and they have usually read a great deal), what the many doctors consulted have told them or failed to tell them about it, and all the treatments and medications they have received. But *Sulphur*, to coin a phrase, is the "pedantic *Arsenicum*," while *Arsenicum* is the "more urgent *Sulphur*." On the physical level also, *Sulphur* and *Arsenicum* complement each other beautifully and can be used interchangeably in many ailments (see Kent's *Lectures* and Borland).

Although pedantry, weightiness and exhaustiveness often characterize *Sulphur*'s presentation of ideas, so also does breadth of vision. Many of the world's most profound and versatile intellects have been *Sulphurs*, and they have produced scholarly works of universal stature

---

* *Sulphur*'s lack of sensitivity is caricatured in one of Snoopy's short stories: "My love for you," says the hero to his beloved, "is as high as Mount Everest, which is 32,000 feet high. My love for you is deeper than the Marianas Trench, which is 12,000 feet deep. My love is broader than [the Siberian steppes, which are 3,000 miles wide] . . . " The last panel shows Snoopy commenting with a rueful look, "Actually, my hero is quite a bore."

and significance. Proceeding from the premise that one comprehensive idea or vision can define and ultimately control all human experience, the strong mind takes an encyclopedic approach to the organization of knowledge, mastering large theoretical concepts and vast fields of technical or abstract knowledge and incorporating them into all-embracing systems in a way that few other constitutional types even attempt.

Massive compendius, and exhaustive commentaries, such as the Talmud, are *Sulphur* in conception as well as, we recall, in style; and Thomas Aquinas whose *Summa Theologica* brought intellectual order and moral design into the formerly chaotic area of theological speculation, embodies this mind at work. His methodical intellectualization of moral and emotional questions of faith and salvation, and classification as to who stands where in the eyes of God and the order of the universe, is the classic antithesis of the *Lachesis* St. Augustine's exposition of the revelatory nature of grace and faith (in his *Confessions*). Karl Marx's *Das Kapital*, which has so profoundly influenced the course of history, yet which is so seldom read in its entirety (being too quintessentially *Sulphur* for ordinary consumption), is another typical work.*

But the type's strength in theoretical understanding and need to build systems is not limited to philosophers and theologians. Johann

---

* The eighteenth-century author and man of letters, Samuel Johnson, provides, perhaps the most graphic picture (almost a caricature) of the constitutional type. He was physically large, red-faced, perspiring, and "stank like a polecat," with scrofulous, dirty-looking skin and unclean, unkempt hair, as unruly as his own unconventional nature. He loved food and was a greedy eater with atrocious table-manners (often stuffing great quantities of food into his mouth with both hands). He was argumentative, overbearing, and heatedly opinionated, at times to the point of insolence.

He was married to a silly, vulgar, unattractive, and vain woman whom he considered the most beautiful and charming creature on earth. While this caused his contemporaries and biographers considerable puzzlement, it is explained homoeopathically by *Sulphur*'s penchant for "seeing as beautiful that which is not beautiful," of discerning virtue in his own possessions.

He was a scholar of remarkable talents, reputed to have "read more books than any man alive" (Adam Smith) and a prolific author in many

Sebastian Bach who, in addition to an almost superhuman output of musical compositions, singlehandedly systematized the principles of functional harmony and elaborated the tempered scale for keyboard instruments, was eminently *Sulphur*.

For our purposes, however, the best illustration of *Sulphur* is Samuel Hahnemann himself. With an explosive temper that thrived on controversy and a mind that boldly expounded provocative and controversial medical opinions, he also possessed a phenomenal memory, exhibiting proficiency in at least five languages beside his native German (French, Italian, English, Latin and Greek) and, if the hagiography built up around him is to be trusted, competence in several others. During the seventeen years of his early professional life, when hounded from town to town by physicians and pharmacists, he supported his large family by translating medical works at night. His knowledge was vast and his scholarship outstanding in several fields. He was the leading chemist of his generation and is considered a minor figure in the history of that discipline; he could probably have been one of the world's foremost chemists had he not chosen homoeopathy. His written style in German rivals that of Luther and others who shaped this language's historical development. According to repute, Hahnemann was able to combine his practice with an extensive literary output by sleeping only every

genres: poetry, biography, essays, prayers, meditations, travelogues, essays, aphorisms, and other literary works. He was also a brilliant conversationalist (as recorded for posterity by Boswell). Best known in his own day as a lexicographer and compiler of the great *Dictionary* (the collecting, classifying, and studying of the etymology of words is an occupation highly congenial to *Sulphur*), his writings and didactic sayings exhibit a distinctly sententious, almost pompous, *Sulphur* flavor ("If a man does not make new acquaintances as he advances through life, he will soon find himself alone; a man, sir, should keep his friendships in constant repair." "To let friendship die away by negligence and silence is certainly not wise; it is voluntarily to throw away one of the greatest comforts of this weary pilgrimage"). He also exhibited a high degree of "male chauvinism" which is an undeniable component of the constitutions of many male *Sulphurs* ("A man is generally better pleased when he has a good dinner upon the table than when his wife talks Greek"), and which has not changed much over the centuries.

second night for long periods of his life.

Furthermore, his case notebooks are highly *Sulphur* in their disorganized appearance, and he was a very fatiguing lecturer. When
teaching at the University of Leipzig, he drove most students away by
his showers of invective against contemporary medical practice or by
heaping on them sententious utterances, and only a handful of faithful
followers continued to come to his class. Then, too, his *Organon of
Medicine* illustrates the dense scholarly *Sulphur* style that needs to be
read at least three times for comprehension.

Most significantly, Hahnemann possessed the *Sulphur* breadth of
vision. He not only redefined the concept of "similarity" in therapeutics and developed a complete philosophy of medicine, to which nothing essential has needed to be added since its inception, even as it grows
in relevance and significance with every passing generation, but by the
provings he was able to make his theories practical and accessible.* The
completeness of Hahnemann's original formulation is seen in the fact
that the only significant theoretical addition was Constantine Hering's
"Law of the Direction of Cure": during the process of cure the symptoms move from the inside of the body outward, from the upper part
of the body downward, from the more vital organs to the less vital, and
disappear in the reverse order of their appearance. But Hering admitted
that this Law of Cure was prefigured in Hahnemann's own writings
(Constantine Hering, "Hahnemann's Three Rules Concerning the Rank
of Symptoms." *Hahnemannian Monthly* I, 1865. 5–12).

For sheer intellectual vigor, endurance, and productivity the mentally strong *Sulphur* is difficult to surpass. Furthermore, he often possesses a messianic spirit, sensing from an early age that something important is expected of him and calling him to greatness. This drive,
together with his intellectual boldness and restless pioneering energy
and a "courageous mood which is ready for great resolution" (Allen),

---

* The homoeopathic "proving" is a technique for ascertaining the
curative powers of medicines by administering them systematically
and in small quantities to healthy human volunteers. The symptoms
elicited by this procedure are the ones which will be cured in an ill
patient by the same substance, and homoeopathy holds that the complete removal of the patient's symptoms means that the "disease" itself
or the disease "cause" has also been removed (see *Introduction*).

permit him to contemplate and carry out schemes of a magnitude that others would not consider possible.*

Not all *Sulphur* intellectuals, however, are movers and builders. Many are impractical visionaries or dreamers whose overambitious plans remain unrealized. Others are strong in conceptualizing large-scale projects but weak in attending to the details that *Arsenicum* or *Nux vomica* love so much. One *Sulphur* patient of solid but moderate musical ability set himself the goal of learning by heart all thirty-two of the Beethoven sonatas. He succeeded in this giant enterprise and was able to plow his

---

* The following cartoon suggests this characteristic (from left to right, *Sulphur, Phosphorus, Calcarea*).

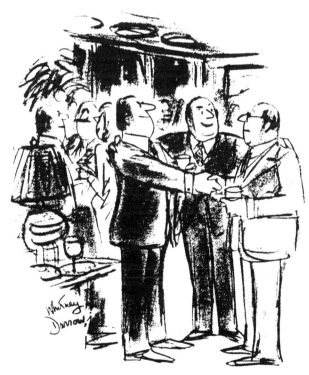

"John, I'd like you to meet one of the people who make the future happen."

Drawing by Whitney Darrow, Jr.
© 1981 The New Yorker Magazine, Inc.

way through the whole opus, but all the sonatas sounded alike. An *Arsenicum* of equivalent musical talent and love of Beethoven would have concentrated on learning two or three sonatas really well.

Or *Sulphur* embarks on some intrinsically worthy and grandiose cause such as raising money for some world-saving mission, learning a Third World language, undertaking to restore a historic building, or translating the works of some oriental poet—without ever completing the job: "*Sulphur* has an aversion to follow up things in an orderly fashion . . . to systematic work" (Kent). In everyday life this trait comes out in the man who never finishes tasks around the house—and will not even pick up his tools. They lie around waiting for him, while he has already started on another project. His triad partner, *Lycopodium*, is better at completing jobs once begun.

Sulphur has been discussed primarily as a male remedy, just as *Pulsatilla* and *Sepia* are female remedies. Naturally, many women also require it, but in them the mental characteristics described above are attenuated and subdued, possibly because they are less "pure" types. It is difficult to pinpoint a typical *Sulphur* female artist, genius, literary heroine or historic figure, while the male sex provides innumerable examples (one of the few female *Sulphurs* that comes to mind is the great pioneer in the philosophy and method of child education, Maria Montessori; her practical and analytical genius, visionary mind, and profound grasp of the learning process argue for the presence of much *Sulphur* in her constitution). For this reason the physician will often prescribe the remedy on the basis of a woman's physical symptoms and modalitites, or during the indicated *Sulphur* time in her process of cure.

An exception to this rule is the woman who exhibits the remedy's troubled or depressed mental symptoms such as: "she has no rest anywhere, neither by day nor night; apprehensive about the future where she sees nothing but misery and suffering; agonizing state; apprehension for [safety of] others [which can trigger off a whole string of imagined catastrophes: see chapter on *Arsenicum*]; she thinks of nothing but anxious, annoying, and dejecting thoughts which she cannot get rid of; cannot do anything so as to please herself; worse evening in bed, hindering her from falling asleep; sleeplessness on account of flow of thoughts; disinclination for everything; finds life insupportable," and so on (Hahnemann, Hering). *Sulphur* is often indicated in such cases.

Pseudo- And Anti-Intellectualism

The polar opposite of the productive type must also be recognized as *Sulphur*—the "lazy" individual described in the homoeopathic texts as, "averse to business; aversion to work; too lazy to rouse himself; sits around all day doing nothing." Instead of earning the family's bread, he reclines in an armchair and thinks his great thoughts or indulges in grand but empty pseudo-intellectual speculation.

This is also the individual who seeks recognition without feeling any need to exert himself for it. He awaits some surprise benefactor who will recognize his hitherto unappreciated talent and raise him to the heights of fame; then he is disappointed at the world's failure to recognize his greatness. Although he considers himself a *génie manqué* (and indeed he might have wasted a fine talent), he is really just a chronic loafer whose will to work has been sapped at the root. This kind of *Sulphur* resembles the apathetic *Calcarea*, with the difference that he harbors pretensions to greatness while *Calcarea* does not.

If philosophically or religiously inclined, this lesser *Sulphur* mind becomes bogged down in futile abstract contemplations. Kent describes him as "studying different things without basis to figure upon . . . philosophy that cannot be followed up," and refers to the *Sulphur* woman who spends her time wondering and worrying "without hope of discovery, without any possible answer, [about] who made God?" In the Middle Ages such fruitless conjecturing as, "How many angels can dance on the head of a pin?" was a *reductio ad absurdum* of the *Sulphur* speculative mode. Therefore, persons with a penchant for ruminating on insoluble theoretical problems or time-wasting philosophical abstractions may require a dose of the remedy to direct their minds to more practical and profitable subjects.

Even though this *Sulphur* can absorb massive amounts of information, his ability to use it appropriately is deficient. He may understand the separate components of a situation, discipline, or method without being able to put them all together. The less experienced *Sulphur* homoeopath, for instance, will take a case accurately and extract the major guiding symptoms, but will still not hit on the obvious constitutional remedy. Or the would-be intellectual is more fascinated with the idea of an idea or some intellectual fad, than capable of understanding a true idea.

When carried a step further, this trait of missing the forest for the trees makes *Sulphur* appear foolish despite his learning. He can be knowledgeable enough but adopts a false perspective or fails in some way to synthesize his information, leading to a lack of judgment which causes this type to be dubbed the "false philosopher" (Kent).*

Whereas the mentally strong *Sulphur* can relate different concepts, and even different fields of knowledge (history, philosophy, economics, science, politics, religion) in an enlightening way, the mentally weak variety is overwhelmed by too much, or misdirected, learning. Losing perspective and lacking focus, his disjointed mind wanders without direction among the various mental disciplines he has only partially absorbed as he seeks a connecting threat that would bind together the confusing phenomena of existence ("muddled in the head . . . and cannot connect two ideas together": Hahnemann). Or he relates disparate concepts and fragments of understanding too readily and inappropriately in an attempt to push forward the frontiers of knowledge. A medical example might be the prescribing of herbal or mineral medicines on the basis of the color or shape of the plant or ore and its supposed resemblance to the disease or part of the body to be treated—known in the Middle Ages as the "doctrine of signatures". Just as *Phosphorus* likes to interpret phenomena in psychic terms, *Sulphur* seeks philosophical rationalizations for the smallest everyday action and fits the simplest event into some overall cosmic pattern.

Yet another type is the one who "despises [formal] education" (Kent). Poorly educated himself, he feels superior to mere "book learning," certain that education has nothing of importance to offer. In the elderly, to whom life has not vouchsafed a good education but who have managed to succeed on their own, this sour grapes attitude ("Colleges and universities only turn out communists and neurotics") may be understandable. But even some younger *Sulphurs* despise the education they were fortunate enough to receive, or turn it down in favor

---

* Typical here was James I of England, who reigned from 1603 to 1625 and was known as "the wisest fool in Christendom" because he lacked the essential quality of a ruler—political shrewdness—despite vast knowledge of history, theology, and law. He was a Scotsman who never understood his English subjects, and his reign prepared the way for the Puritan rebellion and the ensuing Civil War and Interregnum.

of some "beyond learning" philosophy. The type can come up with astonishing observations, viz., "As we enter the Aquarian Age, there is no more room for the conventional sciences; science as we understand it is outmoded"; or, if scientifically inclined, he may say that the humanities and the classics are no longer "relevant," that the future lies with science alone. One such patient hazarded that higher education was valueless because "We are reaching a stage in our understanding and intuitiveness where we will no longer require words to communicate. Words in general, and the written word in particular, are on their way out" (!)

A young and otherwise healthy man came to homoeopathy for migraine headaches recurring almost every weekend (*Sulphur*, as well as *Arsenicum*, should always be considered for the regular Saturday or Sunday headaches of the working man or woman). All his physical symptoms and their modalities, as well as his mental ones, fell between *Sulphur* and *Arsenicum*. The physician was hesitating which to prescribe until the patient began describing his educational background. Then it became clear. For several years he had been an enthusiastic follower of Eastern philosophy. Once he discovered the superiority of the inner over the outer life, he left college to contemplate his immortal soul and past incarnations. He no longer read books, attended plays, heard concerts, or even watched interesting films because, as he complacently put it, he was "beyond all that. None of them have anything to offer me." He then went into a disquisition on the "false linear" knowledge of Western culture versus the "true cyclical" knowledge of the East. Although this latter assertion doubtless contained some truth, the more he talked, the more apparent it became that he would have benefited from an occasional—even if linear—book or symphony. This patient typified what sometimes happens with a *Sulphur*—becoming so lost in his spiritual pilgrimage as no longer to appreciate the richness and variety of human accomplishment.

Sulphur, then, offers the extremes of overvaluation and undervaluation of formal education. Either he cultivates scholarship at the expense of intuition, sensitivity, and human understanding, or he completely disdains it. He begins to feel that he possesses a deeper comprehension, allowing him to dispense with the dearly bought core of classical knowledge that is our heritage as human beings.

What, one may well ask, can the remedy do in the face of such imbalances? We saw earlier that the dry, intellectual *Sulphur* can become more human from the remedy, and it can have the same balancing effect on the individual who undervalues training and education. It can plant the seed of understanding that enables him to shed his pretentiousness and open his mind to possibilities in areas previously shunned. The "linear versus circular knowledge" patient was started on a course of *Sulphur* for the headaches, beginning with the 200x potency and ascending the scale over the course of a year. Within four months he began to suspect that Western culture might have something to offer after all and that he had been underrating it. As he cleverly put it, "I realize that there is less to me than meets the eye. Yet, instead of being depressed, I feel intellectually and psychologically lightened. I am no longer burdened by knowing everything there is to know and by taking myself so seriously." Some months later he started reading the classics and reapplied to his former college. Soon he was enrolled in a humanities program and eagerly immersed in Western intellectual history. He was still *Sulphur*; he still enjoyed expounding at length on the difference between circular and linear knowledge; but his condescension was gone, and he displayed an intellectual humility that had previously been lacking. While such changes often take place as part of the process of growing and maturing, the use of homoeopathic *Sulphur* may initiate or accelerate them.

Old Age and Melancholy

Finally, the remedy is frequently needed for the mental weaknesses and physical infirmities of old age.

A patient in his early eighties was becoming slow in his understanding, both of what he read and what he heard. If asked a question, he was at first uncomprehending and would have to "repeat it before answering it" (Hering); in conversation he was inclined to reiterate the same remarks over and over again. *Sulphur* at any mature age tends to repeat himself, often rather long-windedly and ponderously and in exactly the same phrases: not a word changed, not a comma omitted. Periodic doses of the remedy improved this old gentleman's comprehension sufficiently to enable him to engage rationally in simple conversations, browse through the daily paper, and reread favorite passages of familiar books. The improvement continued until shortly before his death (for mental confusion and loss of memory in the elderly, see, also, *Baryta carbonica*).

Sulphur is also of benefit when old age brings a narrowing and ossification of the mental faculties, when the individual's formerly broader understanding begins to focus more purely on the self. He cannot even attempt to become interested in others, being too absorbed in melancholy reflections or egocentric broodings. When the remedy is administered, the mind and emotions expand again, beautifully exemplifying the homoeopathic view that the mind need not narrow and atrophy with age, but that a person ages because his mind contracts.

A widower in his late sixties was being treated for labored asthmatic breathing. He was dejected, nothing pleased him, and he could not be reconciled to his rather empty, although objectively not difficult, life. His son, who lived nearby, saw to his physical wants and needs. He would have been happy to do more if the father had not been such a burden on the family, selfishly demanding attention (he could talk non-stop for forty-five minutes or an hour at a stretch) yet giving little in return ("indifferent about the lot of others": Hering).

A course of *Sulphur* was prescribed, in the 30x, then 200x potency (with older persons it is advisable to employ the lower potencies). Not only was his breathing facilitated and thereafter controlled by periodic doses of *Sulphur* 200x, but his former more sociable feelings reemerged. He began to appreciate his son better and to take more interest in his grandchildren; and the now healthier ego was channeled into writing an autobiography—for the edification of humanity as well as for his own benefit.

Although this chapter has stressed the creative, energetic, sociable, and buoyant side of *Sulphur*, the remedy (at any age) is often indicated in states of profound depression and anxiety—either alone or to complement the action of another remedy: "profound melancholy; satiety of life; weary of life; longing for death; too lazy to rouse himself up and too unhappy to live; feeling of dullness and gloominess" (Hahnemann, Hering; and Allen has some 40 listings describing *Sulphur*'s despondency, apprehension, and sadness). It is also indicated for the excessively "introverted, introspective" individual (Boenninghausen lists *Sulphur* in the third degree under this rubric) with a hermit-like tendency to withdraw from society. This is hardly surprising in view of Hahnemann's theory of chronic diseases which describes depression and introversion as primarily a manifestation of the psoric miasm.

Sometimes depression is caused by an overtaxed mind, fatigued by too prolonged or too intense study. A *Sulphur* will sit up night after night (like Hahnemann), devouring books in his desire to accumulate *all* available knowledge. One day, however, his mind gives out, drained and exhausted, and he is in despair, having lost his most highly developed faculty, the one upon which he could always rely (we recall that the type tends to cultivate his rational and intellectual side at the expense of his emotions).

At other times a patient is overcome by a "disgust for everything" (Boenninghausen) or "religious melancholy" (Hering). This can happen in the relatively young as well as the older person. He may be devout but finds little comfort in his faith, and his view of human destiny takes on a dark tinge ("embittered": Boenninghausen). For example, religion was no solace to Leo Tolstoy, a writer and thinker whose literary works are permeated with philosophic opinions expressed in true *Sulphur* style—an analytical objectivity that carries the weight and solemnity of papal edicts. With age, as Tolstoy increasingly wrestled with unanswerable metaphysical and moral issues, questioning the reason for man's existence on earth, he was prompted to reject his own great art and the concept of civilization generally. Deciding that the sum total of human wisdom and enlightenment resided in the Russian peasant (?), he dressed in the simplest clothes and tried to become one of them himself. To the horror of his large family, he even tried to distribute his vast land holdings among the peasants. Underlying this socio-political gesture was not only a *Sulphur* nostalgia for the soil and the simplicity of nature, but also its typical anxiety "of conscience" (Kent) or "about the soul's salvation" (Hering).

Patients undergoing such religious or existential crises have been greatly benefitted by *Sulphur* (also *Natrum muriaticum* and *Lachesis*).

In his religious outlook, as in other domains, this type is dichotomous: either profoundly religious or completely irreligious. Thus clergymen and theologians of all religious denominations and spiritual paths will have *Sulphur* prominent in their constitutions. Less well balanced minds, however, can be led astray by religious searchings or by meditation. While other constitutional types can worship or meditate with benefit if properly guided, *Sulphur*'s judgment may become obscured. He will decide that he is "above" human appetites and desires, that his stage of spiritual development places him beyond normal eating, sleeping, or sexual habits; or, conversely, a religious horror at being physically and spiritually "unclean" compels him to undergo rigid cleansing diets or other ascetic regimes. Also, in his impatience to arrive at full spiritual awareness, he may leap too precipitously into mystical or metaphysical regions and lose his bearings, instead of allowing his understanding to evolve toward a higher consciousness in a gradual and organic way. Kent describes these more extreme seekers after the truth as exhibiting a "philosophical mania . . . monomania over the study of strange and occult things . . . that are beyond human knowledge." If *Sulphur* is non-religious, he neither feels any need for religion himself nor understands this in others; the whole religious and mystical dimension is simply lacking in him (*Lycopodium*). He is frankly bored by the subject, by church services and other forms of worship, often falls asleep during them, and feels no need to subjugate his will or behavior to any such higher authority.

The characteristics and cases discussed in this chapter, however, are but drops in the *Sulphur* ocean.* Its range of symptoms and depth of action make this remedy far greater than any description of it—far greater than the sum of its parts. It can act beneficially in virtually any chronic condition or constitutional type. And yet, as we have tried to bring out, the remedy's universal scope of action does not prevent it from possessing its own individual flavor. The physician who can recognize the *Sulphur* slant of mind and emotional shading, who learns at which point to prescribe it, guided by the specific modalities of time, temperature, cravings, periodicity, stages of life, or stages in the healing process will never cease to marvel at its seemingly limitless curative powers.

---

* Although Hering's *Guiding Symptoms* records 93 pages of *Sulphur* symptoms, while Allen's *Encyclopedia of Pure Materia Medica* has 137 pages (both averaging over 50 symptoms per page), these remarkable pictures merely begin to do justice to this remedy.

Pulsatilla

THE remedy *Pulsatilla* is made from the meadow anemone, *Pulsatilla nigricans,* a plant of the Ranunculus family which grows in the plains and pasturelands of Central and Northern Europe and is commonly known as the "wind flower." It is small and delicate, with a flexible stem which bends one way or another according to the direction of the prevailing wind. The constitutional type, found predominently in women and children, is generally delicate and pretty, most commonly of fair complexion, with blond or light brown hair, and a physique that can fluctuate easily in weight loss and gain, with the fat tending to a shapely plumpness rather than the flabby or formless fleshiness of *Calcarea carbonica.*

Like the flower swaying in the wind, *Pulsatilla* symptoms are characteristically changeful: pains wander from one part of the body to another, shift rapidly from joint to joint, appear on one side of the body or the other, with "no two chills, no two stools, no two attacks alike" (H.C. Allen). The circulation is unstable, with a complexion that, like *Phosphorus*', flushes up or blushes easily, and the energy is variable, so that in a few minutes the individual can alter from bright and lively to tired and droopy. Also, like gusts of wind, the pains come on suddenly, then either let up abruptly on first motion or subside gradually; often the patient finds relief in gentle motion—walking or rocking back and forth.* Delicate flower that she is, *Pulsatilla* cannot tolerate the

---

* The remedy has been prescribed successfully more than once for the pain of inguinal hernia, where the guiding symptom was the patient's habit of relieving the pain by rocking his updrawn knees from side to side.

heat of a warm room or the stuffiness of a close atmosphere and requires fresh air to preserve her strength and well-being. She wilts in
the sun, and in warm weather tends to weaken or become irritable,
but a cool breeze quickly restores her flagging spirits. At the same time
she chills easily and needs much covering to keep warm. Finally, just
as the flower grows primarily in dry sandy soil, so the *Pulsatilla* nature
has little need for water; she is thirstless and, even when the mouth
is dry, can go for long periods without drinking. In fact, she must remind herself to drink.

However, the remedy's mental characteristics are usually the most
striking. In this chapter we will examine in detail five seminal mental
characteristics: sweetness, dependence, companionability, flexibility,
and a gentle emotionalism. Most *Pulsatilla* patients will manifest some
combination of these key symptoms.

Sweetness

The personality is agreeable and engaging from the first encounter.
She is "mild, good-tempered, yielding" (Hahnemann), and sensitive
to others' feelings. The children are responsive and "easy to handle"
(Borland), and the adult is easy to get along with. Almost all have a sweet
manner, observable in their pretty facial features, smiles and gestures,
or soft and pleasing voice. In many cases there is a corresponding
sweetness of heart. Delicacy of feeling, consideration of others, and a
gentleness that restrains her from making any comment likely to wound
another's sensibilities all reflect *Pulsatilla's* essential *sweetness*.

Traditionally regarded as a female remedy (Kent points out that
Pulsatilla will be needed in any household where young girls are present), and in these pages referred to in the feminine, it can also be
unhesitatingly administered as a constitutional remedy to boys and men
who manifest the typical sweet and gentle manner.

The type is encountered in the "good," obliging child who seeks
approval and affection. She is not prone to argue, nor does she anger
easily, being basically unaggressive. She tends to play better with her
siblings and to get along better with other family members than the
child who has no *Pulsatilla* in her constitution. She helps out in the
home and is eager to be "mother's little helper" in return for love and
caresses. Even the adult *Pulsatilla*, in her strong need to be loved by
many, remains close to other family members.

The child also knows how to *demonstrate* affection (*Phosphorus*). She comes up with hugs and kisses ("manifests affection by kissing and caressing": Hering), climbs in your lap, cuddles there and sits quietly without wriggling and squirming. In her need to be physically close to those she loves, she instinctively assumes a sweet, acceptable manner and as a result is often the family pet. In the words of the nursery rhyme, *Pulsatilla* is "Friday's child," who is loving and giving.*

When reprimanded, she is terribly anxious to make amends. She lays her head penitently on her mother's shoulder, laces her arms around her neck and apologizes tearfully. No other type can apologize as prettily as *Pulsatilla*, because she is completely sincere, devoid of false pride, and does not bear grudges. She yearns to be forgiven, so as not to suffer withdrawal of the affection she craves.

She also possesses strong peacemaking instincts and from childhood senses the importance of cooperative behavior in any group situation, be it family, school or play. When a cake is divided among a group of youngsters, and one slice is smaller, *Pulsatilla* will accept the smaller piece in the nicest way, saying: "I'll take that one, I don't mind at all!" Since she loves pastries and sweets of all kinds, this is a true sacrifice.

Both child and adult are thus inherently conciliatory and will avoid a quarrel whenever possible. They do everything in their power to maintain good relations and eschew any type of unpleasantness. If a rupture does occur, *Pulsatilla* will bend over backward to restore harmony and even shoulder the blame, since she relies on others' moods to be happy ("sensible to every social influence": Kent). Only *Lycopodium* can approach her concern to get along with others at all times. But *Lycopodium* does so out of principle, and often with condescension, while *Pulsatilla* relates as an equal and from the heart.

Pulsatilla's sweetness and desire to please do not exclude an underlying ability to look after her own interests; it is just that she realizes

---

* Monday's child is fair of face (*Tuberculinum*).
Tuesday's child is full of grace (*Phosphorus*).
Wednesday's child is full of woe (*Natrum muriaticum, Sepia*).
Thursday's child has far to go (*Calcarea carbonica*).
Friday's child is loving and giving (*Pulsatilla*).
Saturday's child works hard for a living (*Arsenicum*).
But the child who is born on the Sabbath Day
Is bonny, blythe, good, and gay."

early in life that sugar catches more flies than vinegar. She likes being fussed over and is content to pass even the simplest responsibilities on to others. To be sure, she graciously thanks those who help her, offering her own affection in return as good and legal tender. Thus she does not take for granted these signs of attention but is grateful for them. For this reason, others do not object to helping her; often they are unaware of the demands she places on them. Consequently, this type can float through life a petted, pampered child. When wielded correctly, sweetness is a highly effective technique for getting one's way!

At other times *Pulsatilla* selfishly expects others to care for her constantly, feels unappreciated if they do not, and can be jealous and possessive of others' affection ("is greedy and wants to have everything for herself": Hahnemann). An idle woman may refuse to take a job to help augment the family income, although perfectly capable of doing so. Perhaps this is why *Pulsatilla* is the only remedy (except *Sulphur*) listed high in the Kent *Repertory* under the rubric "selfishness."

Despite sweet looks and manner, then, she is not all sugar. Beneath the surface mildness lies the resilience of the meadow anemone, swaying in the wind but with roots planted firmly in the soil. The type calls to mind La Fontaine's fable, *The Oak and the Reed*, in which the two are discussing which is the stronger, when a sudden gust of wind smites the mighty oak to the ground, while the humbly bending reed remains unscathed. Prouder and seemingly stronger natures may break sooner than the supple, yielding *Pulsatilla*.

The traditional image of the aristocratic woman of the ante-bellum South illustrates this particular characteristic: the soft-spoken mistress of a plantation, all sweetness on the outside but pliant steel within. Gentle, "timid" (Hahnemann), delicate Melanie Wilkes in *Gone with the Wind*, with her loving nature and fine-spun courage, is a splendid literary example of *Pulsatilla*'s combination of sweetness and strength. And nineteenth-century English literature abounds in soft, yielding, pretty, heroines of uncertain fate, making the female *Pulsatilla* something of a literary stereotype (one need only recall Dickens' gallery of Ada Clare, Lucie Manette, Pet Meagles, Dora Spenlow, Madeline Bray, and others).

However irritating these sweet fictional heroines may be at times, their virtue does reflect an important truth about *Pulsatilla*: her attractive absence of self-righteousness and bitterness. Under duress she does not become bitter because she is neither arrogant nor unduly righteous. She understands the actions of others, however different they may be from her own, and to understand is to forgive. Instinctively sensing why people think and behave as they do, she instinctively forgives them. Another appealing characteristic is her lack of aggressiveness. Even when irritable, she is sensitive and "touchy" (Kent) rather than belligerent.

In everyday life *Pulsatilla*'s sweetness often emerges at her job. It is a pleasure to work with her or for her, as she is open to suggestions and responsive to the needs of a colleague or an employee. At the worst, when she is in charge, her pliancy and lack of direction lead to ineffectualness or dispersal of effort. At best, the easygoing atmosphere of the office leads to high productivity, reflecting *Pulsatilla*'s ability to delegate responsibility, be considerate of others, and respect their ideas. These qualities contribute to harmony and successful cooperation. Her sweetness is also exhibited in the desire and capacity to make life pleasant for her loved ones. The wife of an excessively demanding husband will answer her gruff mate in a soothing manner: "Of course, my love," or "You're so right, darling," "Just as you say, my dear." The more surly his behavior, the more considerate she herself becomes, as if to compensate for his unpleasantness. Only *she* could tolerate such a mate over the years and still preserve a peaceful marriage. Ironically, though, her docility can cause him to react and become all the more brusque and irascible (at times, to be sure, the husband is the sweet *Pulsatilla* counterpart to a difficult wife.)

Yet this obliging woman is not necessarily trampled upon in the privacy of her home. An apparent tyrant of a husband will admit, "I don't know how it is—my wife is compliancy itself, she never insists and never argues, but somehow she manages to do just as she wants, and I have to accept it." And a gentler and more sensitive spouse is so manipulated by his wife, that he laments, "She has a way of twisting things around so that I *always* come out the loser." Even the mildest *Pulsatilla* possesses a quiet pertinacity that ultimately prevails. Moreover, although this chapter stresses the healthy and sociable type, the reverse side also deserves at least brief comment. The classic texts give the following symptoms: "sullenness, very much out of spirits and cross; does not want to talk to anyone; all day long ill-humored and discon-

tented without cause; extremely capricious and peevish about everything; gloomy and melancholy, extremely cross with everything, even
with himself'' (Hahnemann, Hering, and others).

Dependence

The second prominent *Pulsatilla* characteristic is *dependence.* Just
as the flower grows in clusters, so must the human *Pulsatilla* have people around her—not, like *Phosphorus*, for an audience or for stimulus;
not, like *Lycopodium* or *Sulphur*, for someone to impress; not, like
Natrum muriaticum, for someone to help or instruct; nor, like *Arsenicum*, for someone to direct—but for someone on whom to *lean.* She
is not intrinsically weak, but she requires support—just as ivy cannot
grow without clinging to a wall or a tree. Some of her most prominent
fears relate to loneliness: "of being alone, especially in the evening"
(Kent), of being abandoned ("feels forsaken": Kent), of having no one
to love or turn to for stability and protection. "My worst fear is going
home in the evening to a dark *empty* house," is a typical remark. The
remedy should definitely be added to the rubric "feeling of helplessness" in the Kent *Repertory.*

In the young this dependence is manifested in actual clinging: the
child hangs on to her mother's skirt in public, peeping out at the world
from this safe vantage point. Even in the home she may not venture
two steps away from the mother. "Mommy, I love you so much I am
going to follow you around all day," she pipes in her high little voice
as she trails dutifully through the entire round of daily chores. And she
cries when her mother has to leave her. Carried to an extreme (when
ill or when needing *Pulsatilla* as a constitutional remedy) she may be
virtually *glued* to her mother and refuse to be shaken off; she whimpers if her mother is out of sight or when she cannot be held.

Pulsatilla boys may appear girlish in their behavior: fearful of the
dark or of being left alone even for a moment, whining and crying
easily. Although they usually outgrow this stage, they may retain a certain softness throughout life. Some parents feel irritated by this clinging
and ask the physician if it could be changed by a remedy, but others are
quite satisfied with the child who is otherwise "good" and affectionate.

Pulsatilla's dependence does, at times, prevent her from maturing.
Her appealing childlike quality stems in part from a perceptible, almost

tangible, need for support. In her trusting helplessness she is the third of our constitutional types to retain the characteristics of a child ("of rather infantile character": Gutman). *Calcarea*, we recall, retains the child's unformed and undeveloped nature, *Phosphorus* its solipsistic tendencies and free spirit. All three contrast with the more mature constitutional types—*Sepia, Lycopodium, Lachesis*—who, even when children, occasionally seem old or sophisticated beyond their years.

An important symptom is: "first serious impairment of health begins at puberty" (Boericke), which is not surprising in view of the nature's dependence. Puberty is the first stage of true psychological emancipation from the family, which *Pulsatilla* does not seek. She trusts her omniscient parents and does not fight against them to assert her independence.

In her resistance to maturation, she acquires a host of unexplained little aches and pains: last week in the knee, yesterday in the head, today in the chest, tomorrow in the abdomen. In this way she remains reliant on her parents' support, at times even developing into something of a malingerer. Many of her later legitimate ailments, such as chronic headaches, bladder infections, allergies or painful menses, can be traced to a preadolescent or early adolescent period of inception.

In children the resistance to growing up is manifested in one relatively unusual mental symptom: the fear of looking up. Not acrophobia—the fear of looking down from a high place—which is found in many types, but vertigo or fear from looking up at anything high: mountains, tall buildings, the clouds, the sky, or a vaulted ceiling in a church—height and space presumably being associated with growth and independence.*

This symptom was once encountered in a curious adult case. A woman of thirty-five had recently conceived a dread of the skyscrapers in the city where she lived—panicking or feeling faint, losing her balance, and, unless supported, falling whenever she chanced to look skyward. It became so serious that she could not step out into the street alone. Her case history revealed that as a child she had led a sheltered life and then, at an early age, had married an authoritarian husband

---

* Other remedies (*Argentum nitricum, Phosphorus*) have the same symptom, but in the child it is most prominent in *Pulsatilla* (Borland).

(*Pulsatilla* is inclined to put herself in a position of psychological subservience). Recently, however, they had separated by mutual consent, and she was, for the first time in her life, without someone on whom to depend for emotional and other support. It required no exceptional powers to deduce that her fear of looking up was a reflection of her frightening new independence. After several doses of *Pulsatilla* 10M, however, she was able to venture forth alone into the streets, calm and unafraid.

As the child grows into adolescence, dependence begins to be directed away from the family and toward the opposite sex. *Pulsatilla* is attractive to men, being the highly feminine young woman whose whole manner flatters the ego. She is non-threatening and, in her obvious search for a supportive shoulder, makes a man feel strong and indispensable. Men instinctively want to reach out, hold, and protect her.

Time and time again, in a family of several girls, nature seems to favor the mild and self-effacing little Cinderella—the pretty *Pulsatilla* with her dependent and (albeit unconscious) male-flattering ways—with more appeal than her sisters of stronger intellect or character. Indeed, it may happen that several men are willing to protect her. Wind flower that she is, she blows this way and that, not knowing which to choose and wishing she could marry more than one. Frequently she will yield to the most persistent suitor, succumbing to the strongest will.

Since all constitutional remedies embrace their opposites, *Pulsatilla* may manifest "morbid dread of the other sex" (Boericke), "horror of opposite sex; aversion to marriage; imagines company of other sex dangerous to cultivate" (Kent)—or, in the male, "aversion to women; heart palpitations on seeing a woman; fear of women" (Kent), as well as fear of his subliminal homosexual tendencies. But, while these can be encountered, the physician more often finds that, *Pulsatilla*, responding to her simple sensual needs, is easily attracted to men. Tender-hearted and susceptible, she is quite capable of genuinely falling in love with three men in one year. In fact, if one relationship ends, she will immediately get involved in another, even if it is quite unsuitable. The gentle, widowed mother of David Copperfield, who incomprehensibly marries the odious Mr. Murdstone, and Hamlet's mother, Queen Gertrude, who, with even less reason, remarries barely a month after the death of her beloved husband, are simply evincing the typical *Pulsatilla* readiness to turn for closeness and support to the first forceful man who comes along.

This clinging affection may lead the young girl into romantic or sexual liaisons earlier than the typical *Calcarea* or *Natrum muriaticum* who, in this respect, are slower to develop. But, even if inherently flirtatious, once she has found stability in family life, she is entirely fulfilled and remains a faithful, affectionate wife and satisfied mother who enjoys having her brood around her. What the *Pulsatilla* woman basically wants in life is to get married and have children.

Such dependence on the opposite sex is no female monopoly. The man who requires the support of one, and sometimes two, strong women to get through life, is often a *Pulsatilla*. Yet women do not object to such dependence, although other men may feel irritation at the male who too obviously seeks sympathy in his personal problems, is helpless when the car breaks down, and too incompetent even to pack a few boxes in an emotionally upsetting household move. The essentially sweet nature of the son, husband, or brother brings out all their protective and maternal instincts.

Thus the *Pulsatilla* man does give something in return for the support he seeks. Like the woman, he gives affection and offers the opportunity for a warm pleasant relationship, whether as a family member, friend, colleague, or lover. There was much of this remedy, for example, in Felix Mendelssohn. Born to an easy, protected, and privileged life, he was the pet of his affectionate family and famous for his sweet disposition (reflected in the intensely lyrical quality of his music). He could get along with family, friends, and *even* fellow-musicians. Memoirs of his contemporaries attest to his invariable gentleness and absence of egoism—astounding in a composer of his magnitude and, in fact, unique among the great composers. Moreover, *three* good women cared for him throughout his life: mother, sister, and later, his wife. He was so attached to all of them that his mother's death brought on an illness that severely weakened him, while the news of his sister's death shortly afterward caused a relapse and a stroke from which his delicate constitution never recovered. He died at the early age of thirty-eight.

Many a long, happy marriage is due to one of the spouses being largely *Pulsatilla*. There is a well-known joke about marriage in which one of the partners says, "My spouse makes our marriage possible, but *I* make it worthwhile." While the speaker could easily be a *Phosphorus* or *Lycopodium*, it is the yielding nature of *Pulsatilla* which often makes marriage possible (i.e. lasting). A *Lycopodium* might claim to play a similar harmonizing role in the marriage, with the mere difference that he would not be telling the truth, while *Pulsatilla* is.

In her dependence, however, she can place severe demands on the time, solicitude and emotional reserves of friends, relatives, and acquaintances. In family, amorous, and even friendly relationships, she seeks ever more support until, at length, others feel they are captives. At first they want to reach out in compassion, with a "Poor thing, let me help you" impulse—which she allows. But with time this becomes burdensome. In her tender affection she entwines them in chains of velvet, but they are chains nonetheless, and those wishing to withdraw their support are beset by feelings of guilt. *Pulsatilla*'s need for support is so strong and real that others are reluctant to make her assume responsibility for herself, even though the protection she seeks is not necessarily in her best interests. They fear that the ivy can no longer be separated from the supporting wall without being destroyed.

In the adult this dependence may take the form of readiness to subject herself wholly to another's sway—her husband, a parent, or some other authority-figure who takes over the management of her physical and spiritual well-being ("I am *waiting* for someone to tell me what to do!") while offering maximum security. She is happy, or at least content, living in groups, communes or extended families, *sharing* her life and responsibilities with others, and is a good contributing member to her chosen community. Because she is compliant, she abides by the rules. Because she instinctively recognizes the need for tolerance and give-and-take, she readily accedes to the will of the group and lives or works harmoniously with others. This contrasts with *Phosphorus* and *Natrum muriaticum* who enter enthusiastically into group situations with which they are likely to become dissatisfied; either their enthusiasm dwindles or they quarrel with the leader or other community members. Or, sometimes, they just become restless and move on to the next thing: *Phosphorus* casts about for a new intellectual or sensory stimulus, while *Natrum muriaticum* seeks a better solution for her interminable problems.

Because of this dependence *Pulsatilla* is one of the homoeopathic types to benefit most from individual psychotherapy or group counseling. Not only is her nature receptive to guidance, but she also accepts constructive criticism, and her fundamental honesty admits to failings. Furthermore, she needs someone to listen to her woes. She feels much better after whimpering a little and shedding some tears. This remedy is not listed under the rubric "weeping ameliorates symptoms" in the Kent *Repertory* but should be there in bold type—and is found in Boger under "weeping ameliorates." After confiding in another, or pouring out her problems generally ("Having had a long heart-to-heart talk with myself—and with fifty other persons . . . "), she is restored to emotional equilibrium. Predictably, when a homoeopathic class is asked to find volunteers for practice in case-taking, a *Pulsatilla* is invariably among the first to propose herself as guinea-pig.

Although, as the texts state, she can be misanthropic, "suspicious" (Hahnemmann), "afraid of everybody; trusts no one" (Hering), our own experience suggests that the type is, for the most part, trusting, receptive (*Phosphorus*), and looking for guidance; she truly believes that others can help her, so of course they do.

In an interesting case of amenorrhoea this unequivocal trust determined the choice of *Pulsatilla* over *Natrum muriaticum*. A woman in her early thirties, following the lead of the whole female side of her family, was undergoing premature menopause: she experienced hot flashes, occasional spotting, erratic mood swings, and for several years had not had a regular period. She was also concerned about her blood-pressure, which registered in the high-normal range, and about her heart which was subject to occasional mild palpitations.

When the attending physician assured her that she need not feel overly anxious about either, her reaction was overwhelming. 'Oh, thank you for saying it!" she breathed in heartfelt relief, "You are so kind—and I am *so* relieved! Your words alone are so comforting, that my palpitations have ceased already. . . . " At which point her simillimum became apparent. One dose of *Pulsatilla* 1M and, her heredity notwithstanding, in one of those "simple, effective and lasting cures" (Hahnemann) that are the hallmark of good homoeopathic prescribing, her menses were reestablished and remained regular for many years.

But the *Pulsatilla* reliance on others can also make her cling to her illness with a hypochondria born of dependence; and to receive the support of her loved ones, she may even be subject to *sympathetic* illnesses: the mother falls ill when her child is sick, the child when a sibling is ailing, the husband when the wife is unwell. This patient does not seek primarily an effective cure, as that would put an end to the sympathy, attention, and fuss upon which she relies. She presents, for example, with a history of fleeting arthritic pains pointing to *Pulsatilla*.

The physician prescribes the remedy and says encouragingly, "I think we can clear up this problem without too much trouble. Just take these granules, keep away from coffee, and let us see you again in four weeks." Is the patient happy? Not really. She may even be dismayed by the matter-of-fact attitude. She says nothing outright but becomes hesitant, "Yes, but . . . Are you sure . . . Don't you think that maybe . . . I have heard of some doctor who . . . And what if my husband thinks it better to . . . ?" At this point the physician senses that subconsciously she is not ready to relinquish her ailment.

These patients may drift into homoeopathy and out again, even if the results have been good. Sometimes they dislike homoeopathy's infrequent prescription of remedies and encouragement of self-reliance between consultations. Even though improved, they will unexpectedly stop treatment and look for another doctor who offers more continuous emotional support. In their "anxious solicitude about health" (Hahnemann) and in instinctive avoidance of putting all their eggs in one basket (needing an extensive support system at all times) they will patronize several physicians at a time. This is done in a low-key unsystematic way and contrasts with the frantic rushing around of *Arsenicum*, the systematic doggedness of *Natrum muriaticum*, or the eagerness of *Phosphorus*.

If *Pulsatilla* drifts away from homoeopathy, she might call back a year later to say that she feels less well now than when under homoeopathic treatment. "I wish I had stayed with you. I've been thinking that I should come back." Then in a supplicating childlike way, "Will you take me back if I come?" Of course she is taken back. But, again, she might not persevere. Fluctuating in her therapeutic loyalties, she is one of the few types (the others are *Phosphorus* and *Lycopodium*) who will discard homoeopathy during obvious improvement or even after an undisputed cure.

A woman whose four-year-old daughter was cured homoeopathically of chronic upper respiratory tract and ear infections after lengthy and unsuccessful allopathic treatment, returned the following winter to her original pediatrician. When asked why she was again subjecting her daughter to antibiotics she said, "Yes, homoeopathy made her better, but remember we also changed her diet at the same time and took her off milk, which might have had something to do with it . . . Or maybe she was beginning to outgrow the stage of childhood infections, as the pediatrician said would happen." When it was pointed out that despite these reasons her daughter was again taking antibiotics, she said, "Oh, yes, but it is only the second time this year, and we are already at the end of March. And actually, she *did* need *Belladonna* a few times last winter; I don't want her to become dependent on *Belladonna* any more than on antibiotics. . . . " Perhaps the real problem was that the previous winter she had received less sympathy and attention from family, friends, and neighbors with her daughter well than earlier with her daughter ill. As she had no other reason to call upon others for assistance (*Pulsatilla* is truthful and will not invent troubles as an attention-getting device), she preferred the original situation: a sick child with a legitimate claim to sympathy. While this behavior was extreme, even for *Pulsatilla*, many of these patients cleave to their ailments as a way of eliciting emotional support from others.

Finally, the dependent *Pulsatilla* relies heavily on sympathetic approval. Sometimes a dull child needs only to be praised to bring out its underlying brightness and liveliness. Where other constitutional types thrive on obstacles (*Sulphur*, *Lycopodium*), criticism (*Nux vomica*), challenges (*Natrum muriaticum*), strict discipline (*Arsenicum*), and systematic guided instruction (*Calcarea carbonica*), the *Pulsatilla* child and adult blossoms only under continuous encouragement. She even needs others to give shape and form to her opinions, being submissive, easily influenced, and forever fluctuating in her ideas and feelings ("has a great many but vacillating ideas in [her] head": Hahnemann). This is observed in the college student who cannot decide on a major subject and makes up her mind at the last minute depending on which professor she likes at the moment or which has the most inspiring personality. *Pulsatilla* does not trust her own intellectual capacities and lacks confidence in her own judgment. Whatever her innate abilities, she derives security from the convictions and assurance of others.

Companionability

This introduces the third prominent characteristic of *Pulsatilla* — *companionability*. She is inherently friendly and well-disposed toward others. She does not assert herself or impose her ideas on people but prefers to empathize with them, entering easily into all details of their lives, and is always delighted to hear of their children, homes, health and hobbies. After the initial shyness ("bashful disposition": Hering) she relates naturally and effortlessly, making others feel comfortable in her accepting presence (*Phosphorus*). *Sulphur* (although the style is different) is often her male counterpart in sociability, amassing friends and acquaintances as all-inclusively as he collects stamps, coins, and other objects.

The importance of relationships to *Pulsatilla* can be seen during the consultation when she is asked what she would do with a week of free time, if money was no object. She will often express the wish just to visit friends and then search around for something else she would like to do. This is not true of other constitutional types whose responses will vary from a desire to travel and see new places (*Tuberculinum*), go on a shopping spree for clothes (*Lachesis*), spend evenings at the opera or theatre (*Phosphorus*), backpack with a close friend or rent a vacation cottage with her family (*Natrum muriaticum*), just stay at home and *finally* have time to work on his music, painting or writing (*Arsenicum*), spend the time at the seaside (*Medorrhinum*), or bury himself for a week in the Library of Congress (the scholarly *Sulphur*).*

Pulsatilla loves companionship of all kinds: the young and the old, the boring and the amusing, the difficult and the serene, the greedy and the generous. Nor does she relate only to people. She delights in caring for animals, birds, fish and plants—since they all provide companionship.

A five-year-old boy came to the physician for chronic earaches. He was a rambunctious, husky little fellow with nothing of *Pulsatilla* in his looks or outward manner—these boys being usually fair, slender and gentle. So we were surprised to hear from the mother that he defended the very young children at the playground, being known as their "guardian angel" and performing these duties between turns at bat or during pauses in games of kick-ball. If any youngster was teased or mistreated, tears would well up in the boy's eyes and, though he would not fight (*Pulsatilla* children avoid physical skirmishes), for the rest of

---

* These distinctions, of course, are not always clearcut. Many types will add to their primary desire an inclination to visit friends in the evenings (the non-bookish *Sulphur*, for instance, will want to go on an energetic outing or engage in some exciting activity with a group of friends). Man is nothing if not a social creature; *Pulsatilla* in her dependence is just more overtly so.

the day he would hover protectively over the offended party, guarding him from future harm. This symptom suggested *Pulsatilla* which successfully cleared up his ear condition. Parenthetically, if he had been more of a *Sulphur* (as he at first appeared, and which was, indeed, his second remedy), he would have turned red and heated and engaged the offender in a fight, or at least have chased him around the block.

This boy was in no way soft or girlish. He just had the *Pulsatilla* desire to care for smaller, weaker creatures. While this trait is, understandably, found more frequently in girls (who will spend hours caring for their dolls), many a boy doubtless suppresses this aspect of his nature for fear of being considered a sissy. Thus, in any boy who obviously enjoys the company of younger children, or who easily assumes the mother's patient and gentle role in caring for them, *Pulsatilla* is a possible remedy, even if he is otherwise swarthy, robust, and tough.

Pulsatilla's talent for relating to others is undeniably a virtue and a strength. But her yielding disposition and refusal to quarrel have a pragmatic motivation. She has taken pains to cultivate a network of friends upon whom to lean in times of stress; she needs to know that they are *there*, always ready to respond when she calls on the telephone or comes pleading for help and to cry on a friendly shoulder. Thus discord is to be avoided, as it would cut her off from some part of this extensive support system. The childlike quality mentioned earlier as arising partly from dependence can also reflect her instinctive companionability. Maturity, both of understanding and in dealing with problems, usually results from being *alone* at some time in life. By avoiding this prerequisite of maturity she retards the process. But life itself, the great teacher, sometimes takes care of this. The fully self-reliant, independent *Pulsatilla* has usually been forced to spend some time alone, enduring homesickness at boarding school or college, early loss of, or separation from, a parent, a solitary childhood, or some lengthy illness. Having been tested, as it were, she is no longer childlike but may still retain the child's essential sweetness and trust. The homoeopathic remedies perform an equivalent strengthening and maturing role, helping the companionable *Pulsatilla* to be less dependent on others.

Sociability in conversation is one way to spot the type. While less imaginative than *Phosphorus*, she exhibits the same communicativeness or chattiness without undue aggressiveness. She has a naturally civilized manner and an instinctive sense when to talk and when to listen. Occasionally, however, she may go on and on about something, in a non-compelling but insistent fashion, and be hard to divert from her "whims and notions" (Kent). In the physician's office she is apt to keep returning to some one small symptom that is particularly bothering her. Where her health is concerned, she does not distinguish between the important and the unimportant. Everything is of equal significance.

In homoeopathy the most severe or painful symptoms are not necessarily the main criteria for selecting the remedy. The fleeting and apparently inconsequential symptoms are often more important than striking, constant, and painful ones. In asthma for instance, itching of the chin preceding the attack is far more valuable for finding the remedy than the accompanying severe incapacity to breathe. *Pulsatilla* easily discerns these important "strange, rare and peculiar" symptoms for which the prescriber is always searching.* "Yes, doctor, my tongue feels too big for my mouth, are you sure [opening her mouth wide] that it is not broader than usual?" was the guiding symptom to the medicine in a stubborn eczema of the hands and arms where the physician could otherwise find no idiosyncratic symptoms.

Many of these guiding symptoms are found in the section "Sensations" in Hering, where he lists some two hundred, including more common ones as, "sensation . . . as if head between screws; as if ear would burst on sneezing; as if tongue were scalded," and such unusual ones as; "as if cold water were poured down the back; as if roof of palate were covered with tenacious mucus or were swollen; as if worm were creeping up into throat."

Usually this patient can hardly be restrained in the recounting of symptoms. With her trusting nature, she applies literally the injunction to tell the homoeopath *everything* about herself, sometimes in startlingly intimate detail. This characteristic is found especially in the younger generation which likes nothing better than to let everything "hang out." But even dignified elderly persons can exhibit this same childlike artlessness in recounting symptoms that bears witness to their *Pulsatilla* natures.

---

* "The more striking, singular, uncommon, and peculiar (characteristic) signs and symptoms of the case of the disease are chiefly and most solely to be kept in view" (Hahnemann, *Organon of Medicine*, Section 153).

A number of constitutional types evince a similar thoroughness, not to say self-indulgence, in relating symptoms, but each has its own particular way of presenting them. *Pulsatilla*'s style is one of friendly non-compelling communicativeness which always remains highly personal.

For instance, she might describe an arthritic pain as "a painful stiffness in the right knee, with occasional shooting pains which are more severe when the leg is stretched out straight or if I haven't moved it for some time," adding, "Oh, I do so hope you will be able to help me! . . . " whereas the scholarly *Sulphur* will present the same condition as, "The examination of my right knee in multiple X-ray views shows moderate osteoarthritic changes involving the entire knee joint; more so in the medial compartment, the doctor said, and lower femoral-patellar articulation . . . " Both *Pulsatilla* and *Sulphur* contrast with *Arsenicum*'s style, which incorporates both technical and personal descriptions. Even though the latter might be as scientifically informed as *Sulphur* and will also refer to a previous physician's authority, he is less impersonal in his wording. At the same time, *Arsenicum* is more critical and aggressive than *Pulsatilla*. "I have this violent arthritic pain in the right knee joint, which at night becomes completely intolerable, as if I had been bruised or beaten. . . . The last doctor I went to said—for whatever his opinion is worth—that there was no trace of swelling or effusion, but the tearing pain that accompanies the osteoarthritic stiffness . . ." Some *Natrum muriaticum* patients manifest stoic reserve; others describe their physical symptoms to the accompaniment of an extraordinary emotional exposé. *Sepia*'s style can be dreary and complaining, that of *Nux vomica* and the garrulous *Lachesis* driving and forceful, *Calcarea*'s accurate with an occasional note of hopelessness, *Lycopodium*'s detached throughout, begrudging the revelation of each symptom, except when he panics, and then his anxiety resembles that of *Arsenicum*. *Phosphorus* adopts a personal tone, like *Pulsatilla*, and also enjoys describing her symptoms, but she makes lively what *Pulsatilla* makes lengthy, e.g., "My entire right knee feels as if a thousand little demons with red-hot pincers were pricking away at me—for my multiple sins, I guess. And if I stir as much as an iota, they redouble their efforts—this time with hot pokers . . . " (see the relevant chapters for more on this topic).

Furthermore, her companionability may inhibit *Pulsatilla* from ending the interview and leaving the doctor's office. She would love to prolong the visit and talk about her family, her vacation plans, her strange dreams, and so on. She is also one of the constitutional types that calls the physician soon after the office visit to inquire with gentle apprehension, "Do you think you will *really* be able to help my condition?" or "Yesterday I felt a slight nausea after eating some fried fish for dinner—is this natural?" (*Pulsatilla* should avoid fatty, rich, or fried foods, which her digestion tolerates poorly; and if she eats too much or too late in the evening, she will sleep badly or have insomnia). Here again, her style is different from that of the other types who are most likely to call back—*Arsenicum* and *Natrum muriaticum*. *Pulsatilla* seeks encouragement and a closer rapport with the doctor; the other two, while also seeking reassurance, are full of pressing anxiety because they forgot some "important" symptom the doctor *must* know or fear that they misunderstood some essential instruction. *Sulphur* may call back in a couple of weeks with a methodical enumeration of symptoms, "laundry-list" style.

At the other end of the *Pulsatilla* spectrum is the patient who constantly fluctuates in her sense of well-being and is inordinately wishy-washy in describing her state of health. Her account is so confusing that, even after an hour, the physician feels he is getting nowhere. She cannot give accurate symptoms, cannot specify whether or not there has been improvement, and contradicts herself from one moment to the next. When asked how she is doing, she may reply, "I am not sure; I am both better *and* worse—I can't describe it . . . I can't really tell how I feel—How much better *should* I feel to say 'better'?" (this attitude matches the nature of *Pulsatilla*'s physical symptoms: nonspecific indefinite pains that come and go). Yet the prescriber may observe a marked improvement despite the patient's inability to do so.

Flexibility

Pulsatilla's fourth characteristic is *flexibility*, which she manifests in two different ways: through indecisiveness and through adaptability. Hahnemann wrote of the former, "little suited for persons who form their resolutions with rapidity"—an understated way of describing *Pulsatilla*'s chronic *irresoluteness*. Like the meadow anemone which is swayed by every passing breeze, the individual blows one way and another, revealing a habitual inability to make up her mind on matters both large and small. Even when she does decide, she has trouble abiding by her decisions ("changeable, variable": Kent) and is generally fatigued and unnerved by the daily alternatives which life presents.

In choosing which flavor of ice cream, which Matchbox car, or which doll to buy, the child undergoes agonies of indecision, at length crying out in anguish, "Why must I choose only *one?*" To resolve this interminable vacillation the adult may relent and, at the cost of fairness to the other children, provide *Pulsatilla* with more than one. In the physician's office the girl who loves sweets is hard-pressed to say what form of these she prefers. And when the child is really in need of the remedy, changeableness turns into caprice ("child longs for this, now for that, even with good humor": Hering).

Pulsatilla's irresoluteness is seen also in the child who cannot get down to the next day's homework, less from laziness than from extreme "hesitancy" (Hahnemann): which subject should be done first — math or history, English or French? She sees reasons for and against each one and ends by studying none of them unless firmly commanded, "Begin with math." Then she starts work obediently, almost gratefully. Not to be ignored, however, in a child's reluctance to do homework are the *Pulsatilla* symptoms, "headache of schoolgirls" (Kent), "mental work fatigues" (Hering), and particularly, "more indisposed to mental work in the evening than at other times of day" (Hahnemann). It may be recalled that the remedy has strongly accentuated evening aggravation of mental as well as physical symptoms.

With her docile, tractable nature, disliking to make decisions and changing them when she does, uncertain of what she wants and hesitating about what to do, *Pulsatilla* regularly gives the impression of responding to the will of others rather than controlling her own life ("easily led and easily persuaded": Kent). For instance, a seventeen-year-old patient who was accepted into two of the best colleges in the country could not make up her mind which to attend. She weighed and agonized, decided and reconsidered, until on the last day acceptances were due she begged her parents to decide for her. Another young patient of irresolute disposition was invited by two young men to the Senior Prom. Wavering tearfully over which to accept, she resorted to the unusual, but not uncharacteristic of the type, solution of turning them *both* down. In an effort to use the remedy preventively, the following spring a dose of *Pulsatilla* 10M was prescribed a month before the dance. When four invitations came in, she was forearmed. Although there was the usual dismay ("The boys are *all* so nice!"), she sensibly decided to accept the one who had asked first.

Kindness is a factor in *Pulsatilla*'s indecision: she does not want to hurt or offend the rejected party — whether it be a young man inviting her to the prom or a college entrance committee. In a boy or young man it is, surprisingly, the "benevolent" *Sulphur* who will pass up a school dance rather than have to decide which of several girls to invite and thereby offend the others.

Sometimes she continues her "vacillation" (Boenninghausen) between two men long after marriage. Even the one who has chosen correctly may wonder about her selection ten or fifteen years later. She equivocates less out of regret (*Pulsatilla* does not regret) than out of her capacity still to respond to the other emotionally. Occasionally her old vacillation surfaces in a strong internal cry of, "Why couldn't I have had both?"

In daily life her equivocation becomes readily apparent, for example, in a shopping expedition. She handles twenty apparently identical peaches, turning each one over in her hand, before picking four. Or, after spending an inordinate amount of time weighing the merits of different styles of wine glasses, she will ask the salesman, "Which ones should I buy — the short sturdy ones or the taller ones?" The experienced salesman, who is accustomed to *Pulsatilla* shoppers, will confidently pick one style and proffer a convincing reason for it. Sometimes she takes the advice, sometimes she does the opposite. But at least she makes a choice, stimulated by the voice of authority. For a long time afterward, however, she will question the wisdom of her decision. Something in her nature simply hates that final commitment to purchase.

The same happens in a restaurant where *Pulsatilla* must choose from a list of tempting dishes. Menus bring out the worst in her, as she not only takes a long time deciding, but, having decided, invariably changes her mind several times. Here again it is better that someone else order for her, and she will generally be both relieved and satisfied: she is happy to be persuaded by another.

Arsenicum might handle the same number of peaches, examine as many different styles of glasses, and deliberate as closely over the dishes on the menu, but she will do it efficiently. She knows what she wants and does not seek another's advice. Furthermore, *Arsenicum* might spend the whole day looking for a particular scarf without finding anything that is *exactly* right. *Pulsatilla* is different: she finds several scarves that are right, but inclines first to one, then to another. Her vacillating nature is also revealed in games. She can be a menace at the bridge table. In a game where hesitation over which card to play betrays your hand to the opposition, the gentle and well-meaning woman gives her partner apoplexy. This surprises her since she plays mainly for the companionship and pleasant conversation, rarely manifesting a strong spirit of competition or determination to win. Another game not for her is chess — altogether too cerebral and asocial, demanding repeated hard decisions.*

William James wrote in his *Psychology*, "There is no more miserable human being than one to whom nothing is habitual but indecision." This is by no means true. That is a *Phosphorus/Sulphur* male speaking, who cannot imagine the pleasurable agony derived by a female *Pulsatilla* from vacillation per se. It is the same delicious feeling that *Phosphorus* derives from abandonment, *Natrum muriaticum* from discharging a moral duty, and *Arsenicum* from excessive zeal.

Her irresolution is sometimes reminiscent of Buridan's hypothetical ass in medieval philosophy: finding himself equidistant from two sheaves of hay of equal size, he remains rooted to the spot undecided which one to eat, and ultimately dies (poor thing!) of starvation. Similarly, the irresolute *Pulsatilla* finds no reason to choose one college, one ice cream flavor, one suitor over another. She sees virtues in all of them. But, fortunately, she does not starve. The human *Pulsatilla* can, and *does*, voice her dilemma in a way that the mute jackass could not do, and someone invariably turns up to help her.

Indeed, she may happily go through life trusting to another's judgment to resolve her equivocations. Complete and unhesitating trust obviates the need to assume responsibility. In this she differs from *Phosphorus* or *Natrum muriaticum* who choose for themselves from intuition or impulse. It may be the wrong impulse or an erratic intuition, but they are not afraid to plunge in. *Pulsatilla* differs also from *Sulphur* and *Arsenicum* who generally know exactly what they want of life and

---

* A notable exception here, however, was a *Pulsatilla* patient being treated for hay fever who loved playing chess by correspondence with persons in other countries. He could spend days deliberating the next move and additional weeks agonizing over what response to give to potential moves by his adversary. A good game, he stated with relish, could last well over a year (the other side of him was *Calcarea carbonica*).

set out in a beeline to obtain it; also from *Calcarea* and *Lycopodium* who are less aggressive in acquiring what they want but equally certain of their needs at the moment. Of the polychrests discussed in this volume only *Sepia* and *Lachesis* can be as irresolute, but their indecisiveness is sporadic and acute, taking the form of sudden loss of confidence and inability to take the initiative on some big issue. *Pulsatilla*'s indecisiveness is chronic—sometimes more obvious, sometimes less so, but always there.

This trait is generally less overt in men, but the following example shows how it is revealed in the male. A physician wanted to open a homoeopathic practice but could not make himself take the final step. He had studied the discipline in books, attended lectures and seminars, and was quite convinced of the doctrine's efficacy. Yet he continued to waver: "Should I or shouldn't I? When would be the best time? Where is the best location to set up practice? Why should I not continue with what I am doing for a while longer?" He could see the pros and cons of every alternative and vacillated for over two years, before a dose of *Pulsatilla* 50M gave him the necessary nudge. Within a few months he opened his practice.*

Pulsatilla may also be chronically unable to say "No." Her indecisiveness causes her to act against her better judgment, or acquiesce in moves which experience should have taught her to avoid. Thus she finds herself *reacting* in life, rather than actively taking decisions and following them through. Repeatedly, however, patients helped by the remedy state that they feel more confident about issues and definite in their ideas, more in control of their lives, less emotionally dependent, and better able to reach decisions.

One variant of the indecisive type is worth mentioning: the individual who is forever equivocating and asking for guidance but who, in fact, is seldom influenced by the advice so assiduously sought ("sometimes he wants to do one thing, sometimes another, and when he is given something to do, he will not do it": Hahnemann). Advising a

---

* And a notable veterinary case was the champion jumper who suddenly began refusing certain jumps in competition. His rider could never tell beforehand whether the horse would jump or balk. He was not a timid horse, merely indecisive, and a dose of *Pulsatilla* in high potency restored him to his former championship level.

Pulsatilla can be likened to prodding an amoeba: it appears to yield but then lapses again into a fluctuating but obstinate formlessness.

This trait can be seen in the patient who (the mirror image of *Pulsatilla*'s usual flexibility) harbors a "bee in her bonnet" — some irrational fear or conviction from which she cannot be budged despite all evidence to the contrary (the mother who was determined that her child should not become dependent on *Belladonna* was manifesting this arbitrary determination to hang on to such a notion). *Pulsatilla* listens, does not argue, smiles, appears to be persuaded, but refuses to yield an inch where her feelings are concerned. Quite often these whims are centered on health, particularly (as Kent notes) on matters of diet. She conceives the idea that some basically innocuous food such as eggs, cottage cheese, cantaloupe or peanut butter is unfit for human consumption, and *nothing* will deter her from this conviction. Arguing against these convictions can be like trying to make her change her religion.

One mother would not allow her three-year-old son to eat any dairy product. Although he was sickly and nervous, with poor bone structure, she insisted that nothing made from cow's milk could be a "natural" food for a child. This anti-dairy attitude is justified in some cases and is to be respected when applied consistently. Unfortunately, this mother allowed her son to indulge in ice-cream *ad libitum*, claiming that it provided him with the necessary calcium and other minerals (it was hard to discern the logic in all this). After treatment with *Pulsatilla*, however, she relinquished this irrational notion and allowed her now healthier child to eat wholesome dairy products.

Thus, even the irresolute *Pulsatilla*, when convinced she is right, can display a sweet but tenacious determination which, like the stubbornness of *Calcarea*, is sometimes harder to move than the passion of *Lachesis*, the anger of *Natrum muriaticum*, the argumentativeness of *Sulphur*, or the strong and uncompromising opinions of *Arsenicum*.

A corollary of *Pulsatilla*'s indecisiveness is her attractive *adaptibility*. There is little heaviness or pedantry in her nature. She manifests emotional suppleness in her ability to detect nuances of feeling and to sense niceties of thought without needing to have them elucidated. Furthermore, she is remarkably non-judgmental and demonstrates this openness in her aforementioned sympathetic tolerance of all kinds of people and life-styles. This is frequently reflected in her *nil nisi bonum* attitude—that is, she will find something nice to say of a person or say nothing at all. She is one of the least critical of constitutional types.

By not making hard and fast judgments she remains flexible in her relations with others. In difficult or deteriorating relationships, when unable to decide what to do, she lets things ride and trusts that they will straighten out. Indeed, they often do, thus vindicating her passive approach. In this way *Pulsatilla* may fare better than those who quarrel in haste and break in heat, then repent at leisure. The same is true of other stressful situations in life. Her adaptibility enables her to drift with the tide and adapt to cross-currents, instead of fighting them, as more assertive and independent natures are apt to do.

Intellectual and emotional flexibility are also reflected in *Pulsatilla*'s range of taste. She is a great appreciator of all the various art forms, from the classical composers and painters down to pottery, handicrafts and macramé. Receptive to the merits of all, she responds to each in the same openminded way.

When asked what is her favorite art form—whether music, the visual arts, or literature—she will reply, "I like them all," and even be astonished by the question. How can one art form be preferred to another? If asked whether she prefers classical or romantic music, she will give the same somewhat perplexed answer: "Why, I like them both!" She is quite different from the intellectually critical types who have strong likes and dislikes; an art form either coincides with their particular preferences or it does not.* *Pulsatilla* tunes in to all artistic wave lengths—however different they may be from her own. Adapting to the mood of another, she easily relates to any artist's vision.

This is not to suggest that she is indiscriminate. She has inherent good taste, as is evident in her naturally ladylike manner. Her house is cozy and attractive, with plants and pictures and cheerful color schemes which combine in an overall impression of unostentatious taste. The

---

* Here, again, the distinctions can be blurred. Sometimes *Pulsatilla* will express a definite preference, while the more critical *Arsenicum*, *Sulphur*, or *Lycopodium* will claim to appreciate everything. On closer examination, however, these latter are found to harbor a dislike for some particular genre or art form (chamber music, ballet, etc.) or to evince definite gradations in their catholic tastes: "I appreciate all the great painters, but, whereas a few years back I went through a French impressionist stage, now I am beginning to prize the early Italian schools."

same is true of her dress: not necessarily elegant, nor showy, nor in the latest fashion, but "tasteful."

As a creative artist she is generally drawn to the lyrical, not the epic, and creates refined, gem-like works, a splendid example of which is Virginia Woolf's novel, *Mrs. Dalloway*. The whole flow of this tightly-knit and emotionally homogeneous novel's chain of associations has a *Pulsatilla* hue, as the reader lives through the sights and sounds of a day in London, weaving in and out of the minds and feelings of the small group of characters around whom it revolves. Particularly Mrs. Clarissa Dalloway herself, as revealed in her stream of consciousness, is the very embodiment of the type. She must be around people on whose good opinion she depends and on whose companionship she thrives. Acutely sensitive to what others are thinking or feeling, she responds with sympathy and kindness to everyone—her family, acquaintances, servants, and even strangers (a sales girl in a flower store)—wanting them all to be happy so that she can be happy herself. By the same token, she selfishly rejects any intrusive misery (as in the person of her daughter's resentful and pathetically unattractive tutor) which threatens her comfortable, civilized life—and even more her carefully cultivated serenity.

In true *Pulsatilla* fashion, she appreciates the passionate impulses, mercurial nature, and ironic mind of her rejected suitor, the *Phosphorus* Peter Walsh, no less than the emotional delicacy, integrity, and sense of service of her reserved *Natrum muriaticum* husband. Thus she remains reliant on the affection and approval of both. Further, in her finely fluctuating moods, Mrs. Dalloway responds with sensitivity to all external impressions: the sky, the flowers, the sound of a clock striking the hour, the sight of a billowing curtain—all of which strengthen the central *Pulsatilla* ambiance of the novel.

Emotionalism

Pulsatilla's fifth characteristic, *emotionalism*, is marked by fluctuation, self-pity and sentimentality. While less delicately balanced and less impressionable than *Phosphorus*, *Pulsatilla* shares some of the latter's fears: of the dark, of being alone, of not being loved, of illness, of impending domestic troubles. As befits a sensitive type, she may lie awake at night from worry, with some *one* idea running through her mind (*Calcarea*), then awaken in the morning tired and unrefreshed. In fact, the remedy's second emotional low point of the day (the first being the evening aggravation) is in the morning: "very discontented, weeps a long time in the morning after waking from sleep; solicitude about domestic concerns in the morning; anxiety after waking," (Hahnemann).

Pulsatilla has been aptly called the "weathercock among remedies" (Boericke) due to her *fluctuating*, readily swayed nature and her changeable, sometimes "whimsical" (Hahnemann) or "capricious" (Hering) moods. Passive one moment, lively the next, well one hour, miserable the next, she is "easily moved to laughter and tears" (Hering). She can switch from smiling to weeping and back again in rapid succession, or even indulge in both simultaneously (*Ignatia*).

Her "lachrymose disposition" (Hahnemann) is there for all to see. In the physician's office tears gather readily in her eyes, and she lets them fall freely while narrating her troubles ("weeping on telling symptoms": Kent). This is not *Natrum muriaticum*'s reluctant breakdown, with uncontrollable sobbing in spite of all efforts at self-restraint. Nor is it the weeping from rage, anger, or resentment of *Arsenicum, Lachesis*, and (again) *Natrum muriaticum*. *Pulsatilla* is inclined to a gentler kind of weeping, the "mild, submissive form of grieving" (Hering) of a non-combative nature. Less frequently encountered, yet not to be ignored, is her "tendency to inward and silent grief" (Hahnemann).

An exhibition of the nature's gentle emotionalism was encountered in the case of a mother and father, both affectionate and caring parents, who came to the office to discuss the problem of their young son—repeatedly reprimanded by his teacher for classroom misbehavior. As sometimes happens with children of timid parents, he was surprisingly aggressive toward his peers and teacher—ironically confirming Jung's contention that the greatest influence on a child is the unlived life of the parents. Both father and mother had tears in their eyes when discussing the teacher's reprimand (nothing more serious) of their son. In similar circumstances other constitutional types might argue, display anger, ignore the charge or disclaim it, change teachers, or even sensibly strive to improve the child's behavior. But to weep—that was *Pulsatilla.*

She may even effectively use her tears as a disarming strategy, whether consciously or unconsciously. In a domestic quarrel, for instance, she will burst into tears and accept all the blame. "Yes, it is all my fault. I know I'm in the wrong, as always. I can't do anything right—Oh, I'm hopeless!'' All this leaves her adversary with little to do but reassure her that she is not alone to blame, etc.

Ruled by her sensibilities, *Pulsatilla* is essentially non-intellectual. Of course, as with any constitutional type, some are more and some less intelligent, but she generally operates in a highly personal and non-intellectual mode. Mrs. Dalloway, for instance, could not remember whether her husband was on a committee to help the Albanians or the Armenians; they were all the same to her (reminiscent of Disraeli's wife, another *Pulsatilla*, who claimed she never *could* remember who came first, the Greeks or the Romans). What is in question here is the governing principle of the individual's nature, its dominant aspect. Following Jung's classification of the human personality into the four types—sensory, intellectual, emotional, and intuitive—*Pulsatilla* falls squarely, and *Natrum muriaticum* largely, into the emotional category, just as *Phosphorus* is primarily intuitive, while *Lycopodium* or *Sulphur* are intellectual.

Pulsatilla is not interested in facts, statistics, scholarly ideas or theories. Her mind feels more comfortable dealing with the *particulars* of everyday life and human relations. Her indecisiveness, dependence, and non-authoritarian nature lead her, as has already been noted, to be *receptive* to the ideas of others rather than intellectually assertive. The mentality is subtle rather than independent. At best, it is open, supple, and exquisitely sensitive. At worst, it is mundane, with a tendency to expound platitudes. Between the two extremes the average mind possesses socially acceptable ideas and a pleasant and appreciative outlook. Possibly she lacks something in originality.

In conversation she seeks above all to establish a pleasant and comfortable rapport (*Phosphorus*); the intellectual content, the factual information exchanged, can be of secondary concern. Influenced by her emotions, she systematically interprets abstractions and generalities in personal terms—in the light of her own thoughts, feelings, or preferences.

If someone mentions the increased violence in the world, she will remark that, indeed, her Jenny was being increasingly picked on by playmates in the park. Or, discussing the relative merits of boarding versus day school, she will comment, "I would never send *my* son to boarding school. He is not the kind of boy who needs it. Besides, I feel we have too much to offer him here at home."* *Phosphorus* also has a tendency to interpret the objective in subjective terms. Unlike the more conventional *Pulsatilla*, however, she does this with amusing or imaginative observations which, even though reductional, throw light on the subject under discussion.

In all spheres, then—religious, political, or social—*Pulsatilla* tends to bring larger issues down to the subjective level. Her religious feeling, for example, may contain relatively little intellectual or moral questing. With her, religion primarily satisfies an aesthetic-emotional need. She goes to a religious service to pray a little, listen to beautiful music and words in attractive surroundings, and afterwards meet her friends. Religion is just another of the supports that her nature requires.

The other side of this picture, found far less frequently and therefore requiring no elaboration, is described in the materia medicas as religious mania: "with fixed religious notions and misapplications of the Scriptures" (Kent); "with pangs of conscience" (often related to his or her sexuality) or "despairing of the soul's salvation" (Hering). Here she overlaps with *Sulphur* in the male and with *Lachesis* in the female (see those chapters). In such cases the latter two remedies may complement and complete *Pulsatilla*'s curative action.

Pulsatilla's emotionalism can be manifested in a tendency to *self pity*, from the mildest form to the most severe.

The self-pitying note can even be detected in the tone of a baby's cry. It is distinctly plaintive and differs from the angry yell of a *Sulphur* or *Calcarea* baby, as well as from the irritable cry of *Chamomilla*. As Kent points out, the snarling cry of *Chamomilla* makes one want to spank the child, while the pitiful cry of *Pulsatilla* makes one want to

---

* During a college course discussion of Ophelia's character and enigmatic role in Shakespeare's play, a typically *Pulsatilla* girl, pretty, sweet-mannered, gentle-voiced, raised her hand and volunteered, "I can *really* relate to Ophelia."

"Yes," the instructor inquired encouragingly, eager to draw out the hitherto silent, shy girl's ideas, "in what way?"

"Well, my last boyfriend was *exactly* like Hamlet! Let me tell you how he. . . . " She then went on to describe their relationship in such intimate terms that the instructor wished he had not asked.

comfort and caress it.

Later the child may become a crybaby who "whimpers" (Boenning-hausen) and whines a lot, or wails piteously from the smallest scratch—not so much from pain as from self-pity and a desire to be bandaged, kissed, and fussed over. The slightly older child is "easily discouraged" (Hering), feels insufficiently liked, is wounded by teasing, and resorts to gentle tears whenever crossed or reprimanded.

Pulsatilla self-pity is seen in the touchiness of adolescents who are offended when someone looks at them the wrong way and imagine that others are talking or laughing at them behind their backs: "afraid of everybody; considers everyone her enemy" (Hering); also in the young girl who, seeking to arouse sympathy in the listener, weeps while recounting the problems of her social life: that she has no friends and that nobody likes her. The same touchiness is also found in the adult: "weeps when interrupted (!); imagines being slighted or fears she will be slighted" (Kent), "takes in bad part what others say" (Hahnemann). Nursing her ailments and bewailing the world's hardness and inability to appreciate her misery, she can absorb an unlimited amount of comforting and coddling.

At times her very voice connotes self-pity. The sweet and slightly imploring, "Will you help me?—I do *so* need support" announces this constitutional type even over the telephone. Once recognized, this special *pleading* or *plaintive*, even *beseeching*, inflection is hard to miss, being as distinctive as the handshake of *Calcarea* or *Arsenicum*, or the eyes of *Phosphorus* or *Natrum muriaticum*.

Her self-pity may lead *Pulsatilla* to be offended in a situation where another would laugh. Perceptive patients, aware of this sensitivity, have asked the physician, "Please give me more of my constitutional remedy. This last month I have been finding myself strangely low. There is no humor in the air, nothing but clouds and tears, and I constantly feel offended at my husband's or children's teasings and jokes." Later, after receiving *Pulsatilla*, they will say, "I took the remedy and within a day everything changed. Or rather, nothing changed but my attitude toward it. I now find the world entertaining instead of hurting or sad."

The following case recapitulates several prominent *Pulsatilla* characteristics, including this last one. A patient was describing his wife's tendency to offer (in her own indecision) a bewildering variety of choices to guests at dinner-parties: "Would you like your vegetables now or later? And what about salad—on a separate plate from the meat or the same? Should I put gravy on your potatoes, or do you want to take some yourself? . . . " The incident was recounted humorously and not unkindly, but the wife was hurt and remonstrated plaintively, "I was only trying to make everyone happy, to give them just what they wanted. . . . " "But people don't *want* so many choices," the husband persisted. "They prefer to be served food on their plates and not to have to make endless decisions whether to take coffee or sanka, regular or herbal tea, plain or vegetable salt. Just give them something, and most of them will be happy—or *should* be at any rate!" "Oh," *Pulsatilla* mewed. "I guess I *never* will be able to get things right. But I *do* try. And if you would only help me instead of always criticizing, it would be so much easier . . . "

A subliminal self-pity may emerge in subsequent visits to the physician; in an unconscious desire to hang onto her illness *Pulsatilla* eagerly describes what is still amiss. Characteristically these patients *first* tell their little aches and pains to evoke the physician's sympathy; only at the end of the interview do they describe their overall improvement. Some will even reiterate at length how poorly they felt *prior* to the prescription, instead of focussing on how much better they feel now. The physician might be tempted to conclude that he gave the wrong remedy until he asks outright if the chief complaint has improved. One strongly *Pulsatilla* patient who had been regularly hospitalized for severe ulcers of the mouth called two weeks after the homoeopathic prescription to complain about low-grade influenza symptoms which had just started to appear. The physician had to inquire specifically about her mouth to discover that it was entirely free of canker sores for the first time in years.

When reporting progress, the hypochondriacal *Pulsatilla* regularly inserts little "buts" to qualify the unmistakable improvement she at the same time readily and gratefully admits. A woman, responding to the physician's solicitude about her progress, will reply brightly, "No, I haven't had any problems with my periods for two months now," then adds with a little sigh, "but I am *still* worried about the bland discharge in the morning from the inside corner of my right eye. Do you have any idea what it might be?" Or a male patient will say, "Yes, I think [note the "I think"] my prostate condition is better. I have no more difficulty urinating, and my bladder control has returned. But one thing that has been bothering me is this pimple, here on my cheek. See?— Oh, its almost gone! Hmmm . . . imagine that! But I had this spot . . . " and he then proceeds, in a plaintive tone, to describe in detail his erstwhile pimple. It is appropriate to mention here that, just as *Pulsatilla* is of frequent service in "female complaints"—pregnancy, labor, menses and premenstrual symptoms, the hormonal imbalances of menopause, lactation, breast conditions, and in a variety of urinary problems, ranging from tendency to cystitis (involving less burning, pain, or discomfort than in the typical *Cantharis* episode) to a weak bladder with spurting of urine when coughing, sneezing or laughing—so it should not be overlooked as one of the best remedies in complaints of the male genital (particularly affecting the prostate, spermatic cord and testes: Boger) and urinary organs (see the classic texts).

Sometimes in chronic illness of the *Pulsatilla* patient the telltale thread of self-pity can be traced through the entire warp and woof of the case. A thirty-year old woman of gentle and sympathetic nature had a long-standing colitis of such severity as to require strong doses of corticosteroids for a number of years. The case history revealed that she was from a large family in which becoming sick was the only way to get the attention she craved. Her digestion as a child had been delicate, and yet she persisted in eating foods which upset her. Then at night in bed she imagined herself severely ill or dying, with everyone in the family regretting not having treated her with more sympathy. These sad and touching thoughts made her cry, and she was also inclined to feel sorry for herself when asked to do something she did not want to do.

It should not be concluded that self-pity was necessarily the ultimate cause of her complaint. But her attitude certainly nourished her illness and perpetuated it. How the physician wished he could have treated her with *Pulsatilla* when she was a little girl crying herself to sleep! The remedy has repeatedly strengthened the moral fiber of the faint-spirited and easily discouraged, lessening the tendency toward a pitiful concern for self.

Homoeopathy teaches that in chronic illness, and even in some acute cases, mental symptoms precede physical ones. In other words, the individual's emotions, behavior, thoughts, and dreams give the earli-

est outward signs of a deranged life-force.* Since *Pulsatilla* is an extroverted nature that seeks companionship and support, early in the course
of illness she begins to manifest and communicate signs of inner trouble
in a tendency to cling, weep, whimper, whine, and feel sorry for herself. If these warning signals can be recognized and the patient treated
with homoeopathic remedies at this incipient stage, much subsequent
illness and suffering can be averted.

Thus, originating as an attention-getting device or an emotional
indulgence, self-pity can engender not only serious physical problems,
but severe mental ones as well. Leech-like, the trait feeds upon the very
source of *Pulsatilla*'s creative being, imperceptibly eroding her mor-
ale. It prevents her from accomplishing what she could or should do
and from facing up to life's reversals, leaving her with little resistance
to difficulties. In her misery and "weariness of life" (Hering) she then
seeks to gain sympathy and support by employing her arsenal of self-
pity—from the small-arms fire of whimpering and whining to the big
gun of the suicide threat, specifically, by "drowning herself" (Hering)—
like the fictitious Ophelia in *Hamlet* or like Virginia Woolf in reality.

This is not to say that *Pulsatilla* is the main remedy for self-destructive impulses. *Aurum metallicum*'s utter hopelessness, with desire to
throw himself from a height; *Arsenicum*'s frantic fears or despair, reaching a crescendo around and after midnight; *Natrum sulphuricum*'s long-
standing thoughts of suicide with unrelieved depression; or *Nux vom-*

---

* *Pulsatilla* was correctly chosen in a physically and emotionally complex case, involving chronic pain and infection of the male reproductive organs (orchitis), partly on the basis of the following vivid dream
which immediately preceded the onset of the patient's illness.

While walking in a meadow strewn with tiny flowers (anemones?),
he came upon the severed head of a black horse. Realizing that it was
injured, he picked it up, wrapped it in a handkerchief, and slung it
over his arm. He pitied the head and wanted to care for it but did not
know how and could not decide whether or not first to reunite it with
its body. He wandered forlornly in this way for a long time looking
for someone to help and advise him but, finding no one, sat down
and began to cry. The copious tears awoke him out of the dream.

It would be difficult to imagine a more clearly *Pulsatilla* dream.
Among the characteristic features, the type tends to dream of "animals"
(Kent), of "black beasts" (Hering), and also to "weep in her dreams"
(Hering).

ica's desire for suicide but lack of courage, are better known (see the rubric, "suicide," in the Kent *Repertory*). It is just to suggest that, whatever the patient's underlying constitutional type, *Pulsatilla* should be considered whenever there is much weeping and self-pity. The remedy can diminish this self-pity and ultimately cause the patient's life to take a happier turn.

Although the physician's initial reaction to her physical or emotional distress may be a strong urge to help, in time the rush of sympathy starts to dwindle, especially in ailments of a less serious or pressing character. He begins to wish that she would do something about her own problems and not rely so much on others. These thoughts are often intensified by his awareness of genuinely tragic cases sitting in his waiting-room without complaining. His exasperation might even reach the point of wanting to tell her to go away and leave him alone. Professional restraint inhibits the expression of these urges, of course, but if he finds himself harboring such feelings toward a patient demanding sympathy and pity, he should always consider *Pulsatilla*.

Another form taken by *Pulsatilla*'s emotionalism is *sentimentality*, whose groundwork is well laid by her heightened sensibility and lachrymose disposition. By "sentimentality" we mean sentiment for its own sake, the indulgence of feeling, as opposed to true feeling or the ability to be compassionate which, in various forms, is inherent in every constitutional type. She easily sheds tears at all things touching, happy, as well as remotely sad, and the remedy should be added to the Kent rubric, "weeping from joy". "It is not difficult to set off this fountain of tears," is the way one patient described herself; another called herself an "incurable weeper" as, smiling through her tears, she narrated a moving episode in her life.

The tenderhearted woman recoils from tragedy, as well as from any manifestation of bitterness or harshness in people or in art—from whatever upsets her peace of mind. However, a sentimental Victorian type of story, with orphaned children struggling to survive in the harsh world or innocent young heroines striving to overcome the evil designs of rapacious schemers, panders to her softer emotions. Soap operas, cloying romances, tearjerkers on the stage or screen are all aimed at the *Pulsatilla* in women, appealing to their sentimental side. Weeping in sad movies is characteristic of *Calcarea*, *Phosphorus*, *Ignatia*, and others, but emotionalism at the blatantly sentimental, the enjoyment of sickly-sweet fare that would be unpalatable to other constitutional types, is most prominent in *Pulsatilla*.*

And this is despite her inherent good taste. She is quite aware of what is syrupy or gushing in art, but sentimentality satisfies some definite need in her emotional makeup. Weeping from excessive tenderness of feeling is for her a pleasant, luxurious sensation. This is, in part, what Boericke means by "mentally an April day." While referring primarily to the nature's quick changes of mood (laughing one moment, crying the next—as the sun shines through an April shower), it also suggests that, like the April rain that clears the air and leaves the countryside sunnier and brighter, crying to her is a gentle *catharsis* that leaves her brighter and happier afterwards.

Altogether, *Pulsatilla* has a prepossessing and pleasing nature, and, when its softness and malleability are combined with the stronger qualities of other constitutional types, they fulfill a nice balancing function: tempering the aggressiveness of *Arsenicum*, subduing the turmoil or

---

* The artistic expression of rank sentimentality and its undisguised attempt to play on the audience's heartstrings were ridiculed by Mark Twain who cited the following literary specimen: "One lovely morning last week the pearly gates of heaven were left ajar, and white-robed angels earthward came, bearing on their snowy pinions a lovely babe. Silently, to a quiet home nest where love and peace abide, the angels came and placed the infant softly on a young mother's arm, saying in sweet musical strains, 'Lady, the Savior bids you take this child and nurse it for him.' The low-toned music died away as the angels passed upward to their bright home. We wish thee joy, young parent, in thy happiness." On this Twain commented: "This, if I have been rightly informed, is not the customary method of acquiring offspring, and for all its seeming plausibility, it does not look to me to be above suspicion. I have lived many years in this world and I never knew of an infant being brought to a party by angels or by other unauthorized agents, but it made more or less talk in the neighborhood" (*Favors from Correspondents*, 1870). Later, about a passage in a similar genre: "I have read it forty or fifty times altogether with a steadily increasing pleasurable disgust. . . . I almost always get it out and read it when I am low-spirited, and it has cheered many and many a sad hour for me!" (*Hogwash*, 1870).

erraticism of *Lachesis*, moderating the heaviness and rigidity of *Natrum muriaticum*, mellowing the pugnacity of *Sulphur* or the abrasiveness of *Nux vomica*, lightening the discontent of *Sepia*, and softening the arrogance or harshness of *Lycopodium*. Although mild and unaggressive, *Pulsatilla* is by no means weak. There is strength in a sociable and civilized disposition, a sympathetic and sensitive attitude, and even in a yielding and adaptable nature. After all, the massive oak was laid low by the North Wind, not the delicate but resilient reed.

If the homoeopathic physician bears in mind the five basic characteristics just discussed: sweetness, dependence, companionability, flexibility, and gentle emotionalism—he should seldom fail to recognize in a patient the picture of the delicate and beautiful meadow anemone.

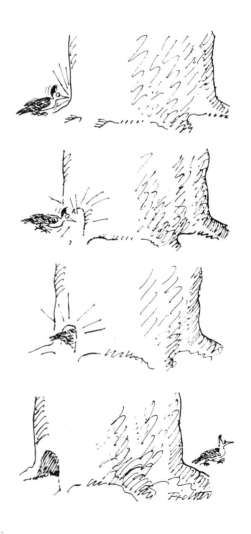

Arsenicum Album

Anything worth doing is
worth overdoing.
— Anonymous

HE above epigraph points straight to the heart of the *Arsenicum album* personality and is a continuing theme in the picture of this strong, projecting, and, at times, immoderate constitutional type.

Made from the white oxide of arsenic, this remedy demonstrates the paradox inherent in the law of similars—the most powerful poisons make the best medicines.*

The *Arsenicum* type is traditionally described as a "thoroughbred"—thin, fine-boned and fine-haired, with delicate skin, aquiline nose, and aristocratic features. The complexion can be pale, almost alabaster (*Silica*), turning dull white, ashen gray or even bluish during sickness. Temperamentally he is a race-horse—nervous, restless, high-strung, "of irritable disposition" (Hahnemann), perspiring easily and profusely, capable of tremendous bursts of speed over short distances, and extremely sensitive to inimical elements in the external environment.

There is also a "farm horse" variety of *Arsenicum*. The patient is squat or square in build with less refined features; the skin is coarser, or dry and scaly, and (like *Natrum muriaticum*) he does not perspire easily; instead his face becomes hot and flushed with exertion, which at times brings on congestive headaches. His movements remain quick, although not

---

* Physicians knew this idea centuries before the appearance of homoeopathy. Paracelsus and others, in medieval and renaissance times, expressed it as *"Ubi virus, ibi virtus,"* meaning "where there is poison, there lies virtue (healing power)."

as precise as in the aristocratic type, and he is not as neat and carefully dressed as the classic *Arsenicum* — although seldom as sloppy as *Sulphur*. This physical variant should be borne in mind, and the remedy should not be overlooked because the patient has thicker skin and a heavier build, or is messier in appearance.

Elizabeth Hubbard presented a third picture of *Arsenicum*: the old dray-horse pulling the milk cart, his head hanging down between his knees, wheezing heavily, with runny eyes and nose, and finding his principal comfort in his feedbag (the *Arsenicum* modality "better from eating": Boger). This picture of misery and broken-down strength is recognized in the patient suffering from a severe head cold, asthma or other respiratory ailment.

Anxiety

All three of these physical types, however, reveal the same *Arsenicum* mental picture. First and foremost is the deep vein of "*anxiety*" (Hahnemann). He is beset with anxieties reasonable and unreasonable, tangible and intangible, major and minor, present and future, visible and hidden. Even when this type claims to be (and is) "depressed," he projects less sadness and dejection than anxiety and frustration, or, in extreme cases, "anguish" (Hahnemann) and "despair" (Hering). His anxiety may be manifested outwardly in some specific worry, or in a general mental restlessness, anticipation of troubles, or a fussy meticulousness. Or it may come out in perfectionism, authoritarianism, and (as indicated by the epigraph) a tendency to immoderation or extremism. The patient is a driven (and driving) person.

In the physician's office, however, the specific which marks nearly every *Arsenicum* patient is an intense concern about health. This is quite a unique feature. His physical well-being, or lack of same, is of endless and all-absorbing interest. He regards his illness with disproportionate dread (for instance, a puffiness under the eyes upon awakening is magnified beyond its real importance), panics at symptoms which others would ignore ("Doctor, you *must* do something about this dry itching on the inside of the fourth finger of my right hand!!"), and, naturally, imagines he has every disease he reads about. Homoeopathy, ironically, in asking a patient to observe and recall his symptoms accurately, often encourages this overt or subliminal hypochondria.

Although convinced that no physician and no medicine can help him—at times to the point of "despairing of his life" (Hahnemann), *Arsenicum* must still turn to someone. Thus he travels from one physician to another, trying therapy after therapy, seeking both confirmation of the gravity of his complaint and reassurance of its curability. A "holistic health clinic," where he can with justification patronize six doctors at once and undergo six different types of treatment simultaneously, is a veritable paradise on earth for *Arsenicum*!. Although hoping for eventual diagnostic accord among his doctors, he meanwhile loves telling each what the others have said (or not said) about him: "My internist tells me that my liver is enlarged . . . but the chiropractor thinks my troubles are due to structural malformation of the dorsal vertebrae . . . A nutritionist I went to found me deficient in . . . But none of them could explain my cold night-sweats . . . " To treat some run-of-the-mill sinus condition he is quite willing to suffer inconvenience and expense, travelling hundreds or thousands of miles to visit an M.D. whom he has heard is "the best" for this complaint. Patients who plow their way through blizzards, who brave tempests and transportation strikes to keep routine appointments with the doctor, are *Arsenicum*. To them no demand is excessive when health is at stake.

Furthermore, while hating to be ill, the type simply *loves* doctors! And how he delights in the process of homoeopathic casetaking! He is drawn to the discipline not only by its results but also by the opportunity to discuss his symptoms in exquisite detail. Whether young or old, his eyes light up as he enumerates his complaints, talking of his "energy levels," "degree of wellness or toxicity," or "optimum fitness." When airing his views on health and medicine, he is like the horse who, feeling familiar turf under his hooves, takes the bit in his mouth, and gallops off unrestrainedly. In an excited voice he will tell of a recent book by some wonderfully insightful physician who has "pointed out to me a number of important problems that I never *knew* I had until I read his book. What an incredible medical mind the man has!"

Sometimes *Arsenicum* seems actually to enjoy his illness. He is devoted to his insomnia, asthma, or nervous disorder and does not intend to relinquish them. For they have served him well: he can discuss them endlessly and invoke them to gain attention or to assert his will. Allen describes the patient who is angered, even enraged, "when spoken to of her recovery, which she considers impossible." An amusing case from contemporary practice was the middle-aged man who came to homoeopathy for inability to throw off an amoebic dysentery contracted in the tropics, whose very first words on entering the office were: "I am a neurotic! I am neurotic about my health and know it; I feel I had better tell you this straight off, so you know exactly what kind of person you are dealing with." For this and his physical symptoms he was prescribed *Arsenicum*, but upon returning two weeks later with his complaint substantially relieved, and when the physician expressed delight at the improvement, the patient retorted, "Don't feel too sanguine about it. My dreams—which, by the way, I interpret with ease—tell me clearly that there are still many problems to solve, and they will take a long time, *I know.*" At times it seems as if this type *needs* an obscure disease, as a way of getting in touch with his deeper self.

   Arsenicum is also fascinated by and sympathetic to other people's health problems, and this topic constitutes a large portion of his conversation. He remembers details of another's health or illness long after forgetting everything else about him, "Oh, yes! You're the person who always sneezes twelve times after drinking orange juice and then has itching ears—now I remember you!" Meeting a formerly sick friend after an interval, he may appear more solicitous about the fate of the ailment than about the friend himself, "What *did* happen to your sore throat? You mean it went away just like that? Of its own accord, without treatment?" he asks almost in disappointment. Or, listening to a baby's normal hungry or angry cry, he will project his own anxiety and say, "Oh, listen to the poor baby crying! He must be so ill, poor thing. I wonder what is wrong with him?" But he also cannot hear of another's ailment, without immediately fearing that he might be developing something similar, and hastening to a specialist to check it out.

   Insistently a woman drags her whole family to whatever doctor she is patronizing at the moment, then supervises everyone in following his instructions and taking the medicines as directed; otherwise she becomes anxious and angry and is convinced they will fall ill (Borland). She is frantic with concern over her child's smallest ailment, even to the point of feeling ill herself, and takes great pains to keep him well. Yet, at the same time, bringing him to the physician and subjecting him to some form of interesting therapy, is an experience of which she would not have him deprived for all the world.

   She sends her friends with almost equal insistence. Thus, for example, they may find themselves somewhat perplexed in a homoeopathic clinic when a month earlier they had never even heard the word.

All they know is that they have been pressured into trying something new. When the physician inquires why such a patient has come, the reply will be, "I'm not quite sure. My friend, Sarah, persuaded me to try homoeopathy, so here I am!" In this way shoals of new patients are persuaded to try new kinds of treatment by (principally female) *Arsenicum* enthusiasts whose own drive for better health carries others along in its wake.

On a more serious level, anxiety about illness causes *Arsenicum* to live in constant *fear*. When in poor health he exhibits a peculiar *frenzied* quality. Rather than abating, his fear crescendos as he rushes from doctor to doctor, working himself into "most intolerable anxiety" (Hahnemann) and becoming so nervous about his condition that he panics at the mere thought of his nervousness. An "agonizing fear of death" (Boger) not only wakes him up at night and makes him jump out of bed in terror but continually haunts him during the day: "he despairs and weeps and imagines no one can help him, that he must die" (Allen). Or he is convinced he is on the verge of an incurable illness—especially cancer: "thoughts of death and of the incurability of his . . . cancerous . . . complaint" (Hering). Even when all tests are negative, and he has no alarming symptoms, the thought that some relative has, or has had, the disease lurks in the back of his consciousness, allowing him no peace of mind.

Typical was the mother of a teenage daughter with amenorrhea. Three doses of *Natrum muriaticum* 10M brought on the girl's menses, but the mother decided to have her tested for cancer ("to detect it early" were her exact words)—despite the gynecologist's assurances that this was not needed. Once the daughter was cleared, the mother—who was perfectly healthy and symptom-free—decided to subject herself to extensive testing ("to make sure that no abnormalities run in the family") and thereafter would undergo barium and other tests every two years with a vigor and insistence that even overruled the reluctance of the internist in charge ("The tests show no malignancy, but of course you can never know for certain, so I feel it is a good idea to be checked up regularly,").

Arsenicum is one of the best remedies for these groundless fears. It also excels in patients with legitimate causes for concern. It can heal the patient of "praecordial anxiety" (Hahnemann) and relieve the accompanying "insupportable cardiac pains" (Hering). It calms the one who has had a heart attack ("acute cardiac failure": Borland), or cancer operation, who "despairs of recovery" (Boericke), and fears a recurrence. It is, in fact, one of the principal homoeopathic remedies for cancer and "maintains the system under the stress of malignancy, regardless of location" (Boericke). It restores cheerfulness and courage, enabling the patient to live more normally instead of in constant dread. On return visits he will say: "My heart occasionally performs a pirouette, and I am still at times constricted in the chest or short of breath, but it doesn't bother me the way it used to. I feel better, eat and sleep well, and enjoy life again for the first time since my heart disease."*

Thus *Arsenicum* is often needed in very serious conditions. The physical and mental anguish which characterize poisoning with this element reveal the conditions which are helped by its homoeopathic preparation: "the most *intolerable* anguish . . . *deathly* anxiety . . . *intolerable* pains drive him to despair and frenzy . . . his anxiety is *indescribable;* continued, long-lasting . . . *excessive* . . . *inexpressible* mental anguish and increasing pain: 'Kill me,' he cries, 'or relieve my pain' . . . *terrible* anxiety flushes up in the evening, after lying down, with trembling and quivering . . . " (Hahnemann, Hering, Allen—author's emphasis).* *

The type is also excessively anxious about germs and contamination. Perceiving pollution and imminent decay on all sides, he combats them every way he can.

Two *Arsenicum* mothers were in the physician's office with their children, one of whom had a cold and the other a cough. To escape from the other's germs, one gathered up her child and took him into a small room adjoining the waiting room, firmly closing the door behind her. Whenever a member of the staff went to the room (used to store remedies), leaving the door momentarily ajar, both mothers immediately jumped up to close it, and it was touch and go who got there first. Later, during the consultation, both delivered scalding criticisms of the thought

---

* The anxious *Arsenicum*'s attitude toward, and behavior during, real and imaginary illness is such a prominent feature of the remedy, and often such an important diagnostic symptom, that we will return to it periodically throughout this chapter.

** A vivid literary description of the anguished mental state and physical torment produced by arsenic poisoning is the suicide of Emma Bovary in Flaubert's famous novel.

lessness of people who bring their sick children to the physician's office and expose others to contamination (!)

Arsenicum is meticulously clean. Even the adolescent boy keeps himself immaculate, frequently showering and washing his hair and feeling compelled to get rid of all the (often imaginary) dirt. Some wash their hands constantly to discourage germs (*Natrum muriaticum, Syphilinum*: Boger). One extreme case encountered in practice washed his hands after every handshake; another wiped doorknobs with a handkerchief before turning them; and Hahnemann describes a (deranged) patient as "seeing nothing but worms and bugs crawling about on his bed, from which he tries to run away." A more usual form of this neurosis is the housewife who, from an acute horror of germs, constantly sprays her house with germicides.

This microbe-phobia, together with the type's intrinsic orderliness, compels *Arsenicum* to wash dishes right after meals. Even when interesting and enjoyable guests are present, he cannot tolerate the idea of unwashed dishes lying around collecting germs and disappears into the kitchen to clean up.

A fixation on cleanliness was illustrated by a woman in her late twenties who was being treated for migraine headaches which came on like clockwork every weekend (*Arsenicum* has strongly accentuated periodicity of recurrence of both acute and chronic conditions: aggravations occurring near midnight or between 1:00 and 2:00 a.m., daily, weekly, biweekly, yearly, etc.). She lived in New York and, when asked how she liked it, replied: "The city itself is stimulating, and we have lots of friends, but it's so dirty! Every day when I come home from work, I have to scrub and scrub, not only the floors, but also the walls. And still they are never really clean. That black grime just sticks there and won't wash off." When asked if she really had to scrub so much, she looked at the physician uncomprehendingly: "The dirt accumulates every day, and I *have* to get it out." And she did. She pondered over her daily battles with the city's soot when going to sleep at night and talked of little else during the day. The remedy relieved her migraine headaches and helped reduce her anxieties about New York City dirt and grime.*

---

* In an extraordinary illustration of Hering's law (see the *Sulphur* chapter), the tips of this patient's fingers turned the color of soot as the

This type also has an inordinate fear of being poisoned by bad food (not surprisingly, in view of the remedy's origins) and will not leave food outside the refrigerator for even a short time, convinced that it will spoil. If a piece of cheese is moldy, he throws it away instead of scraping off the mold—or eating it, like the parsimonious *Sulphur* or *Lycopodium*. The housewife becomes suspicious of something she has just prepared, deciding that it smells funny, or tastes strange, or looks off-color; and, ever on the alert, she threatens to throw away the entire dish, to the horror of her hungry family. If (God forbid!) she has the slightest twinge of cramps after a meal, she is ready to run off to the emergency room. On the other hand, *Arsenicum* is, indeed, the foremost remedy for ptomaine and other kinds of food poisoning (Panos).

The fear of pollution can assume almost superstitious proportions. One patient not only kept an "ionizer" by his side both at home and at work (purportedly to neutralize toxic substances in the air) but never stayed at a friend's house or even went out to dinner without taking it along as a shield. The physician retained an indelible image of this young man transporting his ionizer from house to house and from room to room like some primitive tribesman carrying his household gods from one hut to another.

Arsenicum can also be excessively anxious about the safety of himself and his close ones. The wife is perpetually worried that something will happen to her husband or children, and is frantic if one of them stays out fifteen minutes longer than expected. She imagines some dreadful occurrence and enacts the whole scene in her mind, down to the last detail: "gloomy forebodings (that) something may have happened to her relatives" (Hering). In this she resembles *Sulphur*'s "anxiety for others" (Kent) or *Phosphorus'* "anxiety about her loved ones" (Hahnemann). She will drive her child five blocks to school, when all the other children walk or bicycle, since this is preferable to sitting at

intensity of her migraines diminished—starting with the first dose of *Arsenicum*. Thus the ailment left her body through the extremities; the discoloration of her fingertips persisted for some months until the headaches were cured, and her frenzied concern with cleanliness had relented. This rare symptom was observed by the author in only two other cases: an excessively orderly woman cured of colitis with *Arsenicum* and a germ-obsessed male with severe arthritis treated with *Silica*.

home worrying whether he got there safely. She cannot sleep at night until her teenage children are home from a party and lies awake thinking of all the terrible possibilities.

The male is equally full of fears. The husband never goes off to work in the morning without wondering whether he has kissed his wife good-bye for the last time and never takes a short trip without wondering if he will ever see his children again. Sometimes the type is recognized by an excessive nervousness about crossing the street (Blackie). He hesitates at every corner, even when no car is in sight, then starts across, but, espying a moving vehicle far in the distance, scampers back to the safety of the curb. In today's highly mechanized and increasingly violent society a reasonable awareness of danger is normal in any constitutional type, but in *Arsenicum* the "inclination to be frightened" (Hahnemann) is especially pronounced ("I was born frightened and have lived terrorized!"). Even his dreams are beset with anxieties, "full of cares, distress, fear, and danger . . . of frightening storms, conflagrations, black waters, ... from which he awakes with a cry" (Hahnemann).

Arsenicum's anxiety has a restless, "persistent" (Kent) quality, a terrier-like tendency to worry every issue to death. Or he creates crises everywhere, even while bemoaning his fate to be always faced with problems and difficulties. If not anxious about the present, he worries about the near or distant future. He is not certain when or where the sword of Damocles will fall ("unaccountable fears": Kent), but fall it must, and he is thus alert at all times. His mind is so preoccupied with future disasters ("fear that something will happen": Kent) that the happy resolution of one problem merely leaves a vacuum to be filled by the next.

A patient who had undergone two operations for bleeding ulcers was consumed with persistent fears: first, that he had stomach cancer, then, when ulcers were diagnosed, that he would die from the ulcer operations. When these passed without incident, and he was assured of no malignancy, he began to fear that his wife would die and that he would be left to care for their small children. His wife was happy and cheerful and gave no sign of approaching death. Yet this concern never left the patient's mind, and he even took an extra job at night to have sufficient money to afford a housekeeper in that event (!) But if he had not had this anxiety, it would have been something else: "No one would describe me as carefree and serene," he said of himself. This all doubtless contributed to his serious stomach condition. After a course of *Arsenicum,* however, his ulcers did not return, his digestion improved, and he stopped worrying about his wife's imminent death without developing a new dread to take its place.

Other *Arsenicum* types describe themselves, less euphemistically, as "worry worts" and admit to feeling uncomfortable, even somewhat bereft, when there is nothing to be agitated about.

To control these various hovering fears, the individual devises elaborate safety devices, psychological procedures, and preventive means which leave no room for error. If afraid of burglars, he may sleep with a poker by the bed, even after installing a complex burglar alarm system (*Arsenicum* and *Natrum muriaticum* are the constitutional types who most "fear robbers": Kent, Boger). "In the night he runs around the house looking for thieves; his whole house, also under the bed, is full of thieves" (Hahnemann). One *Arsenicum* patient had a car with special seatbelts; before climbing in he donned a crash helmet, shatterproof goggles, and slip-proof gloves, while a St. Christopher medal hung from the rear-view mirror. With such physical and spiritual safeguards assembled, he could drive off, in relative security.

The housewife who has nightmares about her family going hungry carefully stocks and restocks the basement with food (*Calcarea*). Even if only going away for the weekend, she loads up the refrigerator for a family quite capable of caring for itself.

To safeguard his health *Arsenicum* will carry precautions to amazing lengths, allowing for no exceptions or compromises. Patients will claim that, except for food cooked in restaurants, they have not touched tap-water in five, ten, or twenty years—literally not a drop! This is quite extraordinary, considering the care and concentration required. Along with drinking only spring water, they will eat only unsprayed organic foods, cook only in steel or crockery pots, consume dozens of vitamin pills daily, imbibe numerous herbal teas, and treat sugar as if it were "pure poison." They push themselves mercilessly to run multiple miles, even in the most inclement weather, or in other ways to stay physically fit (in the last century, before jogging became fashionable, *Arsenicum* would "walk further than he needs or can bear": Hahnemann). They may be right, but the effort is disproportionate; one suspects they could achieve the same results using more moderate means.

A seemingly calm woman consulted a homoeopathic physician

for severe menstrual headaches accompanied by cramps, nausea, and vomiting. During the interview she asked if she could take home seven vials of the *Ferrum phosphoricum* which had earlier been prescribed for her son's earaches. "Are you sure you will need *seven?*" the physician asked. "Yes, it is easier that way," she answered. "I can then keep vials all over the house as well as in my pocketbook and in the car; then I'll be able to find the remedy anytime, anywhere, and I won't have to worry." That *Arsenicum* was her remedy immediately became apparent.

Money is another source of concern to *Arsenicum*. Whether or not he has any, he thinks and talks about it a great deal, frequently lamenting his poverty or the high cost of living. His liking for money is stronger than that of most constitutional types, and he can even be "avaricious" (Hering). At the same time he has strong financial scruples. He cannot tolerate being in debt and at great hardship to himself will conscientiously pay off his creditors even when they are not pressing him (in contrast to *Phosphorus*). Like *Sulphur*, he can be tight with the dollar, disliking to spend it even when he has it and claiming not to be able to afford some desirable article or necessary expense. But while *Sulphur* clings to money out of principle and for the satisfaction and feeling of power it brings, *Arsenicum*'s motivation is "fear of poverty" (the remedy should be added to this rubric in the Kent *Repertory*).

Thus, a woman will pin dollar bills to the backs of curtains or slip them into books or sewing baskets, just to have them there in case of need. A child of well-to-do parents will feel obligated to take an unnecessarily burdensome job during high school or college to help defray the cost of his education. Always a conscientious worker, the *Arsenicum* adult develops his talents unsparingly so as to become indispensable at his job. He will even devote evenings, weekends, and vacations to acquiring a second skill or pursuing a hobby, as a second source of income in case of need. He is no mere jack-of-all-trades (*Sulphur*) but rather the master of several, and likes to keep at least two strings to his bow at all times.

These fortifications against an uncertain destiny may be erected unconsciously, or they may be rationally conceived and systematically implemented defenses against what he sees as a hostile environment. As often occurs with *Natrum muriaticum*, some profound insecurity has persuaded *Arsenicum* that hostile forces will bring him down if he slackens his vigilance for a moment. He does not trust to luck or (if religious) rely on God, but depends solely on his own efforts and the safeguards discussed earlier, so that only some unpredictable catastrophe can now affect him. Thus, although he claims to be calm and confident, these elaborate precautions reveal the latent anxiety.

The patient may show no perceptible restlessness, anguish, or fear, especially when the *Arsenicum* in the constitution is mitigated by other characteristics. *Pulsatilla*, for instance makes him more gentle, *Calcarea* less restless, and *Lycopodium* more collected and detached. But *Arsenicum* is a tightly coiled spring, and a certain tension persists in the individual however it may be camouflaged, however self-contained and unruffled the exterior. The hidden worry may be discerned in the expression of the eyes when a sensitive area is discussed—in sudden and ungovernable flashes of fear or anxiety—or in the controlled tautness of the patient's talk and behavior. His smile is a fixed grin, instead of being natural, or he may admit to "grinding his teeth" at night (Kent), that he cannot leave a problem alone, and that he persists in worrying over past decisions: "Did I make my point clear? Did I do the right thing? Did I make the right choice?" (*Nux vomica*). His thoughts keep returning to past business deals, family incidents, and the like, which he examines from every angle, mulling over the different ways he could have improved the situation. Unlike *Calcarea*, however, who worries helplessly about small matters without arriving at a constructive idea, *Arsenicum* usually hits on several viable alternatives.

In some persons the anxiety surfaces only during illness. A self-possessed young teenager, whose calm strength and serenity invariably led him to be elected to positions of leadership in school, presented with a burning weeping eczema on the arms. The condition was not excessively severe, but he was in a panic and for the first time in his life seemed to have lost control of himself. *Arsenicum* was indicated by his frenzied intolerance of the eczema and vocal insistence that it be stopped immediately. When it was administered in medium low potency on a daily basis (skin diseases often respond better, and with less aggravation, to the lower dilutions; for other precautions in prescribing, see Hubbard's *A Brief Study Course in Homoeopathy*), the patient gradually got better.

Fastidiousness

Next we come to *Arsenicum*'s well-known "fastidiousness" (Kent). More than any other constitutional type, except possibly *Nux vomica*, *Arsenicum* is *persnickety*: excessively "anxious about the slightest trifle" (Hahnemann). In his sensitivity to confusion and disorder, he will fuss over the towels on the bathroom rack, hanging them straight and symmetrically, he cannot tolerate a chair not being aligned with the table or a book not replaced in its proper place on the shelf, and is upset if his shoes on the closet floor are not neatly lined up in rows according to color: "the least trifle fills him with care and solicitude" (Allen). He is indignant when cars are parked crookedly, on the lines in parking lots ("Why can't people do it the right way? It's just as easy to park in the spaces") and can spend many hours packing and repacking a suitcase so that everything fits together in a particular way; even when hurrying to leave for the airport, he is still in a twitter about his clothes being folded neatly and socks properly matched (each pair in its own plastic bag). In an admirable but at times excessive concern for tidiness and order he makes his bed and picks up his room as soon as he wakes up in the morning; otherwise he cannot bear to look at it. At work everything must have its designated place and be done in some precise manner, or, distraught, he cannot function properly. In all spheres he is ultra-"picky," and, in his intolerance of everything slipshod, irritated at any clumsiness — dropping a dish, overturning a glass, spilling food — his own as well as another's.

Even without undue neuroses or excess, *Arsenicum* is *meticulous* ("conscientious about trifles": Kent). His finer movements are often remarkably delicate and precise — the handwriting, for instance, is small and beautiful (*Nux vomica*); and whether building a table or painting a fence, cleaning a yard, writing a report, or cooking a meal, his work manifests that particular "finishing touch" — that final polish — that reveals a meticulous attention to detail. The *Sulphur* amateur chef may come up with interesting or unusual food combinations, but is heavy handed with the spices and condiments and serves up his culinary creations in the form of "a rude plenty"; the *Arsenicum* gourmet prepares delicate and subtle dishes and presents them gracefully and elegantly.

In fact, elegance and good taste is the hallmark of this individual. The house is well-appointed, and the decor stylish. Both men and women are well dressed and meticulously groomed. The male patient enters the physician's office with a handsome and well cared for brief-case holding only a few essential papers (it does not bulge like the old tattered one of a *Sulphur*); his elegant—at times finicky—appearance is summed up by Hering as "the man with the gold-headed cane." The woman's handbag precisely matches her shoes and other accessories. This person looks stylish, and clothes sit well on him even when not at the height of fashion.

Arsenicum, too, is the neat and prim elderly lady, spare of build, precise in her movements, brisk and starchy in her manner, whose snippy, persnickety, and at times fearsome exterior conceals a highly developed moral delicacy and integrity.

The type's fastidiousness around the home is discernible in the housewife who prides herself on the spotlessness of her house, and who, as we saw, may even develop various ailments when unable to cope with surrounding disorder, confusion, or dirt. It is also found in the tense, overwrought husband who comes home tired from the office and starts immediately to pick up bits of thread from the carpet, pieces of paper from the floor, wipe flecks of dust off the tables, and look for minor disorders in the household. Altogether he is of an irritable "sensitive disposition; the least thing annoys him and causes him to be angry" (Hahnemann). Nothing, he claims, is done right at home without his supervision ("Why must I do *everything* myself?"). He starts clearing the plates from the table even before others have finished eating—with forks still suspended in mid-air so to speak, and then proceeds irascibly to wash the dishes despite the willingness of his wife and children to attend to this chore in good time. He is *convinced* that no one will do it if he doesn't. But, in truth, despite complaints, both male and female *enjoy* cleaning up the kitchen until it sparkles. If he dislikes the sight or smell of tobacco, the more compulsive individual will whisk away an ashtray to clean it while a guest is still smoking, causing the next ash to drop on the floor. Then, in an exhilarating agony of agitation, he rushes to sweep up the ashes. Such paroxysms of tidying up are, to some extent, a physical outlet for tensions and anxieties accruing during the day, but they also express *Arsenicum*'s generally fidgety, nervous, fastidious nature.

The sicker he is, the more fussy he becomes over minutiae; any iota of disorder intensifies his physical and mental symptoms. The bed-ridden housewife in severe pain will fret over the potatoes not being properly peeled for dinner or a less favored type of soap being used in the washing machine. She is tormented by an open closet door or bureau drawer or (as Kent notes) when the pictures on the wall are not hanging straight (this is also the type who, upon entering another's house, will straighten the pictures on the wall or objects on a table). She becomes dictatorial and demanding, insisting that her every order be carried out immediately and that everything be "just right". The male will stagger out of his sick-bed to search frantically for some particular pair of pliers, emptying drawers and turning the house upside down for hours. Another pair of pliers will not do; he *must* have that particular one, and if he cannot find it, he must know what has happened to it. There is often an element of caprice here also: "When everything is done to fulfill his wish, the least trifle is sufficient to change his mind" (Allen).

One four-year-old, a delicate fine-featured boy with limbs as thin and green-tinted as celery stalks and fine veins showing through his alabaster skin, suffered from severe chest conditions which caused him to spend half the winter in bed. His first symptom of illness, before anything was discernible on the physical plane, was a fussy anxiety. He became upset if the books in his room were not stacked properly, if his napkin was not folded correctly, or if he was eating his cereal with the wrong spoon. He even had hysterics if someone walked up the stairs the wrong way! If he received *Arsenicum* during this incipient stage, either the chest condition was aborted altogether or he had a very light case. This is a fine example of how mental symptoms precede physical ones and of how illness can be averted by homoeopathic treatment during the premonitory phase.

Another facet of *Arsenicum*'s fastidiousness is his use of language; he expresses himself with refinement and elegance. A woman's speech is frequently rapid, clearly articulated, and has a "clipped" quality. But although she may talk as rapidly as *Lachesis* she does not sound as rushed because her speech is more controlled and her enunciation more precise. The individual also takes pains to make himself clear and is a stickler for verbal exactness. If his wife says, "Our friends are buying the house across the street," *Arsenicum* will correct her, "They have signed a contract to purchase the house—that's not the same thing" (the pedantic *Sulphur* may also quibble over verbal inexactitudes). He will leave a note with precise instructions how to get to a certain place together with a beautifully drawn map, adding at the end, "I hope these directions are clear enough and that I haven't left anything out." One patient who brought in an immaculate list of symptoms was asked by the physician, "You never cross anything out, do you?" "Oh, no," was the reply, "If I make a mistake I rewrite the entire list."

In one difficult and confusing case a quirky fastidiousness was the guiding symptom that led to the correct prescription of *Arsenicum*. The patient, a chronically ill woman, appeared to need nearly every polychrest in the materia medica, but the interview revealed a long-standing habit of writing and rewriting personal letters without ever sending them. She had drawers full of undispatched letters. When asked the reason, she replied that it was due to apprehension at not having expressed herself precisely. She then rewrote the letters in order to set forth her thoughts more accurately, but by then the contents were partially outdated, requiring yet another revision, and so on. Few but *Arsenicum* would rewrite letters without ever sending them.

Natrum muriaticum can exhibit a similar anxiety about written communications, but it proceeds rather from a fear of being misunderstood or misjudged; furthermore, he feels guilty about not sending the letter, while *Arsenicum* is unperturbed, feeling that the letter that is not exactly right is better unsent.

No patient is more thorough and meticulous in giving his symptoms than *Arsenicum*. "I've been suffering from low-grade diarrhoea with cramps ever since traveling in Mexico seventeen months ago. I have a complete record of how often I go to the bathroom, at what times, and the type of stool—which is not always the same. By the way, how do you interpret these variations? I've also recorded how long the cramps last. Here it all is, in my diary, if you would like to look at it." He recalls not only the subtleties of every modality and all concomitant sensations, but also the day and hour, even the minute, a new symptom develops. "Your aggravation started a week after you took the remedy?" the physician asks. "No, not a week. A week and a day—eight and a half days actually—because the headache came on Tuesday at 8:30 p.m., and you gave me the constitutional around 10:00 a.m. on Monday of the previous week."

One unforgettable patient brought in a multi-paged report, typed up in neat columns and underlined in coded colors, giving the hourly fluctuations of all his symptoms throughout the weeks since his previous visit.

The Driven Individual

Great *physical* restlessness and anguish in illness is a key to *Arsenicum* (*Rhus toxicodendron, Aconite*). Hahnemann describes the patient who tosses and rolls around in bed: "driven by great anxiety he turns and twists about, finding no rest in any place, continually changing his position." Or he must rise up and walk about: "pacing the floor, he wanders from room to room, to lie, now here, now there . . . from one bed to another" or from bed to couch and back again. Such restlessness is worse upon lying down at night, especially around and after midnight. This well-known symptom can be so intense that the patient's frantic flying around the room can be sensed even in a telephone conversation. Conversely, there can be such weakness and prostration that he is "too weak to toss as much as his anguish and restlessness desire" (Hering).

At times this restlessness reflects his refusal to submit to illness, and certainly these struggles further waste his depleted physical energies and impede his recovery. No one fights a simple 'flu like *Arsenicum* who, in his angry impatience at being ill, clamorously complains that he cannot stand it *any* longer and would rather die than be subjected to such indisposition. But a dose or two of the remedy restores physical peace and emotional harmony. The patient ceases to fight and, submitting to the normal rhythm of the disease, sets out on the path of recovery.

Occasionally *Arsenicum* (in both acute and chronic cases) first allays the patient's frantic restlessness by provoking a collapse. For days he cannot work and can barely move. Thus the medicine compels the overwrought patient to slow down, to rest and sleep, permitting healing to take place. One such case was a concert cellist whose heavy schedule of touring, teaching, and recording brought him to the point of a nervous breakdown. He could neither eat nor sleep, his nerves were shattered, and he had an increased heart rate with palpitations. A dose of *Arsenicum* in high potency sent him to bed for two weeks—a difficult time for all concerned, since he could still muster the energy to telephone twice a day and abuse the physician roundly: "I've never felt so weak in my entire life! How can I be sure I won't die? What if I never get well again?''

The tongue, by the way, is the one organ in *Arsenicum* that retains its full powers throughout even the most severe illness. The patient's "piercing" or "piteous lamentations" (Hahnemann) can be ceaseless (*Ignatia*), and when anxious about his health, he does not scruple to make frank use of his tongue. Some, on such occasions, even tell the physician that they *hate* him and will *never* forgive him for what the medicine has done to them.

The cellist, however, had to stay in bed and comply with the doctor's orders, since he was too weak to do anything else. He got through the crisis somehow and, once it was over, found that he could again eat and sleep and that his heart symptoms were almost gone. Thereafter he was a loyal supporter of homoeopathy. It is a common observation that, after giving the physician an inordinately hard time, *Arsenicum* will usually come around and develop into a dedicated and intelligent patient.

Without the remedy to calm his "no-let-up" lifestyle, anxiety can make *Arsenicum* a *driven* individual. Like one of the Gadarene swine, he rushes headlong to his own destruction, driving himself relentlessly to estrangement from friends and family, to loss of job or ill-health. One young woman came to homoeopathy for persistent eruptions around the lips and ulcers in the mouth, but her more serious problem was her personality. Even though honest, clever enough, and a good worker, she could not hold a job, and the reason rapidly became clear. Her intense way of talking about her work, the incompetence of others in the office, the salary inequities and the uneven distribution of tasks, was reminiscent of Coleridge's Ancient Mariner. The physician instinctively recoiled from her buttonholing manner and critical, gimlet-like eye ("I fear thee, Ancient Mariner").

In general, the piercing blue eyes of *Arsenicum* bore right through his interlocutor. Sometimes their light gleam can be almost mesmerizing, the steel-gray glitter or flashing blue fire rivetting the other's attention. The brown-eyed individual also has a distinctively sharp, bright, anxious-not-to-miss-anything look. This brightness differs from that of *Phosphorus*: while the latter's softly luminous or sparkling eyes seem to envelop their object, *Arsenicum*'s piercing eyes *nail* their object to the spot.

With just such a glittering eye did the patient transfix the physician as she recounted her tale of woe: how all the work was piled on her and how she did twice as much as anyone else. Undoubtedly this was true — since *Arsenicum* simply *asks* to be given more work. But she did not inspire sympathy, and it took many doses of the remedy before this virtually *Arsenicum*-starved individual shed her compulsive manner and ceased frightening others away. In this connection it is noteworthy that this medicine bears repetition well, even when prescribed constitutionally.

The over-zealous, over-conscientious, unrelenting businessman, lawyer, doctor, or broker, who works long hours without letting up and is then unable to unwind, is often *Arsenicum* (also *Nux vomica*). Although he may have accomplished as much as any two other people, he is "dissatisfied all day and extremely vexed with himself because he thinks he has not worked enough and reproaches himself bitterly" (Hahnemann). *Sulphur, Natrum muriaticum* and others possess a similar capacity for work, but it is *Arsenicum*'s driven, compulsive manner that makes him unique — and points to the remedy. *Lachesis* who also exhibits an almost manic energy for work, differs from *Arsenicum* in accomplishing his extraordinary feats without appearing to tire or tax his energies.

A successful lawyer was being treated for alopecia areata (hair falling out in patches). He had no other particular symptoms except one prominent mental one: lately he had taken to working eighteen hours a day, coming home around midnight, then arising at six in the morning to again depart for work. He was not unhappy in his family life but, in fact, perfectly content and wished for no changes. He simply enjoyed his job, like the woodpecker who merrily drills away, non-stop, all day long ("inclined to activity": Hering) and, except for weekend collapses into exhaustion, scarcely noticed the long hours. "I'm one helluva hard worker," he would say cheerfully.* Indeed, *Arsenicum* would not work

---

* As seen by the unchanging expression on the woodpecker's face in the introductory cartoon, although he does things the hard way or to excess, *Arsenicum* considers this perfectly normal.

One ultra-conscientious patient recounted how, as a child, it had

so hard if he did not like it. He is not one to put himself out unless he so chooses, knowing full well how to take care of his own comfort and interests—in contrast to *Natrum muriaticum* who will take on uncongenial or unenjoyable work out of duty.

Arsenicum not only started the patient's hair growing in the bald spots but as a side-effect induced him to come home at least to a late dinner. No previous pleas or reasoning by his wife had been able to reach him. Only the remedy could take the edge off his immoderate work habits and, through a newly acquired awareness, lead him to reflect on his family's needs.

This individual often has trouble finding a happy medium in his work habits. Not only does he love to work, but he loves to *overwork,* however much he may groan about it. The more responsibility is piled on him, the happier he is. Thus he exemplifies the popular wisdom in the business world that a job needing to be done quickly should be given to the busiest person in the office (i.e., to an *Arsenicum).* But while his colossal inner drive creates the semblance of great strength, and he may be as forceful and active as *Sulphur* or *Lachesis*, he is sustained more by "nervous energy" (Borland) than by the true endurance. "I often feel as if I am running full speed on 'below empty,'" was one patient's graphic way of phrasing it. Thus he oscillates between excessive application and total exhaustion; yet, barely recovered from a collapse, starts up again on all cylinders.

A middle-aged man was being treated for recurring angina pectoris. In seeking the source of his latest relapse, the physician discovered that he now held three jobs: during the day he was a computer programmer, he taught this subject at night school, and he sold real estate on weekends. He explained that financial need was his motivation, but his wife objected, "Not at all. The truth is that he is not happy unless he can push himself to the limits of his strength and then despair of being overworked. If homoeopathy could just change this self-imposed frenetic life-style, I am sure his angina would improve" (*Arsenicum* did just that.)

Such patients even have headaches on weekends—when unable to

---

taken her a year to be *finally* convinced that she could make her bed in the mornings without having first to strip it entirely and start from scratch—by simply pulling up and straightening the sheets and blankets.

go to the office to work. Some fall ill during vacations or become restless and irascible while "relaxing" at the beach; they cannot wait to get back to the daily grind.* *Arsenicum* is the only major polychrest *not* listed in Kent's rubric, "aversion to work"; and a decade or more can pass without his taking a day of sick leave from work. When under stress, at a low point in life, or in a state of despair, *Arsenicum*'s most reliable and effective therapy is to immerse himself in work. This is his panacea. For certain individuals work takes the place of an emotional life. Persons who are unmarried without being lonely or unhappy—the spinster who is content with her particular vocation or who tends her home and garden, the bachelor who dreads the day of retirement, the artist who lives happily alone—are often *Arsenicum.* They find in work the meaning and satisfaction that other constitutional types find only in human relations. And a few become so immersed in it as gradually to lose contact with other humans, even developing "misanthropic" (Hering) tendencies—not to be confused with the *Natrum muriaticum* "loner" discussed in a later chapter.

Not that *Arsenicum* is less capable of love and deep emotion than other constitutional types. In fact, both the male and the female can be exceptionally family-minded—particularly strongly attached to their children. He may just not require close human ties. Work affords him emotional self-sufficiency—as it also does for some *Sepias* or scholarly *Sulphurs* and *Lycopodiums.*

The other side of this picture, however, is his need for people ("desires company": Boenninghausen, Kent). Like *Phosphorus* and *Pulsatilla* he hates to return to an empty house and can panic or become frantic when subjected to even short periods of solitude: "dread of death when alone" (Hering), "attacks of great fear of being alone" (Boenninghausen); in fact, *Arsenicum* and *Phosphorus* are the only remedies in bold type under Kent's rubric, "anxiety when alone." But, even here, his craving for companionship surfaces particularly when he is ill, unable to concentrate on his work, and driven to seek distraction in human contact.

---

* Could this be one source of the prominent *Arsenicum* modality, "aggravation at the seaside" (Kent)? It is not the local inhabitants— the fishermen, farmers, or local tradesmen—who are worse by the seaside, but persons on holiday.

His driven quality may prevent him from resting on his laurels and enjoying his own achievements. While *Phosphorus*, *Lycopodium* or *Sulphur* will bask in the glow of success and dine out on it for weeks, *Arsenicum* loses interest once something has been achieved. The youngster, after winning all the tennis medals at the local club or all the school prizes in a certain subject, will drop that interest completely and turn to some new challenge. At any age, his eye is forever fixed on some distant horizon or at least on the next goal. A triumph or success is merely one more step in an endless progression of (largely self-imposed) compulsory achievements. No accomplishment can still this drive because it comes from within and is not satisfied by the world's approval. To be sure, he seeks acknowledgment as much as another and will not turn it down when it is deserved, but this is not his primary motive or principal source of satisfaction. He feels that recognition will only hold him back, while he must ever press forward.

Perfectionism

For what is *Arsenicum* striving? What is the source of his drive? The answer is: perfection. He is the *perfectionist* par excellence. The patients themselves admit it. But perfection is seldom achieved in this world, even by *Arsenicum* himself. Hence his unceasing and unrelenting drive.

The aspiration to perfection is seen even in the child, who is unusually persevering and conscientious: whether in keeping his room extratidy, his clothes immaculate (the more highly strung and super-finicky can become almost hysterical if they soil or spill anything on their clothes), or in painstakingly copying out numbers and letters in his notebook. This often delicate and lovely child evinces much self-discipline and will spend long hours practicing a musical instrument, going over the same exercises again and again until just the right sound is obtained. He may cry in frustration and stamp in exasperation at repeated failures but is ultimately intrigued by the meticulous application this process demands.

As a student, the pale, tired, and sickly *Arsenicum* child or adolescent may still be determined to be first in his class in all subjects. Not content with simply receiving good grades through moderate effort (as *Sulphur* or *Phosphorus* are content to do), he must obtain the *best* grades through superior effort. For a term paper he will read ten books, when three or four would suffice. He will prepare elaborately for every classroom exercise or test, studying the material from every angle; or he will spend days rewriting a three-page short story to make it letter-perfect. Thus the ultra-ambitious and over-achieving individual is often an *Arsenicum.* A college student being treated for asthma explained that he had to *over*-prepare for every examination, since, if he did not know the answer to even one question in ten, his mental faculties were so paralyzed that he could not concentrate on the other nine.

The same striving for perfection is found in the adult who compulsively works on some one obsession, adding to it, redoing it dozens of times, never completely satisfied with what he has done, and unable to cut his losses and go on to the next thing. Typical here is the professor who endlessly rewrites his lectures. He knows that the students cannot appreciate these marginal improvements, but that matters little. He is satisfying his own inner drive for perfection. He could not live with an unfinished product. Knowing that some important bit of knowledge was omitted would prevent him from delivering a good lecture.

This is all emblematic of the nature's immoderation, his delight in overkill. Yet, however serious the physical consequences of such over-exertion, they are still preferable to the anxiety of feeling unprepared.

Thus the *Arsenicum* teacher is the antithesis of the more relaxed *Phosphorus* who trusts to inspiration and can afford to be spontaneous. He also differs from the *Sulphur* lecturer who allows his knowledge to pour out eloquently enough but with little organization or polish, as well as from the original but often chaotic *Lachesis* or *Natrum muriaticum.* *Arsenicum*'s material is invariably well-organized, the presentation discriminating and well-polished. He will often hand out beautifully typed outlines and schedules of his course to which he then adheres to the letter.*

A patient being treated with *Arsenicum* for allergies and hay fever

---

* In further differentiation of teaching types, *Phosphorus* or *Sulphur* can usually improvise on a subject they know, and sometimes even on one they do not know. *Natrum muriaticum* more resembles *Arsenicum*, needing to be overprepared for even the most informal public appearance. But while he overprepares out of shaky self-confidence and a dread of appearing ridiculous, *Arsenicum* is striving for perfection. The inspired *Lachesis* public speaker is a law unto himself (see the discussion in that chapter).

was one of thirty applicants for the post of professor of music history and theory at a local university. As part of the hiring process he had to present a one-hour sample lecture to the faculty, and he resolved to analyze a movement of a Haydn sonata. He arrived with a suitcase containing: 1) a tape of the work for the university audio equipment, 2) his own cassette recorder, together with a cassette, in case the university equipment was not functioning properly, 3) an outline of his lecture and a detailed syllabus of his prospective course for the entire year—in sufficient copies for everyone present, 4) an additional tape reel, cassette, and xeroxed handout of a lecture on a Chopin Prelude in case the faculty preferred that to Haydn. He then proceeded with his lucid analysis and elegant exposition of the subject—every word weighed, every phrase balanced. This was the superorganized *Arsenicum, prepared for every eventuality* and a model of conscientious preparation (he was the candidate chosen).

Incidentally, the taut *Arsenicum* exhibits characteristic nightmares ("care-beset dreams": Hahnemann) about examinations, meetings or appointments, where adherence to a timetable is paramount. He has studied for the wrong test; it was held a day earlier than he had thought (so he missed it); the door to the lecture hall is locked and he cannot get in; he is unable to find the room or the familiar building where a meeting is being held; the elevator keeps going past the floor where he is supposed to lecture. Any dreams of arriving late, of unpreparedness for a journey, of missing trains, airplanes, or an engagement in a fundamentally competent person, can indicate a need for the remedy.

When awake he is also haunted by fears of being late or of missing an event. In his anxious punctuality he takes no chances but starts out early for school, work, or an appointment to allow for delays on the road or losing his direction.

Arsenicum is often encountered in the constitutional composition of the solo performer. Although tense and nervous throughout the performance (unlike *Phosphorus,* who is inherently more at ease on the stage), he is carried to the top by his ambition, ability to concentrate on detail, willingness to practice long hours, and above all by his drive for perfection. This is what sustains him in the arduous, at times slave-like, work of the soloist. Conceivably such a career brings out, or develops, the *Arsenicum* side of the nature.*

In performing, as in other spheres, *Arsenicum* has a tendency to collapse after high achievement or successful effort. The preperformance tension, anxiety, and fear now take their toll ("anxiety when anything is expected of him": Kent), and the taut nerves demand complete rest. He also suffers intensely from the classic *post-creative depression*: the psychological letdown from a resulting vacuum once the intense build-up is over. Where is he now to direct his nervous energy and restless drive? Nothing is left but to fall ill. What is more, even though others may have viewed his performance as a triumph, he measures himself against his own standards of perfection and suffers at the recollection of every unsatisfactory note, gesture, or phrase.

Although self-criticism is obviously necessary in any artistic or scholarly endeavor, *Arsenicum* aspires to more than most persons can attain. His refusal to allow for human imperfection makes him hypercritical of others ("cannot leave off talking about the faults of others": Hahnemann) as well as of himself, and drives him to frustration, anguish and despair. Hence, this is one of the first remedies to be considered for severe self-disdain and self-hatred which, when combined with a despairing frustration, may lead to suicidal impulses "by hanging" (Boenninghausen), with a knife: "a desire to kill himself by stabbing, after midnight" (Allen), or he contemplates self-destruction with firearms, on the ground that it is quicker and less painful. Van Gogh's slicing off his ear in mad frustration, and his subsequent suicide by shooting, are examples of *Arsenicum*'s mental anguish and artistic despair carried to an extreme.

---

* The pianist, Vladimir Horowitz, is *Arsenicum* in his well-known zealous application and determination never to hit a single wrong note during a performance; also in the anxious, almost haunted, expression in his eyes—especially as a young man. The more *Phosphorus* Artur Rubinstein had a twinkling mischievous expression and could hit a dozen wrong notes during a performance without being perturbed, since he was more concerned with musicality than with technical precision. However, in middle age he himself became more *Arsenicum* and was spurred to greater accuracy by the phenomenal example of the younger Horowitz.

Terribly ambitious as he is to achieve perfection and to be "the best," he can display a strong *competitiveness*. Whether in a subtle or cutthroat way, he must constantly prove himself better than others. The student obsessed with grades and who talks about them endlessly is often *Arsenicum*, as is the individual who builds himself up by criticizing others ("disposed to discuss the faults of others": Hering) or who derives a fleeting security from dragging them down. There is room at the top for only *one* person—himself—and he brooks no competition there. This fighting spirit and determination to win, are often displayed in the challenging and resolute expression of the eyes—whether in the young athlete, the trial lawyer, or simply the competitive mother.

In any situation, exchange of ideas, or relationship, he cannot resist being one jump ahead of others. Even within the family, the proud father will say of his son's good report card, "All A minuses, that's wonderful! But when I was your age, I used to bring home all A's!"

The competitive *Arsenicum* can be trendy. Always on the cutting edge of intellectual fashion, he refuses to be left behind in anything. He is always "with it," always keeping up with the newest artistic, educational, health, or medical fad, and sometimes with his aggressive up-to-dateness intimidating anyone who fails to do the same ("Have you seen the latest play by . . . ?" "What! You mean you haven't read the recent book about . . . ?" "Haven't you *yet* tried the new exercise program of Dr. . . . ?").*

The parent who tires others with endless glowing accounts of his children's varied talents and accomplishments is often exhibiting *Arsenicum*'s innate competitiveness. Everything belonging to him or her—

---

* Homoeopaths have speculated why *Arsenicum* is listed only in the first degree under Kent's rubric, "anxiety about his health." Was the type different in the last century? One possible explanation is that the clergy have today been largely replaced by physicians and psychotherapists as symbols of authority and prestige. *Arsenicum*, always sensing which way the wind is blowing, finds his former "anxiety of conscience," to which Kent gave top billing, now superseded by a more timely concern with health. *Natrum muriaticum*, who is also at the forefront of change (with *Arsenicum*) or riding the wave of the future with *Sulphur*, still contrives to remain something of an outsider, eternally on the fringes of society's major culture upheavals.

house, garden, children, job—must be superlative, and better than anyone else's.

Even his illnesses must be special—or more serious than others'. The patient enters the physician's office announcing, "I don't know if you've ever seen anything like this before . . . The three doctors I have already consulted say that I have one of the most complicated allergy conditions they have ever encountered." In fact, the physician may feel that he is doing *Arsenicum* a disfavor by telling him that his disease is not too serious and that he needn't worry. One wonderful old gentleman with a pretty ordinary rheumatic condition confided in the physician with a conspiratorial air, "I am presenting you with a case that is quite unique; and it will probably be the most difficult case you've *ever* handled . . . " Then, as if this were not enough to type him, and unwilling to leave anything to the doctor's imagination, he proceeded to say: "First of all, I am anxious about everything: living, dying, safety, money, my work, health . . . "

Another type of ambitious *Arsenicum*, however, can manifest a disarming *lack* of competitiveness. He will insist (and his behavior bears it out) that he only wants to excel himself and has no objection if others excel also. A child will run home from school all excited that *twelve* members of his class (including himself) got an A on a math test. Or a teacher of ballet who is driving her aspiring daughter to high achievement, will drive her other students equally. She wants them *all* to become great ballerinas. This *Arsenicum* will honestly enjoy and generously applaud a performance or accomplishment superior to his own. He is enthralled by perfection, in whomever it may be manifested.

People are not perfect, human performance is imperfect, nature is far from perfect, scientific theories are always being reinterpreted and supplanted by newer ones, and ideas of ethics and morality in politics or religion are continually changing, so that what is truth today may be falsehood tomorrow. Only in art, *Arsenicum* concludes, can perfection be attained—and, even more important, *sustained.* Not surprisingly, then, he is often attracted to the creative arts. As *Pulsatilla* and *Phosphorus* are drawn to people (and some *Phosphorus* types to the stage), *Sulphur* to scholarship or business, *Lycopodium* to politics and institutions, and *Natrum muriaticum* to teaching and counselling,

Arsenicum, with his drive for perfection, ranks high in the constitutional economy of writers, painters, sculptors, and composers. Even when of other constitutional types, they invariably display a prominent *Arsenicum* streak as well. It is also found in those who might be called "disguised artists": seamstresses, gardeners, hairdressers, surgeons, gourmet cooks, and the like—all occupations requiring a delicate and precise artistic touch to mold something perfect out of the material given.

A fine example of a more purely *Arsenicum* artist is Gustave Flaubert, the nineteenth-century French writer known as an "author's author" for his technical skill and the near-perfection of his style, whose reputation rests on one book: *Madame Bovary.* He worked on this novel for seven years, suffering torments over every adjective, agonizing over every turn of phrase, rewriting every paragraph innumerable times, often spending a week on one page to attain his impeccable prose.* What we know of this strange Frenchman's life fits well the picture of the *Arsenicum* recluse. He was supercilious, uncommunicative, uncommonly sensitive to his surroundings and to most people, despising his fellow humans for their coarseness, vulgarity, inability to appreciate true beauty, and whatever else this supercritical individual chooses to despise in others; but he was equally critical and unsparing of himself. It was entirely apposite that, with his relentless search for the *mot juste,* he should have defined genius as the "the infinite capacity for taking pains."

There must be at least as many different kinds of genius as there are constitutional types. In contrast to the *Arsenicum* Flaubert's "infinite" capacity for perfecting, *Phosphorus* harbors the romantic notion that genius is inspiration, a divine gift which springs forth full-blown, like Venus from the sea foam. *Lachesis* embodies the notion that genius is sublimated neurosis, at times akin to madness. The *Natrum muriati-*

---

* His creative method contrasts sharply with that of his eminent *Sulphur* contemporary, Tolstoy, whose *War and Peace* went through only four rewritings (this fact is well established, since Tolstoy dictated the entire novel to his wife in the evenings). That over 500 characters should have been manipulated and this massive and complex work of history, philosophy, and romance written in only four drafts almost defies belief. *Arsenicum* contrasts also with the *Natrum muriaticum/ Phosphorus* Dickens and the *Lachesis* Dostoyevsky, both of whom turned out masterpieces like hotcakes, regularly every year or two.

cum genius is the distilled essence of suffering, born out of dogged tenacity in overcoming obstacles. The *Lycopodium* genius executes easily what others find difficult; while the *Sulphur* genius accomplishes feats others would find impossible. And we have seen how the genius of *Calcarea* emerges through systematic prodding and coaxing by another person.

Arsenicums who are not creative or performing artists themselves are often avid promoters of the arts. The theater and the ballet, concert halls and opera houses, museums and poetry readings are all packed with appreciative *Arsenicum* audiences. Although other constitutional types are, certainly, also represented, it is *Arsenicum* who most regularly frequents and supports the classical and innovative arts.

As patients these individuals exhibit the same inexorable perfectionism. Striving for absolute health, they spare no pains to achieve it and insist that all around them cooperate in their striving. Indeed, they may cultivate it with such eagerness and ardor as leaves the physician nonplussed. Instead of pursuing their goal merely sufficiently to live a productive life, they allow it to become virtually an obsession or even their *raison d'être*. Thus they are annoyed, even frantic, at the slightest bodily malfunction. Not being in perfect health seems to *Arsenicum* illogical, incomprehensible, and totally unjust.

A seventy-five-year-old gentleman in excellent overall health consulted his homoeopathic physician for a small bony growth on the wrist. He was advised to leave it alone since there was no pain, and he was going to be treated constitutionally, but he was full of anxious concern: "I don't want *anything* on me that doesn't belong there. We *must* get rid of this growth. I can't leave it alone; it bothers me too much. If you can't remove it homoeopathically, I will have surgery."

This perfectionism sometimes leads to "anxious *impatience*" (Hahnemann) at the slow progress of cure (even in serious conditions such as heart disease). *Arsenicum* wants to be well at once—or by next week at the latest—and is exceedingly upset by setbacks, relapses or delays ("I can't stand it a moment longer!" is a key phrase of this type). For instance, a patient will come in for long-standing ringing or humming in the ear (tinnitus). He announces that he is prepared to give homoeopathy a six-month try, but after only two months of treatment with *Ar-*

senicum he becomes impatient and wants to know why his ears still ring in the evenings (formerly they rang all the time). "I don't want to criticize you, but . . . " and he then proceeds to criticize: "How long is the symptom going to last? Why is it still there? Can't you do *any-thing* about it?" he challenges, rather incongruously, since by his own admission the symptom is no longer manifested during the day. If he cannot get cured of an ailment fast enough, *Arsenicum* may become discouraged and convinced of its "fatal termination" (Kent).

An anemic teenage boy was being treated for the complications of protracted mononucleosis. He was blessed with two *Arsenicum* parents who called at least once a day to know why their son, although improved, was not progressing more rapidly (at times they called simultaneously on the two office lines, the father from work and the mother from home). "Could the slow convalescence indicate something more serious, such as leukemia or Hodgkin's Disease?" (*Arsenicum*, incidentally, is one of the most-used remedies in mild or severe anemia: Boger).

In his angry impatience to get well, the individual fights illness so vehemently that he becomes worn out and exacerbates his condition. Whenever the physician instinctively wants to tell an anxiously fretting patient, "Don't be so importunate! Contain yourself, be patient, and everything will be all right. Good health comes with time," he should consider *Arsenicum* as the simillimum.

This trait of carrying a good thing to excess in matters of health is often directed at various kinds of diets (those unending *Arsenicum* diets! what they can and cannot eat!). They almost invariably have strong opinions about food: sometimes correct, sometimes ridiculous. One female patient regularly deprived her children of their favorite pizza and spaghetti during the summer months, claiming that the digestive organs do not function as well in hot weather. Another insisted that they do not function well in cold weather; while a third gave up peanut butter (his favorite food) because, as he decided, it stops all enzyme activity.

With his eyes drilling into the physician and in a quavering voice he talks of "the *quality* versus *quantity*" of his protein consumption, of exactly how *few* ounces of protein he needs to survive, of how he never "pollutes" his body with a mucus-forming piece of cheese (mucus is the horror and dread of many *Arsenicums*). Or, in an extremity of desire for "detoxification" (this is the patient who most fears and talks about being "toxic"), he undergoes rigorous fasts and juice diets over an extended period of time, oblivious to the danger of depriving himself of essential nutrients.* This is the person who, indeed, does not live by bread alone, but also by his interminable theories of nutrition.

Many constitutional types dislike any dietary restrictions the homoeopath may suggest, even if only the elimination of coffee (to allow the remedies to work their best). But *Arsenicum* loves being placed on a diet and will religiously follow the most Spartan regime. He not only delights in nutritional fads, but the necessity of a special diet certifies the seriousness of his condition. If the physician simply advises him to eat a normal healthy diet—avoiding junk food, getting plenty of fresh fruit and vegetables, whole grains, and protein—the patient will be disappointed. This is not what he came to hear. He wants specific, *restricting* instructions. Some proudly bring the physician five-page lists of foods they have scrupulously avoided for months, and even years, because some test or other has shown them to be allergenic.

Arsenicum is, in general, an authoritarian nature which likes to follow instructions, obey (certain select) rules, adhere to timetables, fill out required forms, and in other ways gratify his love for system, precision, and order ("Few procedures in life give me as much satisfaction as filling out forms. It is a clean, precise, self-limiting task, and when you've finished, you don't have to think about it anymore but send the forms away to be read for a purpose, then filed in an orderly manner for present or future use"). One patient stated, when the first dose of the remedy had relaxed his defenses, "I have been feeling disoriented, sloppy, and inefficient ever since taking *Arsenicum*. I would like to recapture my former secure rigidity." He was only partly joking. In fact, this constitutional type is so cooperative and follows instructions so faithfully that the physician must be absolutely precise in giving them. An anxious elderly patient with edema from a heart condition was given placebo pills to

---

* *Arsenicums* are often obsessed with the functioning of their digestive and eliminative systems (*Natrum muriaticum*). They will insist that they need at least three bowel movements a day to remain healthy and consider themselves headed for physical deterioration if they cannot meet this target. Others subject themselves to numberless colonic irrigations. "I am so toxic," one declared with fear in his eyes but enthusiasm in his voice, "that the health clinic tells me I will need three colonics a week for the next two years at least!"

take an hour before each meal while his constitutional remedy was working out its effect. He returned a month later to state that, although his edema was improved, he was unaccountably tired in the morning. Questioning revealed that he had been forcing himself out of bed at 5:30 every morning to take the placebo pills at least an hour before his first cup of tea.

Yet another form of excessive concern with diet is observed in the *Arsenicum* woman (especially) who, although already attractively thin, or even as thin as a rail ("great emaciation; remarkably thin": Allen), feels fat and wants to be still thinner. Indeed, she insists that she *must* lose ten pounds to feel well; that any slight addition to her meager fare will make her bloated, heavy and generally uncomfortable. The classic *Arsenicum* hypochondriac's complaint is "fullness in the stomach after eating" (after all, why *shouldn't* the stomach feel full after eating?). By cutting down on the variety of her foods and progressively restricting her intake ("This doesn't agree with me . . . That is too heavy . . . too fattening . . . ") she succeeds in becoming hypersensitive to an increasing number of foods, and may work herself into an anorexic state that is exceedingly difficult to treat: "having not the least appetite, she . . . gets furiously angry if pressed to eat" (Hahnemann).* Because of the type's self-discipline, the opposite picture, "she eats and drinks more than is good for her" (Hahnemann), is less often encountered.

The remedy however, can encourage moderation and common sense in a patient's eating habits.

Sensitivity to the Environment

An image which particularly suits *Arsenicum* is the E-string on the

---

* As befits the *Arsenicum* picture, anorexics are, characteristically, intelligent and capable persons who are able to exert the tremendous will power and concentration required to stop eating. Also, the type's competitiveness is manifested in the anorexic. Just as he must be "the best" in everything he does, so the focus of his pride and sense of achievement is directed to being "the thinnest" — thereby proving to himself and the world a superior control over his appetite and body. Hence his anger at being urged to eat, as well as his panic, and, at times, hysteria upon encountering someone more emaciated than himself (*Nux vomica* [Boericke] and *Natrum muriaticum* [Whitmont] can display a similar picture).

violin. The thinnest, tautest, and most delicately tuned of all the strings ("oversensitiveness and excessive tenderness of disposition": Hahnemann), it is not only the source of the most sensitive vibrations but also the first to go out of tune. Either it snaps from the least excess of tension, or—if strung a fraction of a millimeter too loose—it plays flat. In just the same way, *Arsenicum* must be perfectly adjusted to function well.

First, the physical environment must be just right. If it is cold, he immediately contracts respiratory ailments: colds, sinusitis, bronchitis, or pneumonia. Along with *Nux vomica, Hepar Sulphuris, Silica*, and *Psorinum, Arsenicum* is among the chilliest of constitutional types, sometimes the chilliest of all, even while liking fresh air. The patient will have *icy* hands and feet and complain that he cannot get enough warmth, even when bundled up in layers of clothes or sitting so close to the fire that another person would be scorched. He can lie like a cat all day in the sun, soaking up its rays. But the more sensitive ones cannot tolerate warmth either, displaying little tolerance of high or low temperatures and feeling really comfortable only within a 3-4 degree range (*Mercury*).

He is also prone to allergies: dust, mold, feathers, horse or dog hair, and cat dander. This constitutional type, which is more sensitive to cats than any other, is perhaps also fonder of them. Patients will put up with endless suffering, including attacks of asthma, rather than get rid of them. Not only do they feel strong kinship with a creature as clean and fastidious as themselves, they admire and respect the cat's precise, elegant, flowing movements, its calm and self-possessed demeanor, and its dignified proud independence.

They may react adversely to specific foods, particularly milk, wheat and sugar; also to cold drinks, watery fruits and certain nuts or seafoods. Ice cream, with its combination of cold, milk, and sugar, can be nearly lethal. Alcohol in any form may give them hay-fever symptoms, with headaches, running eyes, and severe itching in the ears, nose and throat; or it aggravates their other symptoms (*Lachesis, Nux vomica*). They also react badly to coffee, and usually benefit from discontinuing it, being sufficiently highly strung already.

Arsenicum can be sensitive to odors of various kinds: incense, perfume, certain flowers and plants, gasoline fumes, and tobacco (*Ignatia, Nux vomica*: Kent). With the nose of a bloodhound he senses odors long before anyone else (*Phosphorus*). His hearing, like his smell, is extra-acute ("sensitive to noise": Hahnemann). In his state of constant nervous irritability noises of all kinds and any disruption of quiet make him jumpy or angry; music prevents him from concentrating, or even thinking, and he even becomes excessively irritated from the normal background noise of children (*Natrum muriaticum*) or at the aesthetic affront of persons loudly chewing gum. If the dog next door is barking, he cannot work; if church bells strike the hour, he cannot sleep. In short, "everything seems to him too strong and loud, all talk, every noise, all light" (Hahnemann).*

In his extreme sensitivity to his surroundings, even excitement throws him off balance. The child becomes "hyper" from happiness as well as stress and then has trouble getting to sleep. The adult may lie awake most of the night after a good film, an emotionally provocative novel, or a stimulating after-dinner conversation (*Phosphorus*).

Arsenicum, in general, suffers from various forms of insomnia: "anxiety on lying down prevents him getting to sleep before midnight," "anxiety and restlessness waking him after midnight or at 3:00 a.m. with inability to fall asleep again," "great fear . . . or attacks of anxiety at night drive him out of bed," "sleepless from anguish," "no rest by day or night," "so downhearted from continued sleeplessness (for months) that wants to commit suicide," etc. (Hahnemann, Hering, Allen).

---

* A caricature of these *Arsenicum* sensitivities is found in Wilkie Collins' *The Woman in White*, in the portrait of the aesthete and affected invalid, Mr. Fairlie, described as "frail, languidly-fretful and over-refined" in looks, with a "thin, worn, and transparently pale face, high and hooked nose, and white delicate hands adorned with two priceless rings." Upon greeting the soft-spoken hero of the novel in his darkened room with a "Pray sit down. And don't trouble yourself to move the chair, please. In the wretched state of my nerves [I am nothing but a bundle of nerves dressed up to look like a man] movement of any kind is exquisitely painful to me," he then implores him, "Pray excuse me. But *could* you contrive to speak in a lower key? . . . Loud sound of any kind is indescribable torture to me." And a bit later, "I beg your pardon. Do you mind my closing my eyes when you speak? Even this light is too much for them." Finally, this professional hypochondriac dismisses the hero with "I am such a sufferer . . . Gently with the curtains please; the slightest noise from them goes through me like a knife."

Although many of his sensitivities overlap with those of *Phosphorus*, *Natrum muriaticum* and others, *Arsenicum* is distinguished from them by the important guiding modality, "amelioration from external warmth and heat" (Kent) in any form. Hot baths, hot drinks and food, sunshine, a fire, warm applications to the painful or affected area, all bring relief to his symptoms and sensitivities. Some wear heavy socks at night in order to fall asleep, and when the easily awoken individual cannot get back to sleep, he is helped by a heating pad or by *sipping*—not gulping down ("thirsty, for small quantities": Kent)—a hot cup of milk or weak tea. Only certain head and sinus pains are better from cool air, and sometimes he desires the window open at night to feel the cool on his head, while the rest of him snuggles under a mound of blankets.

For the highly strung "E-string" *Arsenicum* to perform well, not only must the environment be just right, but his own subjective condition must also be in tune. External pressures must be precisely offset by his inner tension. Too much pressure in school, for instance, can cause this child to develop headaches, insomnia, facial and other tics, while too little pressure, the absence of deadlines or insufficient intellectual stimulus, may evoke from him a flat and inelegant performance.

A thirteen-year-old boy was being treated for constant fatigue, after-school headaches, growing irritability, and an unusual (for him) inability to concentrate on his schoolwork. The cause seemed to be an absence of stimulus in school. He liked math and French but had not been placed in the advanced class in these subjects. Nor was he inspired by his other courses. He played the clarinet well, but because of his age was in the mediocre Junior Orchestra instead of the excellent Senior Orchestra where he belonged. Thus he was unchallenged on every front. Frequent doses of homoeopathic arsenic helped him through this difficult time, and the following year he was promoted to the fast track in school and to the Senior Orchestra. This increased stimulus had its effect: he blossomed physically and mentally and needed very few medicines thereafter.

This need of a favorable environment for good performance brings back the classic picture of *Arsenicum* as the thoroughbred horse who runs well only under special conditions: when specially fed and exercised and allowed to perform on a graded track suited to brilliant bursts of short-term speed. In such circumstances he will outperform all other breeds; otherwise he may not even place. He does not possess real stamina and endurance but has nervous short-term energy in abundance.

Thus *Arsenicum* is sometimes the discontented (and as a result constantly "complaining": Kent) patient to whom life has not vouchsafed those "perfect conditions" which he needs to succeed and fulfill his potential. But if the environment is right and matches his own inner tautness, he performs beautifully, bringing all his powers of application and his urge for perfection to bear on the subject at hand.

"All or Nothing"

Arsenicum can deceive the physician on the lookout for the classic picture of fastidiousness, as in the following case of a female patient with eczema who had been treated homoeopathically without much success. The condition presented no striking physical features, and the patient was otherwise healthy, so the physician first prescribed *Pulsatilla* for her sweet manner and appearance and then *Sulphur* because he had seen her chronically messy house. Thus *Arsenicum*, with its extreme sensitivity to disorder, had never occurred to him. But he had failed to ask the patient how she felt about her domestic chaos and whether it upset her much. "Does it!" was the vigorous reply. "Every couple of months I can't stand it any longer, blow up, and clean non-stop for two whole days until everything is as neat as a pin. Then I collapse in exhaustion and don't touch the house again until my next explosion."

Strenuous activity alternating with inaction is frequently observed in the *Arsenicum* housewife. She would like her house to be clean and neat, but, because her husband and children disrupt this order and track in dirt, she gives up altogether. If it cannot be perfect, she refuses to do even the minimum—that is, until her frustration with the disorder becomes intolerable, and she embarks on another spurt of frenzied housecleaning.

Another variant of the slovenly *Arsenicum* is the individual who is extra-meticulous in the one sphere which interests him and nowhere else (*Sulphur, Natrum muriaticum*). One memorable female patient used to come to the office dressed as if just released from a concentration camp. Yet her garden, with its beautifully tended flower-beds and shrubs, was a marvel of perfection! Every corner bespoke the year-round toil that she invested in her favorite hobby (landscape-gardening is a prominent *Arsenicum* passion). This was the focus of her fastidiousness, while all other spheres were totally disregarded. By the same token, the eczema patient with the messy house was a superior painter on china, an expert in a taxing craft which demanded hours of concentrated, painstaking application.

This "all or nothing" attitude may lead *Arsenicum* to lose interest in an endeavor once he realizes that he cannot really achieve excellence. Unwilling to compromise with perfection, he prefers withdrawing from the field altogether. The talented pianist will abandon his instrument, knowing that he cannot reach the heights of a Horowitz or a Rubinstein. The gifted amateur painter will never pick up his brush, knowing that he will not be a master. The athlete who has been number one and is then supplanted by another will withdraw from the sport completely rather than be number two.

Such absolutism can lead to wasted talent, as with *Calcarea*, but the highly motivated *Arsenicum* suffers from unfulfillment and frustration, while the unmotivated *Calcarea* is resigned to his lot and dabbles contentedly in something else. *Arsenicum* aims too high, *Calcarea* too low; both may end by defeating their own potential.

On every subject he tends to an "all-or-nothing" response. His tastes are strong, his opinions definite. Generally speaking, he either likes or dislikes a person, respects or disdains him, with few intermediate possibilities. "My present teacher is excellent but the previous one was a fool." "She is a wonderful person, but I can't stand her boorish husband," he states with dogmatic finality, and nothing will induce him to change his mind. Children shout angrily, "I don't *want* to invite Jim to my party. I *hate* Jim! I don't *care* if he is a family friend. I *only* want Peter and Matt!"

To persons fortunate enough to meet his standards *Arsenicum* can be loyal for life; he is sensitive and generous when he so chooses ("gentle kindliness": Hahnemann) but will not waste time on those who fail to live up to his expectations. Furthermore, in his instinct for making distinctions, he finds himself comparing people for their relative worth. "Eleanor is a much better friend to me than Helen ever was," "William is far more intelligent than his brother," are characteristic reactions. He knows exactly who stands where on the ladder of his preferences, as well as in some objective moral hierarchy, and he does not hesitate to tell others. This contrasts with types such as *Pulsatilla* or *Lycopodium* who instinctively dislike ranking people in order of merit and who avoid comparisons. This same attitude is exhibited by *Arsenicum* in the artistic area. He will love oil painting but hate watercolors, love Italian opera but hate German, and expresses his opinions emphatically: "Brahms is by far the greatest composer who ever lived!"; "I can't stand modern poetry!"

Tolerance is not his strong point. He cannot abide incompetence, weakness, failure, ill health, or poor performance. He is quick to call others "idiots" or "crooks" and, to the hypercritical individual, except for himself, everyone is stupid, incompetent, and lacking in integrity (in Kent this trait is listed under the rubric, "censorious," where *Arsenicum* and *Sulphur* are the only two remedies in the third degree). He can also be pugnacious, sarcastic, jeering ("inclined to jest in a malicious manner": Allen), accusatory, swift to put others on the defensive, and his tongue can be as cutting as that of *Lachesis* even though under better control. He may even take enjoyment in "malice" (Hering) and intrigue, or display a "love for scandal" (Boenninghausen); or he is ruthless in asserting himself (*Nux vomica, Lachesis*).

On the physical level this power of destruction is seen in paralyses, malignancies, destruction of the bone marrow (leukemia), inflammations, ulcerations and necroses of the skin, mucous membranes, and other tissues.*

In the consulting room *Arsenicum* can be revealed by his *strong language*—not crude but contemptuous and at times insulting. He will describe as "fools" or "butchers" the physicians who have handled his case in the past and may even launch into a tirade against the whole

---

* In the case of Constantine Hering, *Arsenicum* cured an incipient gangrene—and converted him to homoeopathy. In medical school he was assigned the task of writing an expose of this "New Medicine." While so engaged he accidentally infected his finger in the dissecting room. It became septic and gangrenous, and to avoid amputation he acted on a friend's advice and took a dose of *Arsenicum album*. In his own words, "I owed to homoeopathy far more than the preservation of a finger. To Hahnemann, who had saved my finger, I gave my whole hand and, to the promulgation of his teachings, not only my hand, but the entire man, body and soul." Thereafter Hering adopted as his own scientific credo: "Not to accept anything without proving it, still less to reject anything without trying it."

medical profession ("We all realize that doctors don't know what they are talking about and that most of them are totally incompetent," . . .). The patient who readily criticizes all his physicians, pointing out how often he has been right and they wrong, or who complains that they refuse to acknowledge the seriousness of his condition, is usually an *Arsenicum*: "The doctors tell me I don't have diabetes, and the tests don't show up as diabetes, but you know how ignorant doctors are. None of them ask the right questions, and they never listen to what I tell them. I know I *must* have diabetes because . . . " and so on (*Arsenicum*, together with *Sulphur, Phosphorus*, and *Natrum muriaticum*, is prominent in patients with a diabetic diathesis and has proven invaluable in many cases).

Even in friendly everyday conversation *Arsenicum* may express his views in strong terms. One such patient was commenting to a friend on a Sunday religious service: "Your church is lovely, and the service was charming, but the singing—it was really dreadful! You know, your choirmaster should be shot!" Or a possessive mother, remarking on her infant son's future love life, declares "I know I will want to *kill* his first girlfriend"; or the father of a maturing daughter admits, "I feel like *murdering* every boy she looks at with affection." Interestingly, *Arsenicum* is one of the remedies listed high in Kent under the rubrics, "desire to kill," "sudden impulse to kill."

He is also intolerant of *ideas* not in accord with his own. His is the only "right" way of thinking, and he is quite prepared to ride roughshod over those who do not agree. Even the less intellectually arrogant person will insist in a discussion, "No, you don't understand me, you don't hear what I'm saying . . . ," implying that if you *did* hear, you would perforce concur. Intolerance makes him irritable, or perhaps his irritability makes him intolerant. In any case, he can be "easily annoyed; vexed and dissatisfied with everything" (Hering) or "peevish and sensitive; the least thing insults or angers him" (Hahnemann).

It cannot be claimed that the *Arsenicum* patient necessarily becomes completely tolerant after receiving this medicine. He remains judgmental, discriminating, and fastidious; but, even so, the remedy will help develop in him a magnanimous willingness to concede some virtue to watercolors, German opera, or modern poetry—or to some previously disliked individual, even if he cannot bring himself to appreciate them. In short, he can develop a "live and let live" attitude which was previously lacking. He may not want extensive contact with those misguided souls who think differently from himself, as even the most sociable *Arsenicum* is seldom openhearted with everyone; while polite and cooperative, he is also discriminating and will put himself out only for those he really likes. But in his newfound liberality he is at least willing to acknowledge that there is room on earth for all kinds.

Selfishness

The homoeopathic literature characterizes *Arsenicum* as "selfish" (Boericke), and, indeed, he often views situations in the light of his own interests. But then, as mentioned in the *Sulphur* chapter, each constitutional type has a selfish side which is expressed in its own particular way.

Arsenicum is always watching out for himself. He wants to be sure he is getting his due or his money's worth, and a particular form of his paranoia is the fear that others are cheating or shortchanging him— whereupon he sets up a vociferous protest. Even in the physician's office he may look with suspicion at the small size of the homoeopathic dose ("Is that all? Only ten measly grains? Don't I get something to take home?"). While other constitutional types are surprised or amused by the smallness of the dose, *Arsenicum* may be really perturbed.

He can be relentless in getting "the best" for himself, heedless of the possibility that others might be left with less or worse. He continually seeks special privileges, special attention, special treatment, here again exhibiting a terrier-like persistence in obtaining his desires. He wants exceptions made for himself that are not made for others or constantly feels that what he is getting is *not enough* or *not good enough.* In his striving for more his "desire is greater than his need" (Hahnemann), and maybe greater than he deserves.

This characteristic of always trying to get the most or the best is not necessarily a sign of selfishness. It can be another manifestation of *Arsenicum*'s perfectionism and determination to maintain standards. A quaint illustration was the 93-year-old woman who sought homoeopathic help for her winter bronchitis. She had the type's starchy and tidy look as well as its energetic and sprightly manner. Typical also was the remedy's prominent time modality ("I *love* the early part of the day and am at my smartest and brightest in the morning!"). But the finishing touch was her parting inquiry of the receptionist. Transfixing her with a sharp glance, she asked, "Is that doctor I saw a good one?"

"Excellent. He is one of the best," she was assured.

"I'm glad to know that," was the cheerful reply of the braced-up nonagenerian. "I like to know that I'm in good hands. It's very important at my age."

Sometimes *Arsenicum* is more *pushy* than selfish, never letting up. In promoting his own interests and well-being, he assaults others with demands. Especially the woman (more than any other type) treats the physician as if he were her personal servant. If she wants to talk for an hour about her theories of medicine, the physician should sit there and listen. He must also be at her beck and call any time of day or night, ready to answer all questions, soothe her concerns, and resolve all her problems. Once she has favored the physician with her patronage, he becomes obligated to keep her family functioning at optimum level, the children all doing well in school, and her own mind free of anxieties. If she is not satisfied—for instance, if some family member happens to succumb to the 'flu'—her tone becomes accusatory.

When hiring a servant or employee, *Arsenicum* will press mercilessly for a commitment to perform impossible amounts of work. This egregious pressure does not necessarily denote meanness. Once the conditions have been firmly settled and the boundaries established, he can be a most kind and considerate employer, willing to help out in time of need and retaining employees for years. But at the outset he cannot resist pushing to the maximum.

Every classroom has its *Arsenicum* student who raises his hand at the end of the lecture and requests additional information or further explanations, not because he failed to understand the first time round but because he wants *more*. He is determined to extract every last morsel of information, every shred of the teacher's hard-won knowledge and experience, every last drop of his blood. This reflects, in part, his enthusiasm and eagerness to learn and achieve good results, which is a desirable quality; but, here again, *Arsenicum* can demonstrate too much of a good thing.*

---

* A homoeopathic physician once received a letter from a would-be lay practitioner who was a complete stranger asking for samples of over sixty remedies, each in four different potencies, with the assurance: "I know you do not mind making these up for me, to help set me up in practice, since you are interested in promoting the growth of

He can be selfish with his money, stingily refusing to spend it on a friend or even lend it to him, and also with his time, regarding it as a most precious commodity and aware that it is limited—far too limited to accomplish all that he wants to do. So he husbands it with care, doling it out reluctantly, when and how he chooses and not necessarily according to the needs of others. In daily life this becomes especially apparent on the telephone, where he can be surprisingly curt. He has no time for talk unless he himself has placed the call, and his tone, if not his actual words, will convey this attitude.

The selfishness of *Arsenicum* can make him calculating, regulating his behavior to extract the most from a given situation. Or he may fear to give an ounce more than he has contracted for.* But the positive side is that he carries out to the letter whatever he has contracted to do. In contrast to the intrinsically more generous *Phosphorus*, he is completely trustworthy and reliable.

Furthermore, he will usually not take more than he gives. Unlike some *Sulphurs*, he does not expect favors to run only one way. If he does not intend to reciprocate, he will not accept. He is willing to do his share of work—and more—in any cooperative venture; in fact, he will be one of the first to volunteer and will perform generously and well. But—and there is often a "but" to his giving—he then expects others to reciprocate by helping out when needed (acting "decently and correctly" as he might put it). If the response is not what he considers appropriate, he becomes angry and indignant, and may even peremptorily break off the relationship. Thus, while he might enter a situation calculating "what's in it for me?" he is motivated as much by equity as by selfishness. He is prepared to give much and merely wants

---

homoeopathy." He even considerately included $2 for postage. The physician did not feel he could render this service, but, when returning the two dollars, he did confess to the temptation to send a free sample of high-potency *Arsenicum*.

* This trait was exhibited in an extreme form by an *Arsenicum* tenant who was asked at the last moment by the landlord to water a recently planted bush during the period of occupancy. The response was a letter enumerating several reasons why the tenant could not shoulder this responsibility and concluding with the reminder that it was not specified in the lease!!

a fair return for his outlay. Equity is not always easy to measure, but *Arsenicum* himself knows precisely what it entails.

Sometimes, however, the opposite is true, and he *uses* people; his thoughtfulness and consideration are manipulative, and he drops an acquaintance who has outlived his usefulness. Or his demanding nature may drive him to challenge a friend who has supported and encouraged him in the past with: "But what have you done for me *lately?*" or "What are you doing for me *now?*"

The Commanding General

Whether obvious about it or inconspicuous, *Arsenicum* is a domineering personality. He takes the lead in personal relations, determining their scope and tone, and leaving others no choice but to comply. He is exceedingly easy and pleasant to get along with—as long as he gets his own way (*Lycopodium*). Not only does he balance the give and take in friendship, even in larger social gatherings he often insists on dominating (*Sulphur*). The symptom, "pain aggravated by other people's talking" (Hering), is revealing.* He becomes restless and fidgety, and his headache, sinus trouble, joint, stomach or other pains intensify when he must listen to another person lecture or be present at a gathering where he has little to say (*Sulphur* simply falls asleep when others are talking and *Lycopodium* walks away). The *Arsenicum* teacher, for example, will admit that the most difficult part of his job is the staff meeting, where he must listen to the opinions of others ("Long conferences invariably upset me"). This is due, in part, to the type's physical restlessness ("better from motion, walking about": Boger), but that is not the whole story. When he himself can talk, the symptoms vanish, no matter how long he must remain sitting.

Accordingly, "better from conversation" (Hering) is a major *Arsenicum* modality. Talking in general, and about his symptoms in particular, relieves them greatly and may even cause them to disappear. Hence, also, the prominent corollary, aggravation of symptoms when alone—i.e., when he has no one to *talk* to. Several patients have claimed that they always travel by plane, despite a fear of flying, because of rising panic during long hours in a bus or train with no familiar person nearby

---

* In the Boger *Repertory Arsenicum* is the only remedy listed in the third degree under "aggravation hearing others talking."

(unlike *Sulphur*, *Calcarea*, or especially *Phosphorus*, *Arsenicum* does not easily strike up conversations with strangers). In this he contrasts also with *Lycopodium* or *Natrum muriaticum* who primarily need assurance that they are not alone in the house—that someone is close at hand—and feel no need to engage in conversation.

The domineering *Arsenicum* cannot abide others being in charge and insists on making all decisions himself. Whether in preparing a meal or remodeling a house, others are merely allowed, or expected, to help out by following directions, and the spouses of these types sometimes lament feeling like "indentured servants" who must justify by obedience and submission in work their right to live in their own homes. He takes pride in his ability to grapple with the varied problems of everyday life and constantly gives advice to others. The non-stop backseat driver is *Arsenicum*. He may disapprove of the way the dishes are stacked in the dishwasher and immediately set about rearranging them "better." More generally, he loves putting people's houses in order—either literally (these persons make the best housekeepers) or figuratively, i.e., the secretary will rearrange her employer's files more efficiently or an editor is superb at "whipping into shape" a short story or novel written by someone else.

The exhausted housewife hangs around the kitchen giving ceaseless instructions to the dutiful husband, child, or friend who is trying to be helpful by preparing the dinner. She is also notorious for frantically tidying up her house the day *before* the cleaning woman arrives. Instead of relaxing on this one day, she drives herself into a harassed and irritable frenzy. She offers many justifications for this behavior, but the ultimate reason is her inability to relinquish control. In extreme cases she will follow the unfortunate cleaning woman around, supervising her every step ("You can't leave them alone for *one* minute . . . You never know what they'll do next—or worse, what they'll *forget* to do!").

A single woman, rising in her career as a fashion designer and enjoying her independence, was being treated for Raynaud's disease (circulatory difficulties in the extremities, especially the fingers). She was physically chilly and not overly warm emotionally, but obviously considerate and intelligent. The physician was trying to decide between *Sepia* and *Arsenicum*, both of which fitted her well, and asked if anything in her personal life was particularly bothersome. "My cleaning lady," was the prompt reply. "She is a sweet, honest, reliable person, and after she's cleaned, everything looks fine on the surface. But when I look *close*, I don't like what I see, and that disturbs me so much I can't function at home. I keep asking her to do better, but she doesn't pay any attention. Yet, I don't want to let her go. She needs the money, and she's getting old. So I'm not sure what to do." "Why don't you simply not look too close?" the doctor suggested. "I've tried that, but I can't help myself. Something *compels* me to peer into the dark corners and run my finger along the less obvious surfaces to check for dust." She was given *Arsenicum* 10M and after several doses her circulation had improved, while the edge was taken off her obsessive concern with dark and dusty corners. She later assured the physician that she no longer gave a thought to her cleaning lady's shortcomings.

As an employer *Arsenicum*'s self-drive impels him to drive others. He can be "dictatorial" (the remedy should be added in bold type to Kent's *Repertory* under that rubric) and pushes for *more, bigger,* and *better*. He is furious at incompetence and impatient at delays. He often wants to "dance faster than the music," trying to accelerate the course of events and others' responses to them. He is the boss who needs to run everything himself and have a finger in every pie (*Sulphur*). He is over-anxious, over-watchful, and incapable of delegating responsibility. He checks and rechecks what others have done, tells them what they should do or, if they have done it, how they should have done it differently. He can also be the super-efficient junior colleague or employee who always knows better than his superiors and insists on running the show his own way.

The same superior organizational talent is seen in *Arsenicum*'s other activities. In her well-regulated life, for example, the housewife finds time to do everything, and every minute of her day is accounted for. Although this may require overscheduling, tight deadlines, and rigid adherence to plans drawn up and enforced by her restless energy, she uses the time efficiently, and everything is done well. *Lachesis* and *Sulphur* may display superior energy but are more chaotic and disorganized.

Thus *Arsenicum* is the born Commanding General who loves to issue "marching orders," galvanize others into action, and compel acquiescence in his ideas. Nothing is left to chance or inspiration, no detail is beneath his consideration, as, with enthusiasm enough for all, he proceeds to organize and orchestrate everyone around him. His zeal is infectious and, more than any other type except perhaps *Sulphur,* he can persuade others to modify their lives *here* and *now*. This is all a manifestation of his creative drive, the drive of an artist who must open up and shape new fields according to his own vision—whether dealing with people, events and words, or with paint, clay and stone.

Even the simple cooperative ventures of everyday life are immediately taken over by an *Arsenicum*. In a tone of authority, suggesting little experience with contradiction, he or she lays out the plan of battle, assigning to each individual his or her appropriate role, and expediting matters generally. If 8:30 is the planned departure time for a family to leave by car on a three-week vacation, come hell or high water they *must* leave at 8:30 and not a minute later! The need to orchestrate can be detected in his very voice. Even when gracious and considerate, it is strong, definite, and determined—the voice of one accustomed to command. When displeased or frustrated at his or her loss of control, it can become shrill or strident.

His desire for extreme efficiency makes *Arsenicum* terribly upset when others fail to comply, and his well-thought-out plans misfire. Perfection, alas, has once more eluded him! He does not realize that others do not want to operate with his fanatical precision. They do not derive the same enjoyment from consummating intricate schemes through split-second timing—although *Natrum muriaticum*, whose insecurities also find relief in strict adherence to regimens and time schedules, sometimes resembles him in this respect.* Both types tolerate poorly ambiguity of any kind.

Arsenicum, in short, is unable simply to sit back and let things happen. He must be on top of every situation, seeking to govern not only the present but also the future. Then he panics when things do not go as expected, or if he must adjust to unforeseen circumstances. The slightest deviation from what has been planned throws him completely off balance, making him aggressive, belligerent, and sometimes even irrational. Thus, while there is no denying that a doctor's office often brings out the worst traits of the *Arsenicum* who is already fearful and insecure

---

* *Arsenicum*'s passion for tight schedules and elaborate schemes to implement them is caricatured in the person who, arranging to pick up a friend in the most time-efficient way, suggests, "When I come to your apartment house after work and ring downstairs three times, you jump out the window to meet me."

about his health, any situation of uncertainty about the future will have the same effect. This may be one reason why he enjoys work. His need for predictability and control is channeled and fulfilled—and the outcome is reasonably commensurate with his outlay of time and effort.

The need to dominate his environment emerges full force in the health-conscious person who, we saw, conducts his life in a strictly regulated routine of rest, exercise, and diet, all adjusted precisely to suit his physical and emotional needs. The authoritarian *Arsenicum* likes regulation, authority, and discipline so much that if others do not impose it on him he will impose it on himself. One will insist that his bed be aligned with the head to the North and the feet to the South, in perfect harmony with the polar magnetic forces, for maximum benefit from his essential eight hours of uninterrupted sleep. Another will take his pillow, spring water, and vegetables when he departs for even a short visit with a friend ("Your vegetables have no energy," he tells the startled host). Any guest who (considerately) brings his own food because of dietary restrictions is probably *Arsenicum.* One memorable patient would take not only his own tea, when visiting, but even his own teapot—made from a special clay which, he claimed, was imperative for his well-being.

This may be why he is so morbidly afraid of illness. Aside from a natural fear of pain and death and his perfectionist's frustration at the malfunctioning of any part of his anatomy, he is terrified by the prospect of *losing control* over his own body. Even in minor ailments he panics at the very thought of insubordination by some organ and laments, "I feel I am not in control of my body. I am doing everything I should—eating right, exercising every day, taking good care of myself—but *still* I don't feel well. What *am* I doing wrong?"

By the same token, the healthy *Arsenicum* talks with pride of being always "in control" of his body.

He, therefore, more than any other type, overreacts to the homoeopathic "aggravation," even when forewarned about it. Whereas the effect of an allopathic drug can often be adjusted by repeating or not repeating the medicine or by giving a larger or smaller dose, once the homoeopathic microdilution has been administered, the ensuing chain reaction cannot usually be regulated or arrested by either patient or physician. "How long is this going to last?" he asks in a panic. Or, "I refuse to

282   *Portraits of Homoeopathic Medicines*

put up with this itching rash one minute longer!'' The awareness that the constitutional remedy "takes over" and that he has to submit to its influence, may bother him more than any associated discomfort.

Indeed, *Arsenicum*'s impulse to assume command emerges strikingly in the physician's office. In health matters, as in all others, he not only wants at every moment to know where he stands in the curative process ("I really *need* to know exactly what's going on"), but also to nail down the future with a specific prognosis ("It is *essential* that I be told *precisely* what my prospects are!"). Needing to retain control, he wants to "fully understand *how* the homoeopathic remedies act on the body" or he insists on being given "scientific" names for his various health problems—in violation of two major homoeopathic assumptions: that (1) the action of the remedy is ultimately unknowable and (2) the names of "diseases" are irrelevant, since homoeopathy addresses the ill individual, not the disease. A woman, especially, will be upset and indignant at not being told the remedy prescribed until the following visit.* Sometimes she will just refuse to accept it unless identified: "I *like* to know what I am taking," she explains, with the type's propensity to state the obvious. She will proffer various rationalizations, but the real reason is her need to know the name so that *she* can decide if it is right or not. Curiously, this is the patient who most frequently remarks, "I know that homoeopathy uses poisons as remedies, and I don't want to be given arsenic or something like that!"

Even if the remedy is identified, *Arsenicum* can still be overbearing— questioning the physician's choice or demanding some justification. One persistent patient who extracted from the physician the admission that his wife was receiving *Rhus toxicodendron* (made from the poison ivy plant) for her arthritis promptly made her stop treatment, even though substantial improvement could already be observed. He protested that she was severely allergic to poison ivy and that *Rhus toxicodendron*

---

* In homoeopathy the patient is not customarily told what medicine he is receiving until the next visit, or until the medicine has exhausted its action, in order not to influence his description of his symptoms and their changing pattern. Knowing the name of the remedy, he could readily consult one of the many homoeopathic texts describing in detail the symptomatic changes which that remedy can be expected to produce.

could certainly harm her if it was strong enough to produce a change in her symptoms and physiological state. In homoeopathy, as elsewhere, a little knowledge is a dangerous thing.

Another patient will want to sit in when the physicians are deciding on his remedy: "It's not that I want to control the analysis, you understand, but I want to participate in a discussion concerning *me*. I know myself better than you do, so I think I should have some say in how you analyze me . . . " A third vents her indignation at being asked to step out of the room: "I think it's rude to send me out while you're conferring about me—I don't like people talking about me behind my back. And it's even ruder not to tell me what medicine I am receiving." The homoeopath in these instances feels profound sympathy with Hahnemann's famous retort to a (doubtless *Arsenicum*) patient: "The name of your illness, Sir, does not interest me, and the name of the medicine does not concern you."

In fact, it is a significant victory for homoeopathy when the patient volunteers on a return visit, "I *still* don't understand how the remedies work, and half the time I don't even know what you're giving me, but I don't care anymore. Just keep on doing what you're doing." In other words, once his anxiety to know as much as the physician has been attenuated, once his suspicion of the physician's competence has been allayed (like *Lycopodium*, he ultimately trusts only his own understanding), once he can hand over the reins to another, even if only temporarily, he is is ready to assimilate the homoeopathic philosophy and is on the road to cure.

If he then takes the trouble to read some homoeopathic literature, he will promptly manifest the irresistible urge to take command of his own case and may start to question the physician's choice of remedy or potency: "Why are you repeating *Arsenicum*? I think I am *Nux vomica*. And I think I need a higher potency, to have the remedy's action last longer!". Or, if given three doses to take at weekly intervals for excessive anxiety, he may respond by lecturing the physician on the perils of overprescribing: "These remedies can be dangerous, you know!".

His need to take charge is encouraged by the ready availability of the homoeopathic remedies, and soon after his introduction to the science he may start administering them to himself, his friends, and his family. To give him his due, he is usually quite proficient, even as a beginner, displaying an undeniable knack for this discipline. Whenever the physician finds himself competing with the patient, overtly or sub-liminally, for control of the case, he may be reasonably sure that *Arsen-icum* is prominent in the picture (see also the Appendix).

Intellect and Pride

Arsenicum is frequently endowed with superior intelligence. He is alert, verbally resourceful, sharp at repartee, thinks quickly on his feet, and thrives on intellectual challenges ("mind energetic and fresh": Allen). Not only are the critical faculties well-developed, the mind is orderly, disciplined and at times refined. More often than any other type's it resembles (to use a familiar image) a well-oiled and well-func-tioning piece of fine machinery. The reverse side of this focussed pic-ture is the exhausted or ill patient who suffers from a "crowding of various ideas which he is too weak to keep off, so as to occupy himself with a single one" ((Hahnemann; also *Sulphur* and *Lachesis*).

Not surprisingly, the academic world is populated with *Arsenicums* (together with *Sulphurs* and *Natrum muriaticums*), as teaching fur-nishes them an admirable occasion for dictating to others. Every teacher exerts a certain domination over the minds of his students, but each constitutional type does it in a different way. Some teach by drawing out their students, patiently encouraging even the poorest of them to volun-teer their opinions (*Natrum muriaticum*); others instruct by sparking new interests or performing for their class (*Phosphorus*); *Sulphur* and *Lachesis* talk *at* the students; and any of these types may invite dialogue or controversy, stimulating thought through the Socratic method. The *Arsenicum* style is dogmatic and authoritarian. He lectures crisply and forcefully and lets the chips fall where they may. The good students will profit from what he says, while the poorer ones must fend for themselves. *He* lectures to the brightest, brooking no interruption and not especially interested in the views of others. Since he is convinced that his own opinions are the best, he feels that group discussions are a waste of time. His attitude is that the students are there to learn what the teacher has to give them, not to hear themselves talk (*Lycopodium*'s attitude is similar). However, he is completely dedicated to his profes-sion, unsparingly imparts his knowledge and critical talents to this students, and outside the classroom on a one-to-one basis is a willing and helpful counselor. What is more, his perfectionism drives him to reach every student, and he is genuinely distressed by those who doze inattentively in the back row of the class until with time he realizes that he cannot inspire every student, lowers his expectations, and ceases entirely to be concerned about the unreceptive ones.

He may at times be excessively demanding. A typical *Arsenicum* "five-star general" type was the sixth-grader teacher in a boys' boarding school who suffered from repeated bouts of pleurisy. He was a driver who expected the boys to write intelligent papers on the causes and consequences of the Persian and Punic Wars, to compose sonnets in classical and Elizabethan forms, and to recite long passages from Shakespeare, Milton, and T. S. Eliot "with sensitivity, expression and understanding"—feats generally considered impossible for sixth-grade boys. He could be harsh and irascible, accepting no excuses for poor performance, rewarding those who studied well and disdaining those who did not. When accused of favoring the good students over the bad, he would reply, undaunted, "*Of course* I favor the good pupils. And the best ones I favor the most!" thereby encouraging every boy in the class to strive for acceptance into the elite circle of favorites.

To succeed with this approach, a teacher must be able to inspire and improve the performance of even the dullest child, and this patient did challenge and goad even inferior students to undreamed-of heights of achievement, so that in later years one and all saw him as a formative force in their lives.*

Even in private instruction—language or music lessons and the like—*Arsenicum* can be the sternest of taskmasters: critical, impatient with poor preparation, and chary with compliments. He is most supportive of good work but rarely flatters. "It's coming along," he will comment on a piece of music well performed, or, as the supreme accolade, "It plays well!" He does not aim to discourage, and secretly he is proud of the student who reflects his own good teaching, but, always looking ahead, he wants to elevate him to a yet higher level of achievement.

In fiction the *Arsenicum* cast of mind is exemplified by Conan

---

* *Bryonia* was the simillimum for his acute attacks of pleurisy, but it was *Arsenicum*, prescribed constitutionally, that lessened his susceptibility and prevented recurrence.

Doyle's Sherlock Holmes, the famous sleuth who has become the symbol of meticulous observation, precision in deduction, and scrupulous attention to detail. Holmes is also the confirmed *Arsenicum* bachelor who is devoted first and foremost to his profession. He claims that emotion will only interfere with the carefully cultivated machine-like efficiency and objectivity of his mental processes. His attitude toward Dr. Watson is also characteristic: loyal but demanding and waxing impatient at the latter's occasional slowness and incompetence. "You *see,* Watson, but you do not *observe!*" he continually rebukes his friend.

Then, too, in typically *Arsenicum* fashion, Holmes fluctuates between excess of nervous energy when the chase is on (when he can go for days without food or sleep) and collapse into a state of bored lassitude once the case has been solved. Even his appearance is true to type: thin, pale, ascetic-looking, with a beaked aristocratic nose in a gaunt face; long, sensitive fingers that so beautifully caress a violin; and especially those blue gimlet-like eyes whose penetrating glance overlooks nothing.

Because of these talents as a detective an *Arsenicum* side is encountered prominently among homoeopathic practitioners the world over, whatever their more obvious constitutional type. Along with the fascination with medicine and health and a pronounced intellectual independence goes a Holmesian love of detail and discrimination, also the capacity to make systematic use of skilful observation and deduction. These all attract to homoeopathic practice. Furthermore, the opportunity for rigorous and methodical thinking—for sifting through mountains of facts to extract the essential and making fine distinctions in order to pinpoint the simillimum—appeals greatly to *Arsenicum's* mental fastidiousness.*

The other remedies which figure prominently in the constitutions of homoeopathic practitioners are *Natrum muriaticum* (see that chap-

---

* This source of happiness can be unending. After spending hours "repertorizing" a difficult case, sometimes sitting up half the night classifying and numerically grading symptoms, and assessing their relative importance, then agonizing some more over selecting the most suitable potency, the prescriber can look forward to going through the same process, perhaps with the very next case!

ter) and, especially with the passage of years, *Sulphur* — from constant exposure to, and taking on, the illnesses and problems of others (*Sulphur*, we recall, is the great "cleanser").

Arsenicum has a great deal of pride and even arrogance. "I'm always right," or "I usually know what's going on before anyone else," are characteristic phrases, or he can display a "contemptuous, scornful disposition" (Boenninghausen). Since he must always be right himself, he will blame others when things go wrong (*Lycopodium*). If he botches up a job, he was given wrong advice; if he performs poorly, the teacher taught him badly; if he has given incorrect instructions, the subordinate who carries them out is at fault. Someone else is always to blame for his deficiencies or mistakes. Also, like *Lycopodium* or *Nux vomica*, he has sudden rushes of anger when defied or his authority is challenged.

This pride can take the form of assumption of superiority. He is an instinctive elitist and willing to accept the associated responsibility. Generally this elitism judges people less on birth, wealth, or privilege than on *performance* (although it can be affected by racial considerations and prejudices): he expects others to perform well. Yet, he himself is not exempt from his share of errors and misjudgments. Emma Woodhouse, the heroine of Jane Austen's *Emma,* portrays the type. She thinks her judgment infallible and likes to run other people's lives, even to the point of matchmaking. She is undoubtedly of superior intelligence, with a generous and high-minded character, yet her overbearing manner and her assumption of rank, importance and power lead her to misguided assessments of those around her.

Further, while freely criticizing others, *Arsenicum* himself is intolerant of criticism (*Sepia, Lycopodium*), which at times makes him prone to self-righteous "indignation" (Kent). He wants and needs to be thought perfect and will bend every effort, even scheme and manipulate, to achieve this end. Thus *pride* is another keynote of this character, together with anxiety, perfectionism and a commanding manner.

It can, however, be well hidden by a gracious surface. A young man was being treated for frequent headaches with nausea which built up in the afternoon and into the evening and were so intense that no constitutional remedy prescribed in single doses seemed effective. In

an attempt to discover which of the hitherto marginally helpful remedies could be administered on a more frequent basis he was asked to
reveal more of his inner being and the workings of his mind.* This took
a great effort on his part, as, unlike the more humble and trusting *Pulsatilla*, the proud *Arsenicum* does not enjoy discussing his moral shortcomings or admitting to negative traits, and will often deny his problems to the world, although he admits them to himself; but the patient
was honest and volunteered the following:

"I know that on the surface I appear cooperative and compliant
enough, and that here in this office you find me easy to get along with—
and I am, to a large extent. But I like to control people in subtle ways
and do need a place to express my strength, which I fortunately find
at work. Otherwise, I can become mean and ugly. I get along beautifully
with everyone except those who also seek to manage. Then we clash—
and I mean clash! Even if the struggle remains concealed from others,
I am determined to win out, and I always do. In general, there are few
things in life I cannot accomplish once I decide to do so."

This last characterization is true of many *Arsenicums*. They possess
a purposefulness and directness, an ingrained self-discipline and power
of concentration, that enable them to succeed in whatever they set out
to do. The patient continued, "Also, my outward tolerance is basically
an arrogant person's deliberate adoption of an attitude of amiability and
charity. Deep down I am arrogant and have no scruples or feelings of
guilt about it. I *know* I am more competent and intelligent than most."
This description could equally have fit a *Lycopodium*, but he would
not have spoken of himself in such a frank and self-discerning manner.
The physician rightly concluded that *Arsenicum* was the patient's
simillimum.

The Parent—The Power Behind the Throne

Arsenicum's "commanding general" willingness to take over the
lives of others is strongly exhibited by the female in family situations.
At best she is the "supermom" who balances husband, children, household (and sometimes career) without impairing the interests of any.

---

* In some chronic cases, especially where there has been previous
allopathic drugging, it is necessary to repeat the remedy. And in acute
cases repetition of the remedy is standard procedure.

She is a fair-minded disciplinarian and intelligently supportive parent, with happy, creative, and well-balanced children. But sometimes the "*Arsenicum* mother" so caricatures herself that the phrase has become a byword in homoeopathic circles. Eager to promote her children's welfare, she assails doctors, teachers, friends, and relatives with importunate demands. Her restless drive for perfection may lead her to change her child from one school to another in the middle of the year, yank him out of an extracurricular activity in which he is perfectly content and put him into another, or constantly switch tutors, doctors, baby-sitters, and the like, while frankly indicating to each their deficiencies and the reasons for the change. Like a bulldozer mowing down all obstacles before it, she clears the ground for her children to follow. And woe betide whoever stands in her way!

In the doctor's office she cannot leave even her teen-age child alone but must sit in on the interview, often answering the questions put to him. If asked to wait outside, she pokes her head in every few moments to remind him what to say ("Did you tell the doctor about those stomach aches you had last month?"). But if the physician asks the boy why he has come in, he replies that he does not know. "Well, then, what's wrong with you?" "Nothing." And, indeed, he *is* fine; it is just that his mother imagines him ill and has a list of problems that she thinks should be attended to.

These may reflect nothing more than the child's individual and perfectly acceptable way of functioning. But the mother, with her high expectations, has some preconceived image for the child to fit: "His grades are good enough, but he always puts off studying until the last moment," she complains; or "She is a well-behaved girl but too quiet. I would like her to be more outgoing." The physician's instinct is to tell her to leave the child alone!

Here again she is striving to dominate the future—this time, of her children. The ambitious Jewish mother in the well-known joke who introduces her three sons, aged seven, five, and three: "The oldest is the lawyer, the middle one the doctor, and the youngest is the rabbi!"—is *Arsenicum*.

Naturally this whole parental picture applies to the father as well. It is just that the physician is more likely to encounter the mother.

Sometimes her need for control, overly high expectations, and excessive anxiety can operate to the detriment of the children or lead to a poor relationship with them. This is exhibited in the constant scolder who is impatient with her children, quick to badger them or show her disappointment, critically berating them in that peculiarly *Arsenicum* no-let-up "dentist drill" style, and seldom content with their performance ("dissatisfied and finds fault with everything": Hahnemann). A grown child's common observation about such a parent is, "I now realize that *nothing* that I could have ever done—or been—would have satisfied him/her."

Finally, a different side of the constitutional picture emerges in the doting parent who, although strictly disciplined himself (or herself), indulges a child to an extreme, permitting him to be whiny or rude or constantly to demand attention. This may be another instance of the "all or nothing" syndrome. If the child cannot be perfect, if he is somewhat ornery, intractable, and uncontrollable, *Arsenicum* undergoes an about-face and makes no attempt to discipline him at all.

Thus, the devoted parent of the musical prodigy, rising young ballet dancer, gymnast or athlete, who is willing to spend hours each day chauffeuring him or her to distant lessons, attending competitions, rehearsals, or meets, and who closely supervises the daily workout or practice and constantly prods the child to excel, is most often *Arsenicum*. Graphic examples are Leopold Mozart and Annie Sullivan, the driving forces behind Wolfgang Mozart and Helen Keller. Both were strict and demanding, even though loving, disciplinarians who completely controlled the lives of their charges. Neither for a moment slackened in the task of molding and encouraging to ever greater accomplishment the raw material entrusted to them.

Annie Sullivan and Leopold Mozart manifest another noteworthy aspect of the remedy, a willingness to stay out of the limelight, to avoid center stage. Creating and molding are sufficient rewards in themselves, and the most ambitious *Arsenicum* can be content to remain a force in the background, an *eminence grise* exerting his influence indirectly by shaping the people who shape events. Or even when in charge—on the throne, so to speak—the *Arsenicum* personality may direct affairs inconspicuously and indirectly, unlike the *Sulphur* leader whose influence and power are clearly visible.

A mild-mannered and self-effacing female student at one of the homoeopathic courses, who had been classified by her fellow-students as *Phosphorus/Pulsatilla*, was surprised by the instructor's opinion that she was really an *Arsenicum*. "I am not anxious, aggressive, or tense," she protested. "I am not a worrier and take life easy. I would never consider myself that particular type." But she understood the assessment when it was pointed out that in a quiet way she always took over every situation and became the queen bee. "That's right," she responded with reflective surprise. "In every group I am immediately elected president or chairman, even though I seldom seek the honor. Then I am compelled to organize and direct others. This has happened to me dozens of times." She said this without boasting, in a somewhat wondering tone, intrigued that she had not thought of it before.

The individual is usually conscious of his abilities and, as mentioned earlier, can be boastful, but does not exaggerate his accomplishments. There is a rational basis to his sense of worth. If he says matter-of-factly, "I am a world authority on such and such," or "My son is the best mathematician in his class at Yale," it is usually so, whereas with *Sulphur* or *Lycopodium* it might or might not be. A typically *Arsenicum* succinct assessment of himself is, "I am hypertense, hyperactive, hyperworried, capable, and successful at whatever I undertake."

The Well-Balanced Type

Not every *Arsenicum* is the driving, domineering, anxious, excessively critical, or arrogant personality we have perforce been emphasizing in this chapter (we recall that fear or intolerance of illness brings out his worst traits). He can be the very antithesis: easy-going, exceptionally pleasant to deal with, gracious, and self-contained: "of a calm, firm mind; retaining his equanimity in all events" (Hahnemann).

He is also the naturally cheerful, obliging, and serene person whom few can surpass in charm, wit, or thoughtfulness in friendship and whose high intelligence enables him to perform socially and professionally with a happy ease ("good humored . . . disposed to gaiety . . . has pleasure in entertaining himself with others": Hahnemann). Thus he can be an exceptionally fine individual who reasons correctly, acts with integrity, and whose rational approach to life is supported by the moral rectitude and emotionally unbiased judgment characteristic of the type.

Sometimes this "uncommonly tranquil disposition" (Hahnemann) results from accepting some calming philosophy, and these persons may be deeply religious in a non-demonstrative way. At other times their serenity reflects a deliberate subjection of the instincts. For *Arsenicum* does well whatever he puts his mind to. If his impulse to control is directed at himself, the outcome is a *model of self-control*. In fact, his special aristocratic air and bearing, his dignity, "reserved" (Boenninghausen) or contained manner, and that rare "grace under pressure," reflect a successful cultivation of these qualities and a capacity to control himself at all times. His behavior, after all, is largely motivated by the self-image of perfection he has adopted and which he strives to emulate. That is why he can be virtually the *easiest* of constitutional types to get along with, whether as colleague, parent, child, spouse, teacher, student, or friend. Once he has accepted a given balance of control and submission in a relationship, so that he knows just where he stands and what is expected of him, and as long as the boundaries of the respective spheres of influence are faithfully adhered to by all concerned, he is truly considerate and compliant and gives no cause for friction.

In summary, the homoeopathic physician should consider *Arsenicum* when confronted with a tense, high-strung patient displaying the following symptoms: excessive worry and apprehension over his own or others' health and safety; extreme hypochondria and an undue fear of death; frenetic, driving behavior; perfectionism, fastidiousness, or an over-critical attitude toward others; a demanding, challenging, "bulldozing" manner. A course of potentized arsenic will often appease the patient's apprehensions, calm his fretting over minutiae, modify his tendency to overdo whatever he undertakes, and even subdue any inordinate tendency to regulate, judge, administer, direct, and control the lives of others.

The remedy can also temper *Arsenicum's* inability to be satisfied and too relentless pursuit of his goals; it can encourage him to be less aggressively persistent and importunate with others by becoming less anxious in himself. It can help channel the creative aspects of his drive into the most constructive pursuits. For these are persons who can be counted upon to do things competently, who hold others up to high standards and, when especially gifted, whose drive for perfection has brought humanity so much joy and beauty in the creative and performing arts. They are persons who, through intolerance of incompetence and mediocrity, drive themselves and others to higher levels of understanding or to more distinguished achievement.

Arsenicum demands much of life but can also give much in return. It is the function of the homoeopathic remedy to liberate this individual from self-limiting anxiety and excessive censoriousness, thus poising him for the accomplishments he so deeply desires.

Appendix

The following is a composite of many *Arsenicum* patients and is offered, in particular, as an archetypal example of the anxiety-ridden variety. Few patients will exhibit all of these traits, but everyone will exhibit some.

Arsenicum always makes his presence felt and lingers long afterwards in the physician's mind. The highly congenial atmosphere of the doctor's office encourages many of his traits to blossom forth. In fact, his behavior is often so characteristic that the simillimum is apparent even before he has set foot in the office.

The very voice and manner when he calls for the first appointment—anxiously questioning, insistently demanding, or dogmatically assertive—are a sure giveaway. Even when gracious, he has an unmistakable tone of certainty or authority. At times he sounds impatient. He needs an appointment *immediately*. No, he cannot wait until next week or next month but wants to come tomorrow—or even today. He insists that, although long subject to his particular complaint, he cannot stand it a moment longer! He often sounds (and is) desperate. Furthermore, he may then and there demand to know if his complaint is curable. If the physician hesitates in his answer, *Arsenicum* presses further. "But have you ever had a case like mine which you were able to cure? I know I have an exceptionally difficult problem, but I still need to know how long you think it will take . . . "

Sometimes he drops out after the initial telephone contact, either put off by the lack of a guarantee of cure or, after having telephoned several different physicians that same day (as is his wont), deciding in favor of another form of therapy. But the majority will come anyway. The prospect of exploring and undergoing a new form of medical treatment is irresistible, especially when the therapy offers a chance to participate actively by minutely observing and relaying his symptoms. It is not surprising that these patients form a significant portion of the homoeopath's practice.

Occasionally a long and neatly typed or handwritten letter arrives between the initial phone call and the scheduled appointment, explaining all the patient's symptoms in detail, not omitting the clinical data: "My pulse rate is . . . My blood pressure is . . . The lab tests show. . . . " Frequently the letter will have one, or even two, substantial post-scripts, so anxious is *Arsenicum* that the physician be *fully* informed of all aspects of his case.*

Arsenicum arrives in plenty of time for the first appointment. Being punctual by nature, he expects punctuality from others and may be upset if he must wait. In the waiting room he carefully inspects both the premises and his fellow-patients. Then, not to waste time, he takes out some work he has brought with him, which he opens up with characteristic quick decisive gestures. Once immersed in this, his concentration is not easily interrupted. A mother with children, or a patient so anxious that she cannot occupy herself in this way, will engage the nurse or receptionist in a lengthy discussion about the effectiveness of homoeopathy in general and his or her own condition in particular.

When called, the patient walks resolutely into the office and, sometimes dispensing even with the amenities of an introduction, plunges headlong into a recital of his symptoms. The physician must practically shout, "Whoaaa there! Hold it! Now tell me, what's your name, occupation, date and place of birth?" When reined in to answer such mundane questions, *Arsenicum* obliges, though still straining at the bit, and is soon off again at breakneck speed with his case history.

He of course arrives fully equipped with blood work-ups, lab-test results, X-rays, other doctors' reports, a list of the different medications he has taken since year one, and any other pertinent data. He insists that the physician hear out all this information and then comment on it. Or, if a letter was sent earlier, he may refer anxiously to it to insure that it has been read and fully assimilated: "Did you understand it? Do you feel you have mastered the contents? Would you like to look at it again before deciding on the remedy? I can wait. I don't mind."

But most often he will bring along a small notebook or a sheet with a careful enumeration of symptoms, certain selected ones underlined once or even twice. The very existence of this orderly tell-tale list has already pointed to the remedy, but the patient, armed with his trusty sheet, is determined to conduct the case in his own way and feels uneasy

---

* At the end of one such letter was a third postscript informing the physician, "I used to be a perfectionist, but am not any longer. I have changed. Now I am only terribly concerned about my health." Yet another had a third postscript asking, "Please tell me, do you consider me a hopeless case?"

if the physician does not follow along. He is frustrated if prevented from stating his case in full and discussing each symptom point by point: "I still haven't told you about symptom number eighteen, the strange stinging sensation in my right eye," he says, "and there are a few other things I forgot to write down that you should know about."

At some point he may inquire whether he should take certain complicated tests or other expensive therapy recommended by earlier (allopathic) physicians. If the homoeopath suggests that he wait a while to see if they are really necessary, he may insist that he would rather take them now—that he senses he needs them. And emotionally he does!

The physician rarely has to ask at the end of the interview if the patient has anything to add, as is customary in homoeopathic practice, since the latter himself keeps remembering and coming up with new details. "Wait, I forgot to tell you . . . " or "One more important thing . . . " The closer the end of the visit, the more anxious he becomes to add "just one more thing . . . " after another. This is a classic *Arsenicum* expression and a guiding symptom, especially if the "just one more thing" turns out to be half a dozen. If the physician remarks that he has enough information for the time being, *Arsenicum* may reply, somewhat testily, "I've read that a homoeopath must know *everything* about the patient to prescribe correctly, and I still have a lot more to tell you!"

Even after the interview is over and the patient has finally left the room, he may still stick his head through the door to add, "Wait! I have another symptom . . . " He might even call back later that day or the next morning to rectify any sins of omission or make sure that some point is "absolutely clear" in the physician's mind (lest he misunderstand the case and prescribe incorrectly)—little suspecting that his remedy was quite obvious from the first telephone call.

The more aggressively anxious or hypochondriac *Arsenicum* lingers in the office after the consultation to buttonhole the doctor with more questions and requests for information, more precise instructions, and more detailed explanations of the homoeopathic method. Oblivious of the other patients in the waiting room, he does not consider that he might be taking up an undue amount of the physician's time; where health is concerned only his own interests count. *Natrum muriaticum* might demand the same time and attention but is more aware of others and afterwards apologizes or feels guilty about it.

Sometimes the type is passively aggressive, and this remedy should not be overlooked in the controlled, soft-spoken, and gentle-mannered, but super-tenacious patient who at first seems as dependent as *Pulsatilla* (with the same "imploring" inflection of the voice) or needs as much reassurance as *Phosphorus*. But *Pulsatilla* will remain dependent, and *Phosphorus* will continue to need reassurance, while *Arsenicum*'s urge to take charge reasserts itself with returning health, and he soon becomes independent and self-reliant.

The *Arsenicum* patient over-intellectualizes. Not only does he feel the need to describe every symptom in detail, but he must also assign physiological (or pseudo-scientific) reasons for them. He knows, for instance, that his headaches are "caused" by increased mucosity of the gastrointestinal system; a skin eruption is due to heightened "toxicity" ("I was wondering, for instance, if I am too acid?"); the woman with pains in the lower abdomen is sure that her uterus has dropped, and so on. Or, in his desire to stay one jump ahead of the physician, when asked a routine homoeopathic question such as whether he likes eggs, butter, and pastries, he may reply, "I know you are thinking of cholesterol. I can tell you myself: my latest blood count showed the cholesterol level to be . . . " One woman even announced cheerfully, "You don't have to worry about my cholesterol count. I can sense it myself when it is high." (!)

The intellectualizing *Arsenicum* is further concerned with the "meaning" of every symptom: "What does it *mean* that my upper right arm twitches when I go to bed at night? . . . Why do you want to know if I like the fat on my meat? What does it *mean* if I do? . . . " (*Arsenicum* does "desire fats": Kent; also *Nux vomica* and *Sulphur*—who especially likes butter and bacon). Or, in his need for precision, clarity, and order, he wants to put *labels* on things, which to him is the same as understanding them. At the conclusion of the interview, for instance, after listing dozens of symptoms, he asks what is the matter with him—what he is suffering from. "You have just told me," says the physician. "Yes, but I want to know the *name* of my disease," he will insist. Thus, despite his keenness and curiosity, he may at first have peculiar difficulty understanding homoeopathy. His consuming interest in medicine has furnished him with a copious vocabulary and a full range of concepts, and he wants homoeopathy to be explained in the "scientific" language with which he is familiar. He may try to force the physician to explain—

more than he truthfully can—"how the medicine cures," what it is "going to do" or is "supposed to do," or what it has already done (if this is the second visit). He is rarely satisfied when told, "The medicine is going to cure your illness" or "The remedy will stimulate [or has stimulated] your body's defensive capacities"—which are the only honest answers a homoeopath can give.

While initially *Arsenicum* feels immensely comforted by labels and rationalizations, this is true only up to a point. His critical and goal-oriented nature also wants results, and, if he gets none, he begins to search around for more effective therapies. That is why, having run the gamut of orthodox modes of treatment, and perhaps a series of unorthodox ones also, he eventually arrives at the homoeopath's office— yet with the intellectualizing side of him still believing that names and labels and "scientific" explanations are necessary prerequisites of cure (*Sulphur*).

Thus the days or weeks after the first prescription, before the medicine has had a chance to exert its beneficial effect on the patient, are not the easiest time for the physician. This is when his work really begins. His office is besieged with telephone calls from anxious *Arsenicum* patients wanting to know "What is happening?" and asking more questions than he can answer. Whereas most other constitutional types will withhold comments or queries until the second visit, *Arsenicum* starts to call the very next day, and communications from him continue thick and fast thereafter. As a part of his "homoeopathic aggravation" he may have to work through an increased anxiety regarding his symptoms, which he now notices with *extra* care. Thus, he will not call once for a specific problem, but two or three times. He can also be the most importunate of all types on the telephone: demanding immediate personal attention and outraged by answering devices or even secretarial services. He will leave irritated messages on the answering machine: "Why doesn't anyone in this office ever pick up the telephone? I'm not paying good money to talk to a stupid machine!" Or, if he does not receive immediate attention, "I consider myself a patient person, but I've been waiting two hours for you to return my earlier calls [between 7 and 9 a.m. on Sunday], and my patience is exhausted." Or, "Your answering service doesn't know how to take symptoms; the secretary never understands what I tell her and cannot relay my [full page] message without omitting half the symptoms . . . "

No one telephones at less civilized hours than the panicking *Arsenicum*, to relate some trivial episode. "My cough seems to get worse at night," he will say, calling at midnight or 6 a.m. "What should I do about it?" Or, in the middle of the night, "I'm sorry to bother you at this hour, but I completely forgot your instructions and drank a cup of coffee at dinner. I just woke up and remembered. Tell me truthfully, have I blown the case? Will it stop the action of the remedy for good? . . . "

He even succeeds in tracking down the physician on vacation and calls long-distance on some unimportant matter ("What significance do you attach to my recent 2 p.m. drop in energy?"). Or, with the hypochondriac's disproportionate anxiety, he accuses the physician: "I want you to know that I have broken out into some peculiar hives . . . Nothing like this has ever happened to me before . . . Could you *please* explain to me why . . . "

Even when the results are satisfactory *Arsenicum* may find something to cavil about on the return visit. "Yes, the remedy has helped a little bit," he will say, suggesting that it is not *truly* doing its duty by him. For reasons which are difficult to fathom but may be rooted in dislike of anyone but himself being in charge of his health, he will say, "The varicose vein on my leg feels better, but I don't know if it really was the remedy. I've been exercising regularly and bought a different pair of shoes. So it may have gotten better on its own." Then he adds kindly, "I feel it's only fair to tell you this."

These various extraneous factors may have contributed to his overall improvement; but when a patient repeatedly evinces mistrust of the action of homoeopathic remedies and offers other rationalizations for his improved well-being, especially when they reflect credit on himself, the physician will not err in suspecting that he is dealing with an *Arsenicum* Doubting Thomas.

His scepticism vis-a-vis homoeopathic remedies differs from *Lycopodium*'s in that the latter's "The remedies never work on me" expresses a general distrust of medicines used on himself (for others they work fine, but he himself is exempt), while with *Arsenicum* the remedies seem to work beautifully once *he* has taken over the prescribing—and his scepticism then vanishes completely.

Typical of *Arsenicum*'s general "suspiciousness" (Kent) was the man who, although treated successfully for a chronic eye infection, announced, "I'm not sure that I completely approve of what's happening to me. I used to go to sleep in the dark, and now I want a light out in the hall. I have to know the precise way these remedies may be acting on my subconscious mind, or I don't know if I can keep taking them." Or the mother of the three-year-old girl treated successfully for a chronic bronchial cough who—to show that she was just a little more aware than the physician himself—complained that her daughter's psyche seemed to have been affected by the homoeopathic remedies: "She used to draw her figures plump, now they have become thinner. What is that supposed to mean? Is she undergoing some contraction of her cognitive mode?"

This medical "one-upmanship" which is *Arsenicum*'s specialty makes him distrustful even of those from whom he is seeking help. Despite his fascination with doctors, these latter can sense a definitely suspicious attitude, as if he is waiting for the physician to prove himself. But his assertiveness and argumentativeness are actually a challenge to the physician. He is seeking someone to relieve him of the burden of his medical knowledge which, however he attempts to apply it, still does not make him feel better. He really wants to trust the doctor and be guided by him, to be told exactly what to do. Consequently, after the initial struggle for control, *Arsenicum* can develop into a most attentive and compliant, even while independent, patient. Not only does he follow instructions religiously, but his logical mind will usually respond intelligently to the physician's efforts to educate him in the basic concepts of holistic, and specifically homoeopathic, medicine.

Lachesis

LACHESIS is one of the more complex homoeopathic constitutional types. Although the individual presents vivid physical and mental symptoms, experience is required to understand his psychology and motivations. But once the picture is established, it is hard to miss.

The remedy is derived from the poison of the Brazilian bushmaster, or surukuku, one of the most poisonous and aggressive snakes found in the western Hemisphere (hence its dread name—"the master of the forest"). It possesses inch-long fangs and, when angered, will chase a man and attack him—as few other snakes will do. Constantine Hering, the "Father of American Homoeopathy," discovered the remedy in 1828 (the Swedish botanist Linnaeus, in his classification of the animal kingdom, had earlier named the snake [*Trigonocephalus*] *Lachesis* after one of the three Fates in Greek mythology who measures the thread of life).* He proved it on himself and his students, eliciting some 3,800 symptoms, and in the process of dosing himself with ever higher potencies paralyzed his left arm for life. To obtain the invaluable mental picture we now possess, Hering with characteristic Germanic thoroughness also used the unattenuated form (tincture) of the poison, making his wife stay by his bed for several days, notebook in hand, taking down every word that he said in his delirium.

For several decades thereafter, most of the *Lachesis* in the entire world was made from Hering's single milking of this one snake until in 1868 the homoeopathic pharmacists in America decided that they could not go on diluting the substance ad infinitum and ordered a sec-

---

* The seven-foot snake is now preserved in the Philadelphia Academy of Natural Sciences, entered in the ledger as item #7039 and listed as "*Lachesis Mutus*, collected in Surinam by Dr. Hering."

ond bushmaster to be shipped up from Brazil. When the animal arrived, it caused a sensation in the homoeopathic world: "Lachesis II arrives in America!" was the headline in the homoeopathic journals. Photographs of the snake from different angles were displayed, and its habits and physical dimensions were described as lovingly as if it was a film star!

The interest and excitement were not unjustified. The remedy had swiftly made a strong impact on homoeopathic circles. The dramatic quality of its action had captured the physician's imagination and earned his respect; throughout the homoeopathic world *Lachesis* was by then recognized as one of the most useful and frequently indicated polychrests.

Dualism

Hering's description of the mental symptoms from the first grasped the essential intensity of a *nature struggling against itself,* also the type's erratic moods and behavior: "perfect happiness and cheerfulness, followed by fading spirituality; feels as if she was clear animal right through, whilst all mental power was dormant; voluptuous, irritated state which she fights." Half a century later Kent's discussion of *Lachesis* provided a pointed description of the more advanced mental pathology: "Nothing stands out more boldly than the self-consciousness, the self-conceit, the envy, hatred, the revenge and the cruelty of the man. These things, of course, are . . . an improper love of self. Confusion of the mind to insanity. All sorts of insanity . . . "

More recently Whitmont has presented an insightful analysis of *Lachesis* as the individual who is eager to express his instinctual urges even while laboring under strong repression; the blocked natural energies then find vicarious outlets in some mental overstimulation or physical hyperactivity. Building on the foundations laid by these three masters, we will choose the nature's inherent *dualism* as the theme of our *Lachesis* portrait: that is, its propensity to embrace opposed behavioral tendencies or impulses and conflicting emotions, and the impact of this struggle on the organism.

In *Sulphur* the remedy's polarities are usually distributed among different individuals, who are either the "selfish" or the "benevolent" type; in *Phosphorus* the polarity may be exhibited in the same person but at different times—the opposite emerging with age, hardship, or deteriorating health; in *Lachesis* the polarity can be manifested in the same person almost simultaneously. Within the individual two forces are constantly at war ("feels as if he has two wills": Kent): indulgence vs. restraint, arrogance vs. humility, love vs. hate, faith vs. cynicism—each seeking to overcome the other.

The split psyche is especially disconcerting to the individual himself who can never count on the steadiness of his own feelings and behavior. Sensing that his current mood can easily be overturned by his underlying conflicting side, he fears inconstancies and reversals which he is incapable of controlling.

Complicating the picture is the struggle for supremacy among the three levels of his being—mental, emotional and sensual. *Lachesis* can be a highly intellectual type, displaying a fine incisive mind. The male, for instance, is often as strongly intellectual as *Sulphur* but, rather than spinning webs of philosophical abstraction, gives concrete and more dramatic expression to his profound understanding. In both sexes the strong mind is imaginative and agile, and possesses an almost "prophetic perception" (Hering) or "clairvoyance" (Kent)—the ability to penetrate into the true feelings and motives of another and anticipate the progression of his thoughts and actions, as well as the events that may thence ensue. He judges correctly how others will act and react, consequently the steps to be taken to achieve a desired end. Sometimes he grasps ideas too rapidly for others to follow, seeing with intense clarity that which they cannot yet detect ("quick, rapid perceptivity": Boenninghausen). In the time taken by *Sulphur* to belabor some obvious point or some one big idea *Lachesis* will have seized all the ramifications of a situation, developed a fertile plan of action, and come up with a variety of possible solutions. In fact, he becomes "extremely impatient at tedious and dry things" (Hering).

Yet he is also highly emotional—far more so than *Sulphur*, whose intellect clearly predominates. In fact, the *intensity* of feeling which *Phosphorus* tries to sustain is already present in *Lachesis*—who is often incapable of relinquishing it (the feeling possesses *him,* rather than he the feeling). Finally, the type is strongly given to sensual gratification. This side of him can be controlled, but it is always there, and at times the sensuality is paramount. All three irreducible forces are perpetually battling for dominion, with the patient's body as the war-torn battlefield.

As Whitmont points out, *Lachesis'* primary conflict is between his lower instincts and his higher Ego. The strong animal urges seek expression, but the individual constantly suppresses them for the sake of civilized behavior and/or spiritual growth. Deprived of their natural outlet, the emotions then take their toll on the individual's physical and mental health: "Where *logos* (mind) opposes *bios* (urges), [one] encounters the pathology of the serpent . . . [*Lachesis*] is the unintegrated life impulse, the unintegrated libido," concludes Whitmont.

A pleasant, mild-mannered middle-aged man was being treated for longstanding severe headaches, with nausea and vomiting. The general symptoms pointed to several remedies, but it was difficult to get a clear picture of the headaches themselves because of continuing suppression over the years with allopathic analgesics. To help decide on the simillimum, the patient was asked to talk about himself. He displayed a measured, sensitive attitude toward his family and work, which offered no guiding symptoms. Nothing about him was in the least "strange, rare or peculiar." He was then asked how he felt about himself—if he was achieving what he wanted in life and felt fulfilled? At this point the *Lachesis* surfaced, as he related how he was trying to grapple with his intrusive sensual side.

"My outward life is not me. My inner life—what I think and feel— does not want to be me. I practice my religion but don't know that I really believe in it. Or in what, for that matter, I do believe. I live in a state of constant psychological turmoil, wrestling with sensual urges I both want and don't want to indulge. In fact," he concluded, "I don't know which of my two selves is *really* me—the proper one I live or the lascivious one I repress?" (reminiscent of Oscar Wilde's aphorism: "One's real life is often the life one does not lead").

A dose of *Lachesis* 200x was prescribed, and this remedy was continued in ascending potency for several months until the patient was almost entirely free of headaches. Most interesting to the physician, however, was the gradual and almost imperceptible way the remedy helped reconcile this troubled individual with himself. "I am more at peace with myself," were his own words, "more self-accepting and less tormented by my uncontrolled racing thoughts." There now existed, if not complete harmony, at least a tenuous coexistence between his dominant and subordinate selves.

Any constitutional type may struggle with his instincts to attain a higher personal moral development. What distinguishes *Lachesis* is: 1) the intensity of the struggle; 2) its unremitting nature (it can continue unabated throughout adult life); and 3) his awareness of it.

In fact, this exceeding awareness of the potential inherent in the underlying self may, in extreme cases, compel the individual to confess to crimes he has not committed, to some wickedness or sin in which he has not indulged ("she makes a confession of something she has never done": Kent). This unfounded feeling of guilt suggests that at some level he senses a desire to indulge in moral abandon; he knows he is merely a step away from some erratic flip and that, should the occasion arise, he might be tempted into some reprehensible action. Even though the desire is repressed, its *intensity* makes it almost equivalent to the act itself (it is a fundamental postulate of the mystical outlook that thought *is* action because it puts action into motion). Thus *Lachesis* takes on the guilt of his thoughts, while the unhinged mind mistakes the frightening possibility for reality.

Sleep and Temperature

One symptom suggesting repression is the dominant *Lachesis* modality: *aggravation from sleep*. Sleep is when the unconscious takes over, and emotions which *Lachesis* would rather not acknowledge, instincts which usually lie quiescent, and dreams he cannot control—all rise to the surface. The textbooks emphasize that he is likely to feel worse both in the morning ("feels extremely sad, unhappy, and distressed in mind on waking in the morning; anxious; looks at everything from the dark side": Hering), and also from waking in the middle of the night or even after a nap during the day. He may be reluctant to go to sleep, fearing that when his breathing slows down, or a short time thereafter, he will wake up choking and gasping for air, with an asthma attack, tachycardia, throbbing or sick headache, increased pain of a paralyzed limb (in neuromuscular degenerative diseases), or increased discomfort from whatever is ailing him at the moment.

These individuals may require remarkably little sleep. After staying up half the night socializing, engaging in stimulating conversation, studying, or reading ("without the slightest sleepiness or exhaustion": Allen), and after just a few hours sleep, they are full of energy the following day and give no sign of fatigue. Other patients requiring the remedy, however, complain of "sleepiness without being able to sleep" (Hering), of insomnia until 1:00 or 2:00 a.m. due to mental over-stimulation, of inability to fall asleep again if they wake up after midnight, or of suffering from "persistent sleepiness . . . accompanied by restlessness . . . or trembling and shaking" (Hering). Some of the most recalcitrant cases of insomnia, where the patient can go literally for weeks without sleeping (!) or "does not sleep at night; sleeps only a minute or two at a time during day" (Hering), have responded only to *Lachesis*.

A key symptom of the constitutional type is "mental labor performed best at night" (Hering). Night is when *Lachesis* is most awake and really comes into his own, with heightened acumen and his creative energies reaching their peak. This contrasts with *Arsenicum* who works best in the morning and is incapable of functioning at night. Dostoyevsky, as purely a *Lachesis* male as ever existed, had the remedy's timetable, sitting up all night (when the subconscious is most aroused) and writing in frenzied spurts of near-demonic inspiration to preserve the immediacy and intensity of his insights. Certainly he had to write under pressure because his novels were serialized, but Charles Dickens, who also wrote his serialized novels to deadline, had an entirely different schedule: dealing with external mannerisms rather than (like Dostoyevsky) the subconscious, he sat down every day after breakfast and wrote without a break until two o'clock lunch, in a typically *Natrum muriaticum* unvarying, disciplined routine.

The picture of the repressed individual is further reinforced in the remedy's temperature modalities. Any form of heat, which relaxes the inhibitions as well as the body, aggravates this type: "aggravation from warm bath" (bringing on palpitations, headache, or fainting), "from a warm south wind" (Kent), or in a warm room. In particular, "exposure to the sun's rays" can bring on blinding headaches (Hering, Kent), often centering behind the left eye.

This *sensitivity to heat* may be one reason for the prominent seasonal modality. Of all remedies *Lachesis* is highest in "springtime aggravations" (Kent, Boger). Like the snake shedding its old skin to make way for the new one, the *Lachesis* patient often undergoes a health crisis or purge (symptoms, such as allergies, develop or are aggravated) at this time of the year when the weather begins to get warmer, before taking on new strength.

Conversely, he is conspicuously ameliorated by the energizing cool and fresh air, which he craves, "cold water" (Hering), and by any activity under the control of the conscious mind, such as talking, writing, physical exercise, or eating.

Alcohol and Food

Alcohol, like sleep, brings the dormant instincts and the subconscious mind to the fore. Thus *Lachesis* is often sensitive to strong drink ("worse from alcoholic drinks": Hering), being affected adversely even by very small amounts (e.g., taking communion in church). It may bring on headaches or heart palpitations that keep him awake at night, a red nose or saddle across the nose and cheeks, or an unpleasant flushing of the face. Alcohol may also make the skin feel tight and scaly or aggravate preexisting symptoms (*Arsenicum* can also be sensitive to alcohol, but it usually takes the form of hay-fever symptoms: itching eyes, ears, nose, or palate, with a heavy congested head). Consequently, this patient often abstains from alcohol, either as a simple physical precaution or out of principle, because of its power to elicit the unacceptable urges he has been trying to suppress and to weaken his control over them. Not content with teetotaling himself, he may develop into a temperance movement type who makes drink into a moral issue.

Interestingly, that other stimulant, coffee, which can be so pernicious to many constitutional types, is well-tolerated by *Lachesis* ("desire for coffee, which agrees": Hering). This could be because it stimulates the intellectual and conscious side of the individual, in what could be called a "sober intoxication," rather than arousing the subconscious. Headaches, dysmenorrheas, and other complaints may actually be helped by black coffee, and some patients continue drinking it throughout constitutional treatment without any adverse effect on the remedy— whereas alcohol definitely interferes. This contrasts with the great majority of remedies, where coffee interferes more than moderate amounts of alcohol.

Predictably, the polar opposite is also found in *Lachesis*; he can be ultrasensitive to coffee (*Ignatia, Nux vomica*), developing "headaches [even] from its smell" (Boger: also *Natrum muriaticum* and *Tuberculinum*), or suffering from insomnia after a spoonful of coffee ice cream.

Since alcohol is one of the principal outlets for pent-up emotions, instincts, and sexual energy, *Lachesis* can, not surprisingly, manifest a tendency to alcoholism. Although *Nux vomica* and *Sulphur* are better known as chronic alcoholics, *Lachesis* has been efficacious in "delirium tremens" (Hering) and especially in persons *struggling* against alcoholism, alternately keeping it in check and succumbing to it. It is also a good remedy for those whose physiques have been broken down by alcoholism ("former old topers": Nash), and it has even been prescribed with success for the traumatized spouses of alcoholics, upon whom something of the alcoholic's erratic mental state has rubbed off.*

The individual further exhibits the classic picture of frustrated emotions finding an outlet in food, which has not been sufficiently stressed in the homoeopathic literature. Women, especially, will go on binges and eat until they are stuffed. "I never stop eating," "I never feel full," "I desperately crave something sweet," "When I have eaten 'enough,' it is always too much" are commonly heard phrases. *Pulsatilla* also goes on binges, and these two types differ from *Calcarea* who snacks constantly rather than binging. One of the healthier *Lachesis* cravings is for fresh fruit or cold fruit juices, and many symptoms are alleviated by food: "better eating fruit; generally improved when eating" (Hering).

Insatiable hunger can be triggered by sugar, wheat products, and other substances, and sometimes he can control his appetites only by adhering to a rigorous juice diet for a period of time, or total abstinence in the case of alcohol. Strict control alternating with overindulgence typify the *Lachesis* pattern of behavior. He imposes severe restraints on himself, sensing that otherwise his appetites will have no limit. Fearing the risk, he draws back to the safety of curbing all license.

But this tendency to overindulge can be helped by the remedy, which has the capacity to lessen immoderate cravings. Almost as a side-effect of the treatment of some specific physical complaint patients are imperceptibly weaned from their former excesses. They come back and remark that their addictions, whether for alcohol, tobacco, coffee, sugar, or whatever, have been moderated without any effort or conscious decision on their part.

Discharges

Another manifestation of the blocked *Lachesis* emotions seeking a physical outlet is the symptom, "*amelioration from appearance of discharges*" (Kent) or from "free secretions" (Boger). Draining sinuses or sneezing with coryza will relieve joint pains, and leucorrhea heart symptoms; nosebleeds have relieved asthma attacks, and bowel movements headaches ("I just *love* having bowel movements," "I never feel

* The children of alcoholics will frequently require *Natrum muriaticum*.

as well as when I have a good elimination"). On the emotional plane, tears relieve too intense happiness ("weeping from joy": Kent), and hemorrhages longstanding depressions. Conversely, the patient suffers from "ill effects of suppressed discharges" (Boericke).

This modality is most commonly encountered in the *Lachesis* woman who exhibits severe premenstrual backaches and headaches, fluid retention, weepiness, touchiness, despondency, increased or uncontrolled irritability and anger, which are only relieved once the flow sets in. Patients vividly describe their impatience for the onset of their periods, while some of more rapturous nature tell how they thank God in prayer for every period.

A normally charming, sensitive, affectionate woman may completely change her personality a week or so before her period: "I am not myself. I seem to go crazy and cannot control myself" ("I go/act crazy" or "I completely lose control" are key *Lachesis* phrases in describing the premenstrual mental picture); "I become aggressive with my husband, tyrannical with the children, violently abusive if things aren't going my way. Either I am extravagant, impulsively spending money we cannot afford on clothes and desserts, which I crave, or I feel miserly to the point of refusing to invite even our good friends to dinner." Such behavior may alternate with a taciturn moroseness or extreme depression. A number of variations on this premenstrual theme are encountered, all terminating in the same happy way: with the onset of menses the physical and mental symptoms dissolve as if by magic.

A marked improvement in this monthly pattern can often be observed following the very first dose of *Lachesis*. As one patient volunteered on her return visit, "This month I never even suspected my period was coming on. I was cheerful and relaxed until one day I sneezed, and the menses started—which was the first I was aware of it."

The remedy is frequently required for the hormonal changes and imbalances of menopause. With cessation of the normal menstrual flow (a form of suppressed discharge) the body seeks other outlets, particularly in the form of hot flushes (a surrogate rush of blood to the head), bursting or congestive headaches, hypertension, or severe hemorrhaging. There may also be increase in weight, circulatory disturbances with areas of excess heat and cold, or cutting pains in the breasts or ovaries, especially the left. For *Lachesis* is a left-sided remedy, just as *Lycopodium* is right-sided. Although there are exceptions (such as in sciatica), cysts, tumors, skin eruptions, headaches, and other pains are predominantly left-sided (*Sepia*, and to a lesser extent *Phosphorus*); and any pain or symptom "moving from left to right" (Kent) is a key to *Lachesis*.

At this time, also, the sexual urge receives a final stimulus before decline, leading to the surfacing of disturbing emotions, such as repressed or unfulfilled desires: "the critical climactic period represents the last chance . . . for the juices to flow . . . In this situation the life forces and the emotions produce something akin to the eruption of a volcano" (Whitmont). The sexual energy released in an uncontrolled way may lead to irrational behavior in a woman (here again, "I begin to act crazy" is a common refrain) and, in extreme cases, to true mental breakdown. Finally, the remedy is invaluable for women who have never felt really well since the menopause.

Just as *Lachesis* feels better from physical discharges, so symptoms are ameliorated and he feels emotionally relieved from "mental discharges." During the homoeopathic consultation, when a patient is required to do much talking, the type becomes visibly exhilirated, and remains in this state for a long time afterwards. He can also virtually talk (or write) himself out of a strong anger or deep depression. If is often best to allow him to talk; once all is out, a measure of calm returns. This is in contrast to *Natrum muriaticum* who may be worse after articulating anger or grief; in expressing it, he works himself into a passion he did not previously feel (in a distraught patient this distinction helps to pinpoint the simillimum). In a state of anger, however, *Lachesis* can exhibit extraordinary venom and be extremely spiteful, sarcastic, and insulting (*Arsenicum, Nux vomica*). A lethally wounding or uncontrolled tongue, a tendency to cut people down and leave nothing *un*said, often indicate this remedy. He has difficulty learning that it is sometimes better not to give verbal expression to feelings—that words should disguise thought as well as communicate it. But then the patient might claim that the malicious or biting words are not deliberate but escape of their own accord. He may fight this tendency, but gratuitously tactless or wounding remarks will still slip out in unguarded moments. "Something just *drives* me," "I can't *not* say what I have the urge to say," "I actually have *no* control" (to return to a familiar theme), are characteristic confessions.

Loquacity

This introduces the well-known *Lachesis* characteristic—*loquacity*.

Instincts and emotions denied a normal physical expression may find a surrogate in excessive verbosity. An unending flow of words is the classic sign of an emotionally unfulfilled or creatively thwarted personality. Mental hyperactivity compensates for the "heavily repressed emotions" (Whitmont), and inhibitions are released in an "unusual desire to be communicative" (Allen). This characteristic is more pronounced in the female, probably because up until recently the sexual and creative energies of women have been more suppressed than those of men.

Lachesis frequently expresses her thoughts in a rush of words, as if hurrying to catch up with them before they slip away. Once started, she cannot control her pace; she cannot *slow down* ("hasty speech": Boenninghausen; "much rapid talking": Hering). The patient may talk so fast that the physician will ask her to decelerate, since the tongue moves quicker than the ear can catch—certainly than the hand can write.

Also, once started she can hardly *stop* talking ("wants to talk all the time": Hering). When the subject is of particular interest to her, there is no arresting the torrent of words and associations. The physician recognizes *Lachesis* in the patient who sits erect, looks at him with a sharp and penetrating glance, and, allowing no interruption, not only pours forth her list of symptoms but digresses into various related and unrelated subjects—her family, work, theories about homoeopathy, opinions gleaned from the latest book she has read or trip she has taken—with one idea breeding another. A simple question, such as whether a specific symptom is better, is likely to provoke a torrent of explanations and digressions in reply. She will bend one's ear, even over the telephone. The loquacity of the male is usually lower-keyed. Although he, too, at times sounds rushed, and is equally *exhilarated by conversation*, he is less a mountain cascade than a steady stream of water from the tap: a compelling voice that goes on . . . and on . . . (also *Sulphur*).

Individuals of either sex can use language with dramatic effect. The orator who stirs up an audience with his emotionally charged language, the preacher who can penetrate straight to the hearts of his listeners, the teacher whose delivery carries a note of ecstasy, or merely the person who is carried away by his own eloquence, talks with extreme facility, and conveys passionate conviction—all are frequently *Lachesis*. Whereas *Natrum muriaticum* attracts by his high moral character,

Phosphorus allures by his responsive nature, *Arsenicum* breeds respect for his competence, *Pulsatilla* elicits protective instincts, and *Sulphur* awes by his fund of knowledge—*Lachesis fascinates* his willing or reluctant interlocutor by his "animated" (Boenninghausen) and imaginative talk and his creative approach.

The complement of *Lachesis* articulateness is the patient with speech defects. The remedy, as Hering notes, has helped many cases of stammering, stuttering, inability to enunciate certain consonants, or inability to move the tongue easily in the mouth (it gets caught on the teeth, for instance, or trembles when the patient tries to protrude it for examination). The child with a lisp is usually *Calcarea*, the adult quite often *Lachesis*. Or the patient, without being an alcoholic, exhibits the latter's slurred speech and difficult articulation ("thick tongue, blunders and stumbles, only partly finishing words": Kent—also *Natrum muriaticum*). There are also some interesting pointers regarding the mouth. Sometimes he has the habit of flicking his tongue out over the upper lip, to lick it as he speaks, at other times he "darts it in and out" (Kent); sometimes he spits when talking, at other times small bubbles of saliva gather at the corners of his mouth. Or there can be a certain hypnotic quality to the movement of the lips and mouth when he speaks.

The *Lachesis* mind sometimes works so fast ("rapid thoughts": Kent), with the tongue following so closely behind, that in conversation he anticipates the other's train of thought, jumps to complete his sentences for him, and literally takes the words out of his mouth. This can be an irritating habit. Even though *Lachesis* may be perceptive and accurate, the other may still feel like crying out, "Let me say it myself, for Heaven's sake!"

The quick flow of words does not, however, always denote a strong mind. The racing of unorganized thoughts may rather reflect the intellectual or psychic confusion of a person out of touch with reality. The manic state, with its obsessive incessant talking, often requires this remedy. Or a stream of words conveying little of consequence may represent the automatic responses of a simple mind.

Jane Austen's *Emma* presents one of the finest literary examples of the simple-minded *Lachesis* in the "rambling" (Hering) unselfconscious free association of the amiable, chatty, pathetically grateful, and ingratiating Miss Bates—a middle-aged spinster whose life has been thwarted by financial stringency, inferior social status, and the need to care constantly for an invalid mother. In the following passage Miss Bates has just arrived at a dinner accompanied by her niece, Jane Fairfax:

> "As the door opened [Miss Bates] was heard: "So very oblig-
> ing of you—no rain at all. Nothing to signify. I do not care
> for myself. Quite thick shoes. And Jane declares—"Well! This
> is brilliant indeed—excellently contrived, upon my word.
> Nothing wanting. Could not have imagined it—so well lighted
> up—Jane, Jane, look—did you ever see anything? . . . So
> obliged to you for the carriage!—excellent time—Jane and
> I quite ready—Never were such neighbors. I said to my mother
> 'upon my word, ma'am—' Thank you, my mother is remark-
> ably well. Gone to Mr. Woodhouse's. I made her take her
> shawl—for the evenings are not warm—My dear Jane, are
> you sure you did not wet your feet?—It was but a drop or
> two but I am so afraid:—But Mr. Frank Churchill was so
> extremely—and there was a mat to step up on—I shall never
> forget his extreme politeness—"

Miss Bates' prosings also reflect the *Lachesis* tendency to leave sentences uncompleted. Like the snake's tongue that darts from one side to another, the mind darts from thought to thought in disconnected phrases: "rapid change of subject, jumps abruptly from one idea to another" (Hering). A word in the preceding sentence reminds her of another idea, and she strikes off on a new tangent, then may or may not return to conclude the initial thought ("half-finished sentences; she takes it for granted that you understand the balance": Kent). Occasion-ally *Lachesis* gets lost in her multiple threads of dangling thoughts and will draw herself up saying, "Now where was I? What was I saying?"

A *Phosphorus* patient described her troubles in the small travel agency where she worked; while she loved meeting new people and getting free vacations off-season, she found her employer singularly dif-ficult to deal with: "She is generous enough and well-disposed towards me, but the lack of sequence in her talk makes her almost impossible to follow. She will say, 'Don't forget to call Mr. Norton who wants tickets for—Oh, and by the way, did you arrange that flight to Venezuela for that nice man who—Which reminds me, don't forget to—Oh, no! I think you've already taken care of that—Haven't you?' I have become pretty expert at guessing at the unfinished sentences, although only the other day I booked Mr. Norton for Paris instead of the Bahamas. Is there anything homoeopathy could do for her?'' The physician suggested that she offer her boss a dose of *Lachesis* 1M, and on the return visit the patient, her eyes alight, stated that the remedy had worked miraculously: now her employer never left a *single* phrase unfinished. Due allowance had to be made for her *Phosphorus* enthusiasm, but many times a single dose of the medicine has modified a patient's volubility or disconnected mode of talking—even if not quite as drastically as claimed by this patient.

Alternately, *Lachesis* is rigidly single-minded and impossible to deflect from her chosen course. She appears not to hear when her interlocutor interjects some comment into the flow of conversation, even if it is in response to an apparent question. When the physician asks her something during the office interview, the patient either simply goes on without replying or says, "Let me first finish my own way," and only then is willing to comply with his mode of questioning.

To sum up, the snake poison should be considered in any case of overhasty speech or incessant verbal flow—whether from alcoholism, premenstrual syndrome, suppressed emotion or sexuality, the manic state, the onset of menopause (at which time a previously silent woman will suddenly become talkative)—or simply in a healthy, outgoing, vital, but voluble individual.

A laconic type of *Lachesis* also exists, although less easily recognized. This is the person who silently takes in everything around him, only periodically throwing out trenchant remarks. "Like the ever-watchful snake" (Gutman), he lies coiled and quiet but is ready to strike. Economy of expression, pointedness of speech under an unassuming demeanor, a laconic manner concealing an incisive mind, or the ability of children to use words with keen penetration (with the sharpness of the "serpent's tooth")—can all indicate *Lachesis* in the picture (also *Arsenicum*).

Although more usually the child is jumpy, hyperactive, and an incessant talker, a willingness to listen quietly and observe can also mark its style. Shyness, reserve, and sensitivity mask an intense inquiring mind and eagerness to learn, especially through *conversations* with others. And once launched on a topic of interest, the usually laconic child pours out everything he or she knows in an unarrestable rush of well-formed phrases.

Hering was the first to comment on the *Lachesis* sensitivity to language, more than once alluding to the patient who "makes speeches in very select phrases, uses exalted (or elevated) language, exceedingly particular about the language she uses, often correcting herself after using a word and substituting another of similar meaning." He was writing about the mentally deranged, but a heightened consciousness of language and care in its use may also be observed in the healthy, intellectually-minded individual. Patients will affirm that the symptoms, "weeping from reading" and "weeping at soothing poetry" (for the former of which Kent, somewhat surprisingly, lists only the two snake poisons, *Lachesis* and *Crotalus horridus* [rattlesnake—the right-sided *Lachesis*: Boericke], and for the latter only *Lachesis*) reflect an appreciation of the beauty of the language even more than a *Pulsatilla*-like sentimental response to its content.

Sexuality

The sexual drive is usually strong in both the male and female ("amorousness, amativeness, great excitement of sexual desire": Hering), with "many voluptuous thoughts" (Allen), and patients testify to the eminently satisfying sexual performance of their *Lachesis* partners. But if this high sexuality is not satisfied, it may become an obsession. Without the calming effect of a normal sex life, deep depression may set in (*Natrum muriaticum, Staphysagria*). Alternately, the patient may exhibit manic behavior with sexual passion "excessive; exalted to the highest level; perfectly insatiable; and release from all inhibitions" (Hering). The constitutional type is also high in various sexual disorders or irregularities, including homosexuality ("aversion of men to women," "falls in love with a member of her own sex": Kent), abnormally strong attraction of older men to preadolescent or early adolescent girls, or of older women to men who could be their sons.

At times an aura of controlled or restrained sexuality emanates from the *Lachesis* patient: "a thick smell of repressed . . . and sultry . . . sensuality" (Whitmont). It may be expressed in the eyes: by a particular kind of level, penetrating, compelling (and occasionally disconcerting) look from under half-lowered lids which is immediately felt by the opposite sex. In the sexually deprived individual (whether by choice or from force of circumstances), the still active sexual feeling may be revealed by an exaggerated disapproval of the whole subject. He or she is hypersensitive to sexual references or innuendo, has an aversion to off-color jokes or linguistic crudeness (*Natrum muriaticum*), and may even regard sex as degrading—something that humiliatingly drags man down to the animal level ("aversion of women to marry": Hering).

The middle-aged or older woman leading a strictly virtuous life may be excessively concerned with others' morality, heatedly asserting that relaxed sexual morality and promiscuity are the causes of the downfall of society. If advised not to worry about others' sexual behavior, but to be content with doing what she thinks right, she is shocked by what she takes to be a callous attitude. How could anyone *not* be concerned? But, in fact, *Lachesis'* extreme disapproval of sexuality or a puritanical concern with "moral standards" often reflects a perverse preoccupation with the subject and fear of her own repressed sexual nature. This judgmental attitude may also conceal a subliminal *regret*, a disturbing feeling that life is passing her by and denying her certain fundamental experiences.

In biblical and mythical tradition the serpent symbolizes both sexuality and the higher realms of knowledge: "the serpent is the image of the primordial, autonomous, and impersonal life energy underlying and creating existence and consciousness . . . the urge to taste life, to learn and grow through tasting life" (Whitmont). By thus containing within itself the seed of spiritual development, sex to the dualistic *Lachesis* mind takes on the attributes of religion, and this individual seeks in sexual passion the mystery and revelatory fervor usually provided by religion. Thus the remedy immediately comes to mind for any patient who tends to confuse religion and sex.

A historical example of seeming inability to judge where spiritual love ends and sexuality begins was Henry Ward Beecher, the brother of Harriet Beecher Stowe (who wrote *Uncle Tom's Cabin*). The founder and for fifty years the revered pastor of the Plymouth Church in Brooklyn, New York, he was a charismatic pastor to his flock and the possessor of a fine rhetorical talent and many high ideals: preaching Abolition from his pulpit a decade before the Civil War and collecting money to buy the freedom of runaway slaves. But in an excess of Christian love he seduced the pretty wives of his two best friends and faithful financial backers. The tremendous ensuing scandal rocked the whole of American society, and there were several interminable lawsuits. Whatever one's view of his sexual peccadillos, they without doubt represented a truly *Lachesis* confusion between religious and sexual love—where love of God, love of humanity, and love of the opposite sex begin to blend and are no longer distinguishable.

Religion and Beliefs

Lachesis is intrinsically a religious nature and requires some strong faith or spiritual commitment as a convenient outlet for his superabundant emotional energy and susceptibility to "ecstasy" or, in extreme, to "trance-like" states (Hering). The Deity is an almost concrete living presence with whom he establishes communion, as well as a practical guide to morality and ethics in the interminable warrings of his psyche; and those of philosophical bent enjoy nothing more than heated discussions about the "nature of God," or "good and evil," lasting well into the early hours of the morning.

When asked if he shares his problems with others or keeps them to himself (a standard homoeopathic question), *Lachesis* will reply, more often than other constitutional types, "I do neither. I tell them to God and need no one else," or words to that effect. His fortitude in ill-health or other trials frequently issues from this unshakeable faith. He is also the wise, exceptionally fine individual of high moral or even saintly character, who is well aware of the paradoxes and weaknesses of man's nature. He has been tried by fire and emerged victorious from his internal struggles and doubts, reaching a level of compassion and serenity that little can affect.

Conversely, the mental and emotional problems of a *Lachesis* often stem from misunderstood or misapplied religious fervor. He is beset by religious fears ("fear of being damned": Hering), dreads falling under Satanic influence ("thinks she is under superhuman control": Kent), or sees evil all around and is convinced that God will punish everyone, including himself, for their sins.

In some individuals intensity of belief goes with narrowness of outlook, yielding a "dogmatic" (Boenninghausen), rigid, or even "bigoted" (Borland) outlook. The female adherent of a minor religious sect who actively imposes her beliefs and life-style on others is expressing *Lachesis* impulses, as is the middle-aged man, formerly a sybarite and rake and now satiated by overindulgence, who adopts a strict religious discipline to control the now unacceptable side of his nature; also the individual who turns to religion out of profound grief or disappointment; also the person raised in a strict religious atmosphere, who has broken away from it, yet continues to bear the marks of an ingrained dogmatism.

Since a strong impulse in one direction suggests an equally strong one in the other, the most passionate and militant atheists will often be *Lachesis*—individuals who bitterly and cynically hate (and *Lachesis* can *hate* more intensely than any other type, except possibly *Natrum muriaticum*) anything to do with religion, its institutions, or God Himself. Even during the initial interview with the physician, patients express bitterness against their former religion and use the slightest pretext to revert to this pet aversion. Actually, at some level, whether they are pro or con religion hardly matters since vehement denial gives their life as much focus and meaning as does faith.

The Jesuit-trained Voltaire, the most vocal exponent of eighteenth-century Enlightenment (whose *Lachesis* nature can be deduced from his voluminous letters and the comments of his contemporaries on the deliberate public show he liked to make of his life), who spent the greater part of his life attacking the Church with his sharp tongue and wicked pen or fulminating against the existence of a moral or benevolent Deity, betrayed by this lifelong obsession a *Lachesis* fascination with the subject. The story that he begged final absolution on his deathbed may be apocryphal, but it would not have been out of character.

Thus *Lachesis* will be either an exceptionally enthusiastic and devout member of his chosen religion, or, if more independent and anarchic in tendency, may argue vehemently that organized churches and religions, entrusted with *preserving* fervent religious impulses, actually discourage spontaneous and meaningful communion between the individual and God by reducing revelation to dogma and mystical experience to rites and rituals.*

---

* Martin Luther's protest that lead to the Protestant Reformation can thus be seen as a passionate *Lachesis* reaction against Thomas Aquinas' intellectualization of the direct communion between man and God and the Church's over-institutionalization of faith.

The same intense emotionalism marks *Lachesis'* convictions and beliefs in other spheres than religion.* His actions and reactions can be motivated by an *exhilarating hatred* of some particular ideology, idea, or even individual. The schoolgirl, for instance, may cultivate an intense dislike of some teacher, family member or schoolmate. There is no apparent reason; the person has done her no harm; it just appears that her intense emotionality seeks a negative release when denied a positive one. Not surprisingly, she may be subconsciously fascinated by the object of this seemingly unequivocal and articulate hatred, although she cannot admit this even to herself. Thus, she will manifest intense dislike of some particular subject or extracurricular activity in school. Then, the following year, she performs a typical *Lachesis* flip and becomes enthralled by, or excels in, that very subject or activity.

Lachesis thus needs constant grist for his high-powered emotional mill. If there is insufficient passion or religion in his personal life, this intense nature will seek an alternative in moral indignation or righteous despair.

A woman came to homoeopathy for her encroaching pterygium. The yellow membranous growth had spread from the inner corner of both eyes and was now covering a good quarter of their surfaces. While this is an unusual condition in American medical practice today, the patient's prominent seasonal modality—springtime aggravation of asthma and hay-fever tendencies—together with her mental nature quickly pointed to the remedy.

She could talk about her physical ailments without undue anxiety (*Lachesis* often exhibits fortitude in the face of even the most serious illnesses). What really distressed her, as emerged during the consultation, was the dreadfully perilous state of the world. Every morning she would pounce on the *New York Times*, avidly read it through, and then despair of the future. Granted the *New York Times* (or any other news medium)

---

* For example, Sigmund Freud held in horror anything carrying the taint of religion, but its place in his thinking was taken by sexuality, and he expounded his views with a dogmatism which allowed no deviation from the true doctrine (see the chapter, "Sigmund Freud," in Carl Jung's *Memories, Dreams, and Reflections*). Indeed, Freud's heavily sexual psychology, with its basic premise that religion, spirituality, cultural and artistic activity are largely sublimations of sexual neuroses or repressed sexuality, has a truly *Lachesis* coloration.

is full of important and serious problems, but if it affected her so greatly, why did she continue to read it? especially as she could do little to alter matters. Yet, horrified, fascinated, indignant, she read on.

The remedy prescribed was *Lachesis* 200x, and she was recommended to undergo a month's abstention from all news, especially the *New York Times*. She initially balked at this suggestion, claiming that being deprived of this favorite stimulus would in itself make her ill, but she eventually yielded to the physician's advice.

Within two months her pterygium had receded, she had been weaned from her *New York Times* addiction (she could now take it or leave it), and she no longer viewed the world in terms of imminent Armageddon. Altogether, she had a far healthier outlook on life, serenely accepting the things she could not change and saving her energy for those she could.

The *Lachesis* intensity of feeling or conviction is encountered even in the intellectually sophisticated and highly educated. An Oxford graduate who worked in the news division of a radio network sought homoeopathic help for a full-blown case of shingles (herpes zoster) on his scalp, neck, and torso, with severe neurological pain. *Ranunculus bulbosus* and *Rhus toxicodendron* are almost specifics for this condition, and the two remedies did alleviate his symptoms substantially, but the shingles kept relapsing despite intervening doses of *Sulphur*, so the physician had to probe further. Fortunately the patient presented an almost finished portrait. The eruption was left-sided; he feared going to sleep because he often woke up in increased pain; and he was a "night person," choosing to work the late shift. Yet, *Lachesis*-style, even after little sleep he could function well.

To confirm this picture with deeper mental symptoms, the patient was asked about his hobbies or interests outside work. He turned out to be obsessed by the moral-political question of whether a complete collapse must take place in Western society, and the latter have to undergo a Stalinist form of repression (or equivalent tragic episode), to acquire the political maturity and moral understanding that guarantee a viable and effective democracy. "Cannot mankind," he lamented, "learn from history so as not to be condemned to repeat it?"

The physician attempted to comfort him: possibly his pessimistic political analysis was not applicable to the West which, having undergone its Renaissance, Reformation, civil wars, and Industrial Revolution, need not relearn the harsh lessons of recent Russian or Chinese history. But this made him even more excited. Reassuring phrases were not what he wanted. Contradicting a strong-minded *Lachesis* or arguing with him is futile—he should rather be encouraged to release the pressure of anger and indignation which has built up inside him. At any rate, the patient was convinced that Western society must undergo a socio-political "Fall" to be spiritually prepared for an enlightened Democracy (Redemption).

Such passionate eloquence was surprising in a reserved, correct Englishman to whom the physician was a complete stranger, even while it corroborated the choice of *Lachesis* as the remedy.

After a couple of weeks of treatment, his shingles cleared up entirely, but what became of his intense political views and fears is unknown. Once cured, he never came back again and later returned to England. The pure *Lachesis* is not a clinging hypochondriac. His vision encompasses far broader issues than his own health, and, if successfully treated, he stays away from doctors.

This patient exemplified the *compelling* quality of *Lachesis* beliefs. The type can be so forcibly struck by some particular conviction as to reject the possibility of a dissenting one. He forgets to take into account that different people are ready for different revelations at different times in their lives; or that they may espouse their own particular philosophies and thus be closed to others. His own vision *must* be, always *has been*, and always *will be* true for all mankind, and he proceeds to apply it to humanity in a Procrustean manner.

Dostoyevsky and Freud have already been mentioned as typifying the *Lachesis* mentality. They fit this constitutional type also in their intensity of feeling, amounting virtually to revelation. Both saw themselves as prophets, and did indeed venture into previously unexplored regions of the soul, opening up new channels of thought about the subconscious and ushering in the profound twentieth-century interest in psychology. The works of both exhibit the sort of intellectual seductiveness and lucidly compelling subjective style typical of *Lachesis*—leading the reader to believe that the theories propounded embrace the whole truth and not just a segment of it. The intellectual *Sulphur*'s strength, it will be recalled, lies in the analytical objectivity of his style.

The reverse side of this absolutist picture of strong faith and in-

tense convictions is the chronic sceptic. Constantly sensing two opposing forces in himself, this *Lachesis* subtype becomes acutely aware of
the duality and consequent neutrality of all phenomena. Typical here
is Hamlet, whose sinuous mind dissects motives, actions, and ideas in
a passionate moral-philosophic quest, coming to rest in the relativism
of "there is nothing either good or bad but thinking makes it so."

With a proclivity for constantly reexamining his own motives this
person might reason as follows: "When I help a fellow human, I appear charitable in the eyes of the world, but inwardly I am proud of
myself. Perhaps I do it merely to elicit praise rather than out of true
kindness. And, by the same token, when I do something reprehensible,
I later sincerely repent and thus become morally better. So I no longer
know whether I am a better person when doing good but thinking
proud, or when doing wrong but repenting." Then, after a moment,
with yet another twist of the mind, "Yet I wonder whether I am *truly*
humble and repentant when I think I am, or am only indulging in a
pretense of humility . . . " and so on. This circular and ultimately futile
(as well as psychologically debilitating) self-analysis, which leads to motives taking on the attributes of their opposites, is well symbolized by
the image of the snake eating its own tail.

Thus the *Lachesis* patient may wonder in his bifurcated mind if
he has not actually incurred needless grief by putting up with a difficult
situation, or by restraining himself from licence, out of loyalty to some
higher ideal, and if he would not now be in better health if he had been
more selfish and self-indulgent.

Moral turmoil and intellectual conflict are hardly specific to any
one constitutional type. But when mature patients question their religion
or vocation, or experience doubts about their ideals, marriage, or personal development ("sudden doubts arise about truths of which he had
hitherto been convinced": Allen), a *Lachesis* pathology may be suspected. Even basically non-*Lachesis* types often require the remedy
when passing through some profound disillusionment or reassessment
of their lives. That is why it is considered one of the "mature" remedies and why many patients (especially women) need it at some point
in their mid-life passage.

To resolve moral or intellectual ambiguity some individuals accept
a strict behavioral framework or deliberately limit their understanding
or beliefs. *Lachesis* may deal with moral conflict by rejecting mental

elasticity, emotional suppleness, and awareness of paradox, refusing to acknowledge or be aware of aspects differing from his own convictions.* Or he might do the opposite; lacking a strong commitment, he intensifies his relativism or cynicism. He resolves, for instance, that the institutions of civilization are intrinsically worthless, if not actually evil. The institution of marriage, for example, theoretically established to preserve love, serves only to destroy its sincerity and spontaneity (compare this to *Lycopodium*'s viewpoint); while the defect of public institutions, he maintains, does not lie in administrative or legislative flaws which can, after all, be remedied (the *Lycopodium* viewpoint), nor yet in the individuals making up the institutions who can be changed (the *Natrum muriaticum* viewpoint), but in the very nature of the beast: they end by perpetuating themselves rather than the values for whose protection they were initially established.

This *Lachesis* nihilism—the type's innate "suspicion" (Hering) and mistrust—is essentially a projection of his own inner conflicts onto the world at large. If man is weak, selfish, and easily corrupted (as he knows one side of himself to be), how can these characteristics not be compounded in institutions where, notoriously, "the scum rises to the top," or where the weight and impersonality of numbers obliterate all that is moral and ethical in the individual?

A third type vacillates between extremes of intellectual rigidity

---

* Toward the end of his life Dostoyevsky followed a policy of deliberately limiting his understanding. Disturbed by the subversive impact of his works, he stopped writing fiction altogether. The ideas and moral precepts in his novels had a way of turning against themselves, suggesting the opposite interpretations of those he had originally intended and undermining the moral values he had set out to defend. Instead of continuing with the second volume of his intended trilogy, *The Brothers Karamazov*, for which a detailed outline had already been completed, he concentrated increasingly on his *Author's Diary*, which presents the complex philosophical issues raised so subtly in his novels in a less ambiguous, even simplified and bigoted, form. He died quite suddenly a year or so later from a pulmonary hemorrhage—a condition for which *Lachesis* is one of the major remedies (also *Crotalus horridus*: Kent). Could his sudden death be interpreted as a dramatic example of "ill effects from suppressed [mental] discharges," from not having allowed his genius full play?

and scepticism, with both mental attributes residing in the same person. This divided personality, with its erratic shifts of attitude and behavior, resembles a small sailboat tossed and buffeted in a gale and tacking first to starboard and then to port in its attempt to stay afloat and steer a course to harbor.

The Child

Only a mature mind can experience moral conflict, be aware of paradox, or appreciate intellectual relativism, and *Lachesis* children can be sophisticated beyond their years where intellectual or moral issues are concerned. These children (mostly girls, who mature more rapidly than boys) are often said to have been "born old" because, from an early age, for better or worse, they possess something of the wisdom of the serpent.

The youngest *constitutional* case treated with *Lachesis* in our experience was a four-year-old girl with severe temper tantrums.* Usually of peaceable disposition, she had suddenly undergone an inexplicable transformation and would strike out at her siblings like a veritable snake. When reprimanded, she lashed out at her parents with verbal venom: "You are animals—nothing but *wild* animals—you are worse than animals. Animals at least love their young and don't punish them like you do. You are not only animals but *real beasts!*" (note her feel for the distinction between the two words). She was beside herself and carried on like this for days. At one point, when her rebelliousness and intense negativism provoked the threat that Santa Claus would not be kind to her at Christmas, she responded with the defiant declaration: "I don't care! I hate Daddy, Mommy, God, *and* Santa Claus!" Yet, the internal struggle was quite visible: "I want to be good. Part of me wants to be good and tries hard, but *something* in me *makes* me bad. I hate the bad part, but I can't help it . . . " she would sob, as if some inner force was driving her to destructive behavior.

Since this resembled Hering's *Lachesis* symptom: "she feels as if in the hands of a strange power; feels as if she is charmed and can't break the spell," or Kent's "she hears commands . . . that she must carry out," the girl received a dose of *Lachesis* 10M. Her parents reported

---

* The remedy, of course, is used in many acute conditions of children: earaches, sore throats, "strep throat," boils, etc.

that an hour later she came down from her room and announced quietly and simply that she was over her temper tantrums and would behave herself thereafter ("I will be good forever"). Indeed, she lived up to her word, and the temper tantrums never returned. Whatever the nature of the destructive force that had to be purged, the one dose of *Lachesis* did it effectively.*

The second case was a nine-year-old girl brought to homoeopathy for epistaxis and excessive bleeding from small cuts and scratches (*Lachesis*, like *Phosphorus*, has an affinity for the hemorrhagic diathesis: "Like all snake poisons, *Lachesis* decomposes the blood, rendering it more fluid; hence a haemorrhagic tendency is marked" [Boericke]). She was a bright, pretty, high-strung girl, *Phosphorus* in appearance and outward behavior, but beneath the attractive surface lurked serious behavioral defects which emerged both in school and at home. In class she was an intriguer, inciting others to defy the rules; and while they were often caught red-handed, she herself cleverly eluded punishment. She thought of hateful, even insulting, ways of angering her parents (once urinating on their birthday presents to her), regardless of the consequences. She also stole money, jewelry, and watches, and even tormented the family dog, biting his tail until he yelped in pain.

This is not *Phosphorus*, but *Lachesis* testing her surroundings: "What will happen if I bite the dog's tail? Can I steal? What happens if I challenge my parents?" The *Sulphur* boy steals to test his nerve and boast of his manliness, or to satisfy his instinct for accumulation; the *Lachesis* girl who steals tells no one and is testing her power for "evil" (in *Lachesis'* own terms), to see if she can get away with it. When the patient was reprimanded for gratuitously hurting the defenseless dog, she replied in self-justification, "I'm not all bad. He's old, fat and half blind, and no one in the family paid any attention to him till I treated him unkindly. Now everyone feels sorry for him and is nicer to him." At age nine she had arrived at a sophisticated dualistic awareness that

---

* A similar case of violent tantrums cured with one dose of a homoeopathic remedy was with *Tarentula hispania*. In addition to articulating her struggles of conscience with a strange maturity, this young girl darted frenziedly like a spider from corner to corner of the room. These two virulent animal poisons seemed almost to exorcize the possessed children.

every action contains the seed of its opposite; just as good actions carry a potential for evil, so cruel actions may have a potential for good.

Furthermore, the patient's alert eyes had a *Lachesis* expression, a quick, darting quality in their sidelong glance (*Lachesis* can also peer out sideways from under the brow or through half-lowered lids); and her penetrating gaze was mistrustful ("suspicious look": Kent). A course of the medicine in ascending potencies caused a profound change in this girl, deflecting her audacious and defiant energies from trouble-making into constructive academic endeavors.

A third case exhibits quite a different facet of the constitutional picture. An eleven-year-old girl came to be treated for after-school headaches and a persistent urinary complaint: frequent micturition on going to bed at night, with little passage of urine (she would have to jump up a dozen times during the first two hours). There was nothing specifically *Lachesis* about her symptoms, nor did any other remedy particularly come to mind. True, she experienced "disturbed areas" of heat and cold (Nash) and was always either shedding her clothes or bundling up, but some of the modalities contraindicated the remedy. It was one of those hopelessly characterless cases.

Otherwise, the patient was an obedient, sensitive child and received in turn *Pulsatilla, Calcarea, Natrum muriaticum, Sepia, Nux vomica, Sulphur*, and *Tuberculinum*—all to no avail. Her urinary trouble and headaches persisted month after month. The physician, therefore, probed more deeply into her mental symptoms, returning to the subject of her school. In taking the case of a child much can be inferred by his or her way of discussing or *not* discussing this subject. For the first seven visits the girl was somewhat *Natrum muriaticum/Calcarea*: reserved in her answers, low-key, and reluctant to impart much information. Then, on the eighth visit, she abandoned her control, and everything she had heard or learned just flowed out of her—as if she could never say enough and never say it all!

Especially *Lachesis* was this girl's fascination with the moral problems raised by the study of medieval history: the paradox that the Christian ideals had both beneficial and detrimental effects, the moral ambiguity of the Crusades. She was intrigued by the issue of whether the age was ultimately progressive for European civilization, spreading culture, learning, and civilized behavior, or regressive—breeding ignorance and superstition? All these truly difficult concepts the child sensed and was trying to understand—no wonder she had those after-school head-aches! Furthermore, the way she so clearly articulated these questions (under the surface shyness of the type there often lies a reservoir of knowledge), even though they must have first been formulated by her teacher, argued for a *Lachesis* mind. She received a dose of the remedy in high potency, and her condition improved. Further doses eventually cleared it up completely.*

Relationships and Love

The classic homoeopathic literature, which of necessity emphasizes the characteristics of ill patients, stresses the mistrust, jealousy, malice, vanity, and hatred which *Lachesis* manifests in his relations with others. But since the present portrait aims to give the healthy and attractive aspects as well, the amiability, generosity, moral "firmness" (Boenning-hausen), and nobility of the type will be accorded equal weight.

Devotion and self-abnegation can be displayed by this individual to a very high degree. Physicians and nurses will devote themselves to energy-draining patients in a spirit of sacrifice that is wonderful to behold! Sons and daughters will care for afflicted parents with unpar-alleled devotion. The altruism of these courageous souls shows little subliminal self-pity (*Pulsatilla*), little desire for Promethean effect (*Phosphorus*), even less resentful dutifulness (*Natrum muriaticum*). They discharge their responsibilities with saintly submissiveness and seem-ingly without thought of recognition—sustained by the conviction that the Lord will provide strength and help. Others, full of principle, will act with noble renunciation in some personal matter. One patient, only moderately well-off herself, believing that the inheritance she received from her late husband more correctly belonged to his children from his first marriage, conveyed it to them. If praised for their virtue, they hardly understand what is meant, taking for granted that no other be-

---

* The following summer this slip of a girl spent most of her vacation outlining and typing up with two fingers a twenty-page "History of the Middle Ages," which was remarkably *Lachesis* in appearance as well as execution. Not only were the well-marshalled thoughts pre-sented in all their paradoxical complexity, but the crowded, single-spaced pages had no right-hand margins. She had so much to say that the words virtually ran off the pages, leaving the reader to guess at the last few letters or syllables.

havior is possible. The same selfless devotion can be directed to a cause that they indefatigably promote at the expense of their own interests.

Lachesis is also *loyal* and strongly stresses this quality in personal relations. Once he chooses a friend, partner, or protégé, he will strive unstintingly to preserve the relationship and benefit the other, and in professional and business life he will lay great store by group solidarity. A woman's loyalty may take the form of successfully furthering her children's education or her husband's career (*Arsenicum*), but she will also be exceptionally hospitable and kind to any person once numbered among her friends. However, she is likely to demand the same loyalty of others—at times to the point of endangering relationships, since they may not possess her emotional energy or the desire to give as much in return.

A *Lachesis* woman can exhibit the sweetness of *Pulsatilla* and the emotional sensitivity of *Phosphorus*. She will say nothing unkind of anyone and be extra-thoughtful of others, always endeavoring to bolster their self-esteem. Her liberality and friendliness can even be a little indiscriminate, in that she will treat everyone with the same emotional generosity, and sometimes she is even smothering in her sweetness. But, although "sweet," she is not "soft." She will fight back when provoked, especially when her territory is threatened. Mild, yielding *Pulsatilla* backs away from conflict while *Lachesis*, the snake, draws herself erect and is prepared to strike.*

What is more, she can combine extreme bluntness of manner with an almost clairvoyant awareness of the feelings of others and sensitivity

---

* Different as these two remedies are, their projections in patients can overlap to a large degree. A common scenario has a sweet, soft-spoken woman seeking relief for headaches, menstrual disorders, or inability to tolerate the sun. Her physical symptoms are evenly divided between *Pulsatilla* and *Lachesis*, and a discussion then ensues between the two attending physicians, one male and one female, over which is the correct remedy. The male physician, responding to the patient's femininity, will insist that the sweet woman is *Pulsatilla*, while the female will sense the subliminal "sharpness" and claim that *Lachesis* lies beneath the sweet exterior. The guiding symptom is sometimes supplied by asking the patient how she reacts to criticism or opposition, especially in the home. The former is more likely to withdraw weeping, feeling intensely sorry for herself. The latter will retaliate vehemently, giving toward them. Her understanding seems at such times uncoordinated with her behavior. She can also be direct and forceful in what is traditionally regarded as a masculine way, while her incisive mind is capable of giving offense. In conversation she may appear brusque, or she continues her own line of thought rather than responding to another. But it eventually becomes clear—from her having taken steps to help—that, even while appearing not to listen, she has intelligently understood the other's concerns and that her digressions, while disjointed and seemingly unconnected with the subject at hand, were not entirely purposeless. Thus, even though not always gentle, the generous, creative, and "vivacious" (Kent) *Lachesis* can be exceedingly likable.

The Jekyll-and-Hyde aspect of the *Lachesis* character creates an ambiguity which eludes simple analysis: this is the individual on whose "true" nature no two observers can agree.

The charming, generous, considerate man will suddenly turn crafty and manipulative—and then become kind and enchanting again. The woman who to some observers appears a hurricane of energy and commotion is seen by others as a gentle summer breeze. Or the formerly obliging, loving, and reasonable family member becomes harsh, rash, or irrational, in an abrupt reversal of her usual mood. An adolescent girl will spend hours helping a slower friend with her homework but then attack her venomously on some slight provocation. Hostile feelings which had hitherto lain dormant suddenly become dominant. Her behavior is quite incomprehensible to the non-*Lachesis* victim who does not understand what motivates her former "best friend." This constitutional type, incidentally, forms strong adolescent (and adult) friendships and is highly possessive of her female friends—insep-

---

no thought to withdrawal, and incapable of verbal self-restraint.

The opposite, however, should also be taken into account. Since there is always an element of subjectivity in a physician's response to his patient (i.e., the male, we saw, responds to the *Pulsaltilla* in a woman, while a female picks up more readily the *Lachesis* side), and since the patient, in his turn, is subject to mood alternations or responds to pressures from the environment in a way that affects his nature, often the physical symptoms and modalities are the more "objective" ones. They, then, become of primary importance in a given case and serve best as guides to the simillimum.

arable from them, protective of them, and insisting on their unwavering loyalty. Her behavior and jealousy make it appear as if she, indeed, "falls in love with a member of her own sex" (less frequently, *Lachesis* adolescent boys display a similar possessiveness toward one of their own sex).

As a rule, discord, quarrels, and fallings out do not upset him as they do others. Like *Sulphur* he can put personal unpleasantness behind him and go on optimistically to the next thing. In fact, *Lachesis* derives energy from conflict and at some level thrives on it. Combative confrontations, like the earlier-mentioned strong passions, are grist to his ever-churning emotional mill and spur him on to even higher levels of performance.

The individual with high ideals will try to suppress any vindictive or manipulative instincts. One friendly, direct patient—with *Lachesis* well hidden beneath a *Pulsatilla* surface—told the physician that she hated gossip and intrigue above all things because she was aware of their power to influence and hurt others. As a young girl she had easily succeeded in turning members of her family against one another, and she now so despised that manipulative part of herself that she vowed never again to give free play to her cutting and influential tongue. "I used to find it difficult, at times," she concluded, "but now, whenever the urge becomes strong and persistent, I just take a dose of *Lachesis* and the urge evaporates."

On the other hand, *Lachesis* in high potency can bring to the surface long-buried emotions and behavior. One kind and soft-spoken male patient suffering from arthritic pains told the physician that he had made remarkably nasty comments to everyone for several weeks after his first dose of the remedy. "I used to be wittily malicious, with an instinct for the jugular, but I thought I had put all that behind me. It is frightening," he added, "how easy it is to be sarcastic, to spot another's weakness, and then laugh at his expense. Better find me an antidote to the remedy quickly—or else give me back my arthritis!"

Aware of his own capacity to act underhandedly, *Lachesis* can be highly suspicious of the motives and integrity of others: "he attaches the most hateful significance to the most innocent occurrences" (Allen). Mistrusting everyone, he suspects that others are out to harm him or plotting his downfall ("imagines he is being followed by enemies who are trying to hurt him": Hering). For example, a sixteen-year-old girl being treated for menstrual complaints (severe migraine headaches two days before the onset of menses and an intermittent flow), who was bright and attractive and trying to be ultrasuccessful in her studies and extracurricular activities, could talk of nothing but her friends' intrigues, vindictiveness, and envy of her accomplishments. This clearly mirrored her own feelings and behavior which, in self-justification, she was projecting onto her classmates. The snake poison cured her physical problems and also attenuated her somewhat paranoid attitude.

Many remedies display suspicion (see the rubric in Kent), but to summon up one of those fine distinctions in which homoeopathy delights, *Arsenicum* and *Lycopodium* are mainly suspicious of another's understanding or competence, trusting only their own. *Pulsatilla* suspects the sincerity of one who expresses solicitude ("You say you care, but do you really?"). *Lachesis* is more suspicious of another's motivations and behavior and always fears betrayal.

In his embracing of opposites the individual may combine hotheaded impetuosity with cool, clear-sighted deliberation, or overheated intellectual passion with a cold and trenchant logic. In a woman, an incisive "masculine" mind coexists with an emotional feminine disposition; or else a dictatorial decisiveness alternates with bouts of painful "irresolution" (Kent). At crucial moments she hesitates or procrastinates, demonstrating helplessness, weakness, dependence (like *Pulsatilla* or *Sepia*) or autocratically changing her mind. She seeks counsel, yet refuses to do as advised.

But, whereas with *Pulsatilla* and *Sepia* irresolution is a form of weakness—a sign that the individual is not in control of her destiny—with *Lachesis* it can be a form of control. A graphic example was the strongly *Lachesis* Queen Elizabeth I of England who used her indecisiveness to wield power and retain her throne.

She could never decide whether or not, or whom, to marry; advisors and retainers regularly fell in and out of her favor; she was undecided whether or not to take decisive steps against the Roman Catholics and Mary Queen of Scots, or what stance to take in the religious conflicts seething on all sides; whether to sign treaties with other countries or declare war on them. She shamelessly and autocratically reneged on personal commitments and in state negotiations. This vacillation drove her advisors to distraction but contributed to her survival, both as a person and as a ruler, during the dangerous and strife-torn times in which she lived and reigned.

A further dichotomy is exhibited in the nature's capacity to be simultaneously straightforward and deceptive. On one hand, he has definite ideas, and an assertive intellectual integrity prompts him to take a firm stand when they are challenged. Even though occasionally deceptive in smaller matters, on the larger ones and with respect to important values some essential part of his nature remains true and incorruptible: "Myself I may contradict, the truth I may not" (Montaigne) is this type's conscious or unconscious creed.* He can be scrupulously honest; some even give the impression of over-aggressive honesty or bluntness, perhaps cultivated to overcome the subliminal dishonesty which chronically threatens to surface. On the other hand, *Lachesis* may, indeed, protest his honesty too much. His "I cannot lie," "I always tell the truth," "I never deceive," disguise a certain deviousness—which sometimes surprises the individual himself. His mind operates so sinuously or erratically that he finds himself acting underhandedly without so intending.

However, *Lachesis* can also be an accomplished liar. With a powerful and "vivid imagination" (Hering), he can get into positions where one falsehood leads irresistibly to another, as he succumbs to an intellectual intoxication. Mere facts fade into insignificance, and veracity yields to verisimilitude during his gripping accounts. Such imaginative outbursts are not only a technique for releasing his unsatisfied energies or dormant instincts in intellectual activity, but also reflect a certain "artistic pride" (Clarke) and conviction that a story worth telling is worth telling well! Incidents are presented in elaborate detail, full of the "authentic" touches which, purportedly, only truth can supply, but which, in his case, are the product of a fine imagination.

Yet, although *Lachesis* may resort to boastfulness, hypocrisy (speaking with the serpent's "forked tongue") or mendacity, he does not deceive himself. Being in close touch with his subliminal side, he has few

---

* Voltaire, for example, for all his notorious mendacity and lack of scruple in personal matters, fought unrelentingly for political justice, personal liberty, and freedom of thought and speech; he was intrepid in opposing every type of despotism, obscurantism, prejudice, or shortsighted ignorance; and he tirelessly defended the oppressed of all societies, such as the persecuted Huguenots and the enserfed peasantry.

self-delusions—here contrasting with *Lycopodium*. He also contrasts
with *Phosphorus* who, charming others into his version of reality, ends
by charming himself. "The serpent knows itself," is an old adage, and
Lachesis knows full well what is what. He does not always choose to
act on this awareness, but it is there.

A characteristic form of the type's self-awareness in a well-balanced
patient was exhibited by a middle-aged woman who came to homoeopathy for chronic sore throats.

Located approximately midway between the brain (intellect, reason,
restraint) and the heart (passions, instincts, unrestraint), i.e., symbolically
where the conflicting mind and emotions meet, the throat is one of the
remedy's most vulnerable areas (with eight pages of symptoms in Hering's *Guiding Symptoms*). The *globus hystericus* or "lump in the throat"
syndrome, experienced when the patient is under severe emotional
stress, could be considered a physical manifestation of the patient's attempt rationally to control his rising passion, anger, or hysteria (*Ignatia,
Natrum muriaticum*): "The *globus hystericus* is a typical response for
the throat, when the ego has difficulty holding its own against the invasion of emotional and especially sexual forces" (Whitmont).

The above patient had a history of tonsillitis in childhood and presented with such typical *Lachesis* throat symptoms as: larynx sensitive
to touch, better from eating but aggravated by hot drinks, with pain
extending into the ear when swallowing, feeling of constriction in throat
as from a lump ("When I swallow, I feel as if I am passing over a mountain!"), pain starting on the left and moving to the right. Mentally, however, she manifested no dualistic struggles and showed no sign of repressed emotions. She resembled *Phosphorus* in being sensitive and
sympathetic, and *Lycopodium* in being attractively cool and detached.

But, when questioned about her inner life, she showed the typical
Lachesis honesty and absence of illusion. For instance, when asked if
she was sociable and outgoing, she replied: "I suppose I could be considered so. People bring their troubles to me, maybe because I am a
good listener—although my husband says I can't be because I talk too
much myself." Asked if her husband was critical of her: "A bit," she
answered, "but just look at me! Here I am fifty-five, overweight, with
no special talents or good looks. You can hardly blame him for finding
some little fault with me." Actually, her husband was an excessively
grouchy and disagreeable man who consistently made life difficult for

her; yet the patient never referred to this during the entire course of treatment. When asked if she was selfish or generous, "I like to consider myself generous, and I act the role of a generous person. Occasionally, however, I astonish myself by lapsing into what can only be called extreme selfishness. When I feel possessive about someone or something, or perceive an infringement on my territorial rights, the measures I take in defense can actually be quite frightening." Finally, asked if she considered herself tolerant or critical of people, she replied: "It's hard to say. I'm constantly amazed at the way my friends and family behave. Not at all the way I would. But then, I dare say, they are just as often amazed at me and *my* behavior." Her honest comprehension of herself and lack of self-delusion were in this case the guiding mental symptoms to *Lachesis*.

Even the adolescent, when confronted with unpalatable truths about himself may say, "At first I was angered by, and totally denied, them. But then I decided to try to understand why the person said I was [arrogant] and what exactly he meant by it. And I now see that there was legitimacy in his assertion, if one interpreted my behavior in a certain way. So I am actually *grateful* to him for pointing it out to me. I can now work on changing myself . . ." and so on.

But a patient can also be devastated by awareness of his subliminal side. Seemingly healthy individuals confess to a fear of losing their mental balance from the pressure of excessive self-restraint: "I'm always in conflict, always holding myself in, or holding myself back; I don't know how long I can go on this way." Nothing in their outward behavior indicates such a danger, but *Lachesis* himself senses with disturbing clarity the warning signals of loss of control and fears an erratic reversal.

In the patient verging on nervous breakdown the fear of losing his mind is accompanied by feelings of unworthiness, of having committed some evil, of horror at the sinfulness of the world, or at his or her heightened sexuality. The woman confesses to an almost irresistible urge to indiscreet behavior or a humiliating show of emotion, and wonders if she will be able to withstand the impulse when it seizes her. The man is tormented lest antisocial elements of his previously restrained sensual side suddenly overcome his reason. He fears that his energies, if released, will explode in all directions. At such a moment, when the scales are tipping from restraint to "the point of breakdown of control" (Whitmont), and the patient is aware of treading a thin line between the two, *Lachesis* can come wonderfully to his aid and right the delicate mental balance (also *Ignatia*). This is also the time when the remedy can best be observed and understood—when both sides of the nature come to the fore.

The *Lachesis* ability to embrace contrary emotions is often displayed in the love relationship. This passionate nature can alternate between love and hate more suddenly and violently than any other— reversing within minutes and then just as suddenly switching back again. One would say that the opposite emotions coexist except that the dominant feeling of the moment so entirely *possesses* the individual as to leave little room for ambivalence. Then again, these emotions may not really be opposed, since in this type both proceed from the same source of intense feeling (both Dostoyevsky and Freud, for instance, insisted on the closeness, if not actual oneness, of love and hate).

Not all *Lachesis* individuals oscillate between the two. For instance, he can be the most devoted of husbands, throughout his whole married life directing all the intensity of his sexual and emotional nature toward one woman (*Natrum muriaticum*). An example of this attitude was the otherwise healthy elderly patient being treated for a severe undiagnosed, non-specific pain in the groin. He had been through a barrage of tests which had revealed nothing, but the fear of cancer was at the back of the patient's mind. To find the simillimum the homoeopathic physician had to be guided by the patient's mental symptoms. Among other things, he said that in all his years of marrige, he had never *for one single moment* regretted marrying his wife. In fact, he woke up every morning and went to bed every night "thanking God for the blessing of a good marriage." This was very touching and obviously true, as his wife was like a religion to him. But he was also very possessive about her, not liking her even to say a good word about another man. Hearing this, the physician gave *Lachesis* 200x. The pain went away after two doses, and no one was ever to know what had caused it.

This picture of single-minded devotion is even more common in a woman. She can be passionately in love with her partner for life, even through the most difficult times (we recall that she is the faithful wife who stands by her alcoholic husband). Yet she is not herself always easy to live with, being often unduly possessive and subject to unfounded ("insane": Hering) jealousy ("as foolish as it is irresistible": Kent). She is suspicious of every letter or telephone call her partner receives and fearful that he is deceiving her every time he comes home late. Even if not cross-examining him or making a scene, she nurses a gnawing and unrelenting dread of betrayal that allows her no peace of mind. And if she thinks she has been spurned or betrayed, the humility and selflessness of love quickly turn into their opposites—unbearable humiliation and uncontrollable jealousy. These characteristics may only surface premenstrually, at which times she can indeed not be wholly responsible for her behavior. The injured *Lachesis* can then, like Medea in her rage, act on violent impulse, or say something venomous, heedless of the consequences. Romantic jealousy can even bring on epileptic seizures (Boericke; also *Hyoscyamus*: Kent).

The well-known jealousy is by no means limited to the object of sexual love but can extend to friends, siblings, colleagues—even parents—causing headaches, hay-fever, asthma, dysmenorrhea, skin eruptions, and other pathology. One adolescent girl's violent hay-fever attacks, to which she was subject only in her own home, were traced to jealousy of her youthful and pretty mother who usurped all her father's attention. Or a picture of jealousy sublimated into friendship, then undergoing a sudden reversal, often attests to *Lachesis* in the constitution.

The individual may also be possessive of his ideas and jealous of a competitor's professional success,* and many of these various forms of jealousy have been significantly helped by this remedy. At times, however, what appears to be jealousy is really anger or indignation at

---

* An example from history was Francis Bacon's gratuitous denunciation in court of his friend, the Earl of Essex, whom he had counseled and advised for years and from whom he had received many favors. It was doubtless motivated by jealousy of the Earl's success in ingratiating himself with Queen Elizabeth while he, Bacon, had not. In his moving reply to Bacon's damaging evidence during his trial for treason Essex cried out in his defense: "I call forth Mr. Bacon against Mr. Bacon." He was invoking the now subordinate loyal and noble side of his former friend and mentor to testify against the now dominant betraying side. Interestingly, the fascinating and forever ambiguous Lord Bacon with his darting glance was described by contemporaries as "reptilian" and possessing a "viper's eye."

a colleague's straying from the true path and branching out on his own. *Lachesis* demands ideological as well as personal loyalty or solidarity (typical here was the relationship of Freud to his prize pupil, Carl Jung).

Power

At the root of many *Lachesis* self-torturing relationships (and of a good portion of his physical pathology) lies a wounded and oversensitive "pride" (Hering). The "arrogant" (Kent) or vain individual wants to be recognized for some extraordinary achievement in life. If he cannot make his mark in a positive manner, he may in frustration make it negatively. Thus the theme of revenge often crops up in his conversation, and candid patients will say, "I'm going to manipulate him into a corner just as he's manipulated me," or "I've got her in my power, and she'll be sorry for what she did. I'll get back at her if it's the last thing I do."

He can be a formidable opponent when feeling threatened or seeking to assert himself ("malicious, vindictive": Kent). A man in his forties suffering from constant pressure in the sinuses had been, in his view, unjustly demoted from a high position in a corporation he had helped establish. He was talented and could easily have found an equivalent position in a rival firm but was determined to stay on in his subordinate capacity to wreak whatever vengeance he could: "I'm going to force them to respect me again," he told the physician with a hard dangerous look in his eye.

Lachesis 10M was prescribed, and the patient was asked to return in a month. By this time his sinuses had cleared (stringy, green, rotten-smelling mucus poured out for several days in copious quantities), but, what was more important, his energies had been redirected along constructive lines. He had decided to leave the old company and form his own, where he could run everything himself. The homoeopathic physician cannot always gauge what else beside the remedy might have changed the patient's attitude, but change there was.

This patient revealed another aspect of the type. While "egotistical" (Kent) and full of disdain in his former job, in his new company he was kind, patient, humble, and unassuming. Parenthetically, the *appearance* of "humility" in a powerful, prominent, or influential person frequently conceals inordinate pride kept hidden or under control in a predominantly *Lachesis* or *Arsenicum* personality; *Sulphur* and *Lycopodium* openly parade their power. Once satisfied, this individual's dominant power-hunger turned into its opposite and brought out his dormant magnanimity. Lord Acton wrote: "Power corrupts, and absolute power corrupts absolutely," yet *Lachesis* in a position of power (whether in the world at large or only inside his family) frequently demonstrates the reverse: restraint, integrity, and humility vis-a-vis those whom he is leading or supervising. These can take over and all but obliterate his original selfish impulses.

When not in a position of power *Lachesis* can be rebellious, arrogantly intent on doing what he pleases, scornful of authority, and prepared to defy the rules and regulations. An English teacher sought help for a "constricted feeling and cramplike pains" of the heart (Hering), as well as bursting or pulsating headaches.* She was at present unemployed but confident about finding work. "I never have any trouble in this respect," she assured the physician. Nor was it surprising: she projected intelligence, vitality, and an obvious love of inspiring others through her charismatic manner. Yet she had never held any teaching position for more than three years. The reasons she gave were: unreasonable supervisors, jealous colleagues, unsatisfactory contractual terms, or her own restlessness: "I am like a potted plant that needs to be transplanted every few years." Further questioning and some reading between the lines revealed a different pattern. The first year she was the general favorite, the fair-haired child admired by all. The second year she would begin to weary of the prescribed curriculum and start to instruct as she liked, not as was required. She brilliantly reproduced the alternately pleading and threatening tones of the headmasters: "We want less of your impassioned discourses, Madam, and more of the fundamentals of English grammar—and more of Melville and Milton. Our children have to get into the better colleges, as has been the tradition

---

* "Some symptoms are valuable because of the frequency of their associations, and when such is the case their concomitant relation becomes important. The cardiac symptoms are frequently connected with headache symptoms in *Lachesis* . . . A weak pulse, or the pulsation felt all over the body, is more or less associated with violent *Lachesis* headaches" (Kent: *Lectures on Homoeopathic Materia Medica* Lachesis).

of this school for seventy-five years." Yet she would ignore instructions, continuing to teach as inspired, discussing the writers she preferred, flaunting her power and influence over her admiring students, and all the while displaying an "I don't care what you or anyone thinks of me" attitude ("scornful mood, without being vexed": Allen). In short, she behaved so provocatively — even autocratically — that her dismissal was assured. At the same time, her dedication to her vocation and devotion to her students were clear to see. She simply could not tolerate being in any way compelled or directed in her work.

Many constitutional types do not well tolerate authority, curtailment of their freedom, or pressure by others to perform or conform. But in *Lachesis* the intolerance of psychological restriction finds its physical counterpart in a sensitivity to pressure on any part of the body and in particular around the throat (Gutman points out that the snake's neck is its only really vulnerable part: "any firm grip on the neck leaves the most poisonous snake helpless"). The woman dislikes tight clothes or jewelry around the neck and will wear open-necked blouses and dresses or constantly tug at a turtle-neck sweater as if to lessen the constriction there. The man will loosen his tie and unbutton his collar: "cannot bear shirt or neckband on throat" (Hering).* Even the bedclothes pulled up around the neck at night may cause him to feel nervous, uneasy, or choked (the *Lycopodium* or *Calcarea* dislike of pressure is manifested physically by a reluctance to wear belts or tight clothes around the waist or hypogastrium). Yet sometimes the patient, whose "abdomen is [also] sensitive to the [mere] weight of clothes" (Hering), will not object to a tight belt because *hard* pressure does not aggravate. In fact, a number of his pains are relieved by hard pressure (*Bryonia, Ignatia*); a sore throat, for instance, is better from the pressure of swallowing solid foods, while empty swallowing or the swallowing of liquids aggravates. Aggravation from light touch or "oversensitive to touch" (Kent) combined with amelioration from hard pressure always suggest this remedy.

Whitmont notes that this physical symptom symbolizes the underlying psychic condition: "When you are pressed or hit psychologically, you bound back, but when the soft approach is used, you are 'touched.'

---

* In an intriguing coincidence, Hering's congenital dislike of tight clothing around his neck was intensified by his proving of *Lachesis*; this has since been regarded as one of the key symptoms.

Your feeling overrules your defenses and comes forth. This is what the *Lachesis* person's repressed life feelings and emotions cannot afford . . . But hard pressure improves because [you] respond with a tightening and shaping up to pressure . . . " An analogy can be made with the above-mentioned springtime aggravation. Why should the spring aggravate more than the heat of summer? The answer could be that the softer stimulus is more aggravating than the firmer one. As the weather starts to become warm, certain instincts are awakened and dormant emotions are aroused in the classic "spring fever," while *Lachesis* "tightens up" and puts out defenses to the heat of summer.

On the intellectual plane, this positive response to pressure may explain why he works well to deadlines. In contrast to *Calcarea, Pulsatilla,* or *Silica,* who react to pressure, respectively, by "tuning out," weeping, or timidly withdrawing, "hard pressure" and emotional stress stimulates the *Lachesis* mind and brings out the best in him. *Arsenicum* and *Natrum muriaticum* also respond to firm pressure, but it must be of a consistent, regulated, and predictable kind, whereas *Lachesis* reacts best to intense sporadic pressure.*

A not uncommon expression of the *Lachesis* intolerance of confinement is the woman who resists marrying the man she truly loves, and with whom she may be sexually involved, out of fear of the psychological restriction of marriage. The symptom, "aversion to marry," may thus reflect an aversion, not to sex, but to the emotionally binding commitment of wed*lock.*

As befits the person who likes power, *Lachesis* may exhibit a concurrent fascination with money, the symbol of power. He enjoys talking about wealth—more about rich people than about money per se

---

* It is significant that Harriet Beecher Stowe, who had the same strong *Lachesis* vein as her brother, wrote her only significant novel under conditions of extreme hardship—sickness, financial stringency, emotional trials—when she was only able to work at night, after having discharged her family and household obligations. She herself claimed that the story came to her "almost as a tangible vision" and that it was not merely inspired, but "written by God" (in a *Lachesis* "*trance-like*" state?). Certainly, her subsequent nine novels, written under relatively easy conditions, after *Uncle Tom's Cabin* had made her fortune and reputation, were unremarkable.

(for example, the prices of things)—and is almost as fascinated by the wealth of others as by his own. But he does not necessarily hang on to his wealth (*Arsenicum, Sulphur*); nor is he cautious about money (*Sepia, Lycopodium*). Money to him is to be *spent*, not accumulated. He can be the soul of liberality and rash generosity, even squandering his substance, in part for the feeling of power it gives him. *Lachesis* women may go on enormous shopping sprees for clothes; although almost all women like spending money on dress, in this type it can become excessive and uncontrolled.

Money is also there to be risked: thus, *Lachesis* is more prone than others to become addicted to gambling. Even in living-room card games he is carried away with the exhilaration of risking his pile of chips. In contrast, the competitive but more cautious *Arsenicum* plays in tense and deadly earnest even when only a few cents are at stake.

Vitality

Notwithstanding their scepticism, moral relativism, and internal conflicts, *Lachesis* individuals exhibit such unquenchable vitality that others instinctively describe them as "intense," "hyper-excited," "addiction-prone," "overstimulated," "obsessive," or "passionate"— not solely in the sexual sense, but also for knowledge, experience, understanding, passion for a cause or a faith—passion for life itself!

This type's incredible energy is manifested physically and emotionally in ways already mentioned: strong pulsations all over the body or in some part of it, racing heart and throbbing head, little need of sleep, intense attachments, a strong sexual drive ("emotionally and sexually charged": Whitmont), and mentally in a high level of intellectual activity: the mind races, with "increased power of originality in all mental work . . . writes with the greatest freedom and increased vigor about everything that he knows" (Allen); "no sooner does one idea occur to him [when writing] than a number of others follow in quick succession" (Hering). In fact, his creative energy can take on an ecstatic quality: "a state of exaltation which induces desire to compose intellectual work" (Clarke). In everyday life, the more he does the more energy he generates. He may accomplish so much on the job that it takes three persons to fill his position when he leaves or retires. He is never fatigued, never slows down, and his day seems to contain more hours than other people's.

A familiar figure, for example, is the *Lachesis* school teacher who not only adores her work but never wearies of the same subject, bringing to it every year a freshness drawn from her own unabated enthusiasm. She has so much to say that she can never finish the class on time. If she has thirty tests to grade, they are all given back the next morning. Term papers are corrected with equal alacrity, the perceptive comments on every page revealing that hers was no perfunctory reading. She will have stayed up all night reviewing them. But in class the next day she is as full of dynamism as ever, showing no sign of sleeplessness and with seemingly unlimited attention for even the most demanding student. Watching *Lachesis* operate at full throttle, the observer can only wonder where all the energy comes from.

Voltaire, who worked 18-20 hours a day (and night) on his varied writings and a correspondence that ran into the thousands of letters, and who dictated so rapidly that his secretary could hardly keep up with him, at age sixty-four said of himself: "I am as supple as an eel, as lively as a lizard, and as tireless as a squirrel." And so he remained for another two decades (to be sure, this energy must have been fortified by his lifelong habit of consuming up to forty cups of coffee a day).

When the *Lachesis* energy, passion, and fertile ideas are properly *channeled*, his creative output is unsurpassed. All too often, however, for all his fine capacities, he falls short of true distinction because he attempts too much to do any one thing perfectly: "he wishes to do a great deal, begins many things; need of being busy, without . . . perseverence" (Allen). His creativity is *chaotic* ("cannot perform anything in an orderly manner": Allen), and his inspiration erupts in sporadic bursts, so that the quality of his output is erratic—original but unsystematic. This contrasts with the orderly *Arsenicum*'s consistent level of performance.

This inextinguishable vitality is observed in the consulting room. Patients with terrifying illnesses or personal tragedies—problems that would devastate or overwhelm the ordinary individual—still face life with blazing intensity, with energy and spirits quite unsubdued. In fact, one hardly believes they feel as poorly as they claim: like *Phosphorus*, *Lachesis* patients can be much sicker than they appear. Not only does their vitality remain undiminished in the face of adversity ("I feel as if I've been in combat all year, but I'm feeling great anyway"), at times it seems as if the more trying the circumstances, the higher they soar in a kind of manic reaction to stress. In general, both mental and physical illness in *Lachesis* take on a restless overstimulated quality: the patient is wakeful, "wants to be off somewhere" (Clarke), doing something more than usual, talking all the time—and these are all impulses which generate energy.

His dynamism can actually be conveyed to others. The patient's very presence in the office is stimulating and invigorating, and even after a 5 p.m. consultation the physician feels reenergized, as if he could effortlessly start his long day all over again.

This is part of *Lachesis*'s problem. His energy is so plentiful, his vitality so strong, that he cannot handle it constructively, cannot direct it so as to avoid harming himself ("Sometimes it scares me how much energy I have. I don't know what to do with it, how to control it!"). Patients requiring the remedy describe an augmentation of their ambition, feeling of power, and drive for accomplishment, even while experiencing a need for enhanced control of their impulses.

However, the "shadow" side of this vitality is also encountered— in the patient exhibiting "complete dullness, apathy, despondency, wanting in comprehension, satiety of life with longing for death, hopelessness, loathing of life" (Hering); also an aversion to all mental activity: "dilatory, cannot accomplish his usual business, inability for abstract thought; a kind of loss of ideas" (Allen). It is as if his vital force has been simply switched off. In a physical correspondence, the remedy has helped in serious breakdowns of the body's immune system.

The *Lachesis* heightened assertion of life can also be perverted into a powerful self-destructive force, taking the form of alcoholism, drug-addiction, a perverse determination to undermine his own success just when things are going well, or sudden and irresistible "suicidal impulses" (Hering) which erratically supersede the carefree outlook of an hour earlier. Or the individual begins to destroy his relationships with others by unrelenting demands and overpossessiveness. Fearing the loss of friends or loved ones, he coils himself around them, thereby forcing them to seek escape from his too heavy and enveloping emotions and ultimately bringing about that which he fears most.

Impersonality and Humor

This special vitality could contribute to the curious aura of *imper-*

sonality which emanates from the *Lachesis* patient, as though on some emotional level events do not affect him as they do others. To all appearances he possesses neither the excessive vulnerabilty of *Natrum muriaticum*, the hypersensitivity of *Phosphorus*, the clinging dependence of *Pulsatilla*, the emotional fragility of *Ignatia*, the faint-heartedness of *Silica*, nor *Arsenicum*'s agony at losing control of his health and fate. These factors—which elicit, even command, the physician's emotional involvement—are usually missing from *Lachesis* whose tribulations are intellectually intriguing but do not rend the heart. He does not elicit pity because he does not demand it.

It is not that he is insensitive to emotional trauma or suffering. On the contrary, the remedy is frequently employed for "complaints resulting from long-lasting grief or sorrow; from disappointment in love; after vexation, loss, etc.," (Hering). Although *Natrum muriaticum*, *Ignatia*, and *Staphysagria* are better known for these conditions, *Lachesis* should never be overlooked. This individual suffers and may even pay a heavy physical or mental price,* but he *appears* to maintain distance between himself and his troubles, displaying a philosophic acceptance of the part he is fated to play in the inevitable ebbs and flows of this world. Such acceptance of trials and tragedy—as if he were an observer in a drama larger than himself—is partly what gives him the capacity to endure hardship; and the pathos of some especially courageous severely tried souls has a "luminous" and "distilled" quality that renders it objective and detached. With time the physician develops a sensitivity for this *Lachesis* "impersonality"—which should not be confused with *Lycopodium*'s detachment and emotional aloofness, where events simply do not traumatize or overwhelm him.

An impersonal approach to oneself favors a humorous attitude, and,

---

* Whitmont suggests that the high incidence of cancer in menopausal and post-climacteric women may be the price paid for their unfulfilled lives: "*Lachesis* is the penalty for the unlived life" of women of correct "Victorian" morality. By suppressing sexual urges they sever themselves from normal emotional growth, leading to unnatural growth in the form of tumors. *Lachesis*, to be sure, is a major remedy for cancer in middle-aged women, and thwarted sexual passion is frequently found at its source.

notwithstanding the misfortune of a given situation or ailment, in *Lachesis* a touch of the ridiculous is often blended with the pathetic. Even though feeling genuine care and concern, the physician may still find himself laughing at the extraordinary picture — even caricature — he (or more often, she) presents.

Sometimes the patient herself encourages this impression by playing up the comic side of her hardships and emphasizing the absurd. She may deliberately create distance between herself and her mishaps through humor (perhaps, in her sensitive pride, to ensure that others are laughing *with* and not *at* her). One patient said of herself, "My last name is Strange. I am a Miss Strange. I was born on April Fool's day, and absurdity has marked me for her own. My life has been one long parody of what a life is meant to be." She then proceeded humorously to relate the series of extraordinary misadventures and bizarre calamities that seemed to shadow her at all times. Perhaps the nature courts these mishaps, or perhaps the cast of mind is particularly attuned to extracting the ridiculous from the variety of daily experience ("witty, facetious": Boenninghausen); or perhaps the reverse is true, that an unrelenting series of mishaps and ludicrous disasters leaves a *Lachesis* stamp on the individual. In any case, fate not infrequently seems to confer on these persons more than their share of semi-farcical, semi-tragic adventures.

Indeed, humorists and satirists frequently exhibit *Lachesis* characteristics ("tendency to mock, ridicule, satirize": Hering), as the type is quick to sense the absurdity of situations, to spot what is ridiculous in others' behavior, and to perceive weaknesses in their use of language. He may be the jokester whose relentless wit — with one quip or jest following another in a humorous commentary on the happenings of everyday life — compensates for a difficult or even tragic life. After all, the humorous and tragic outlooks are complementary expressions of the conviction that worldy things are vain and worthless. Thus, a grim or bitter attitude may underlie his humor. Whereas the wit of an *Arsenicum* or *Lycopodium* seems to proceed from his command or control of the situation, the joking of *Lachesis* is more that of the victim, of one who has been defeated in some way and for whom wit is the only outlet from an intolerable or unalterable situation. Conversely, the apparently serious individual who always has "a laugh up his sleeve" (Hubbard) and is ever ready with a laconically humorous comment may also be *Lachesis*. Raised to the level of art, *Lachesis* humor reveals a profound awareness of the tragicomic irony of life.

Mark Twain, whose humor so often contains a strain of "misanthropy" (Kent) or bitter pessimism ("Why is it that we rejoice at a birth and grieve at a funeral? It is because we are not the person involved.") is a fine example of the *Lachesis* type in his person and his literary work. The passionate inner struggle that dominated his tragedy- and comedy-filled life made him both a cynic and an inveterate moralist, predictably sermonizing most strongly against his underlying self.

He could not abide moralizing in others and repeatedly criticized his fellow-authors for it, yet much of his own writing is marred by too heavy or too passionate preaching, more fit for the pulpit than for the press. At the same time, *Lachesis*-style, he questioned with relentless irony the ethical assumptions of the age and society in which he lived. Few passages in literature present the ambiguity of conventional morality more charmingly than the scene where Huckleberry Finn, feeling obliged to turn in the black man, Jim, as a runaway slave, finds his "educated but deformed conscience" contending against his "sound heart" (Twain) and ends by lying to the pursuers and diverting them in the wrong direction:

> "They went off, and I got aboard the raft, feeling bad and low, because I knowed very well I had done wrong, and I seed it warn't no use for me to try to learn to do right; a body that don't get started right when he's little, ain't got no show—when the pinch comes there ain't nothing to back him up and keep him to his work, and so he gets beat. Then I thought a minute, and says to myself, hold on—s'pose you'd a done right and give Jim up; would you felt better than what you do now? No, says I, I'd feel bad—I'd feel just the same way I do now. Well, then says I, what's the use you learning to do right, when it's troublesome to do right and ain't no trouble to do wrong, and the wages is just the same? I was stuck. I couldn't answer that. So I reckoned I wouldn't bother no more about it, but after this always do whichever come handiest at the time."

Furthermore, Twain ridiculed literary sentimentality (see the *Pulsatilla* chapter) but was himself not entirely free of guilt, particularly in his later writings. Also, while a true democratic American who abhorred whatever smacked of class privilege, he enjoyed nothing more than being courted by the aristocracy and royalty of England and Russia when he visited those countries. He despised material greed and in numerous works denounced the "damned human race" for its worship of money. Yet he was himself fascinated by wealth and made certain to marry the richest heiress of Elmira, New York, where he was living (the way he sought his future father-in-law's consent to the marriage is classic: Twain, "Have you noticed anything between your daughter and myself?" Father-in-law, "No, I haven't." Twain, "Well, look sharp and you will"). Furthermore, he had the *Lachesis* inability to resist a gambling venture and embarked upon several get-rich-quick schemes that inevitably collapsed. He spent money lavishly and was generous to friends in need, going through several large fortunes during his lifetime.

Few can excel Twain at his best in laconic style and incisiveness: "Clothes make the man; a naked man carries little or no influence in society"; "The reports of my death have been greatly exaggerated"; "Wagner's music is better than it sounds," or, when asked to comment on the Christian idea of Heaven and Hell, "I would rather not voice an opinion. I have friends in both places." However, he was also responsible for some of the worst writing of any major author. For the emotional chaos which often characterizes *Lachesis* can, we recall, spill over into the intellectual area, and the damage is compounded by this type's inability to call a halt. Thus Twain can be verbose and repetitious, hammering away endlessly at his pet ideas and, in typically erratic *Lachesis* fashion, swinging back and forth between writing of genius and thoroughly second-rate prose. Even within the same work passages of brilliance are swamped by the prolix and undistinguished.

Twain lived to a ripe old age (his particular addiction was cigars, not the more destructive alcohol encountered in such *Lachesis* humorists as Ring Lardner or Walt Kelly) and remained true to type until the end of his life, never slackening his passionate struggle to reconcile the moralist and the cynic in himself or to integrate his tragicomic viewpoint.

At times the odd *Lachesis* mixture of the pathetic and the ridiculous is entirely unintentional. A common example is the bustling and commotion-causing female friend or relative who offers assistance too eagerly and incompetently, all to the accompaniment of ceaseless or absurd chatter. These unfortunates definitely "turn people off" despite the best of intentions. The more self-conscious patient will remark: "My friends avoid me. I can't seem to get along with anyone at my job. Although I work better than other people, I don't get the promotions or raises they do. So I realize there is something in *me* that is doing this. Apparently I have a communication problem." Strictly speaking, it is a personality problem. They estrange others by too much intensity, too much talk, too much interference and imposition of self.

Furthermore, too much stress, unrelenting internal conflict which the individual can neither comprehend nor control, loneliness, spinsterhood, and the like may bring on a slight "mental derangement" (Hering). These persons are able to function in the world but are still somewhat peculiar. Their "aura of impersonality" precisely reflects a lack of contact with reality and with themselves, as they "laugh sillily" (Kent), talk "irrationally" (Boenninghausen), and behave in semiautomatic responses. All that mental and emotional energy has, sadly, never found an adequate field for expression and turns on itself, causing a psychic imbalance.

In conclusion, much *Lachesis* disharmony arises from the struggle between the individual's opposing selves. Within this divided psyche gratification competes with moral or intellectual restraint, scepticism with devotion, emotion with reason. The warring factions are not easily reconciled, and the physician thus finds himself dealing with a conflicted or tormented personality seeking some "oneness" in himself, some wholeness within which to resolve, or at least reconcile, the conflicts and clashes of his dualistic nature.

True harmony may elude him until he finds firm ground in a worthy faith, dedication, or discipline providing a higher spiritual or mental integration. But meanwhile the homoeopathic remedy may assist the patient in turmoil to find a workable balance between too-rigid control and over-indulgence, between suppression and overstimulation. And the two sides of his nature, each seeking supremacy, will then no longer feel in perpetual strife, but can coexist in a more peaceful, albeit at times still precarious, state of truce.

Natrum Muriaticum

*N*ATRUM *muriaticum* is sodium chloride or common table salt, an everyday substance which possesses a number of unique properties. Salt absorbs, retains, and condenses; it also crystallizes and preserves; and salt brings out the taste of other foods. These properties are manifested both physically and mentally in the patient needing *Natrum muriaticum*.

Retention

On the physical plane, *Natrum muriaticum* retains water and other bodily fluids in several different forms. The individual may not perspire freely, or else perspires only on certain areas, such as the forehead, or in certain circumstances—such as when eating. Sometimes he is subject to urticaria or hives, or red blotches particularly around the face and neck, as a substitute for perspiration when under stress or during physical exertion; and the adolescent or adult acne, or excessively dry or oily skin, that so frequently call for *Natrum muriaticum* are graphic evidence of the individual's faulty elimination of waste products through the skin. This remedy is one of the best for obstinate cases of amenorrhea, especially when caused by long-standing emotional stress; and a guiding symptom is commencement of menstruation only in the late 'teens. It is also invaluable in various edemas, whether due to poor elimination of urine or (in women) to pregnancy or the premenstrual syndrome; it is used in severe constipation (three to four weeks can elapse between bowel movements), particularly when accompanied by depression or inability to express emotion. Finally, it breaks up retentions of mucus, as in obstinate and painful sinus congestions.

Natrum muriaticum also "retains" physical pain, especially the different types of headache. Whether "splitting," "throbbing," "hammering," accompanied by nausea or vomiting, whether "bursting," coming on in paroxysms or due to hypertension; whether congestive, neuralgic, anemic or menstrual, whether low-grade or severe, once these headaches develop, they may continue unrelenting day after day. At times they are caused by eyestrain and are accompanied by blurring, blindness, aching, and zig-zags before the eyes.

The characteristic *Natrum muriaticum* "retention" is encountered in the mental sphere as well. From youth onward, impressions are absorbed deeply and retained tenaciously. On the positive side this makes the individual compassionate, sensitive to another's wants, loyal in affections, strong in attachment, and appreciative of past kindnesses. All too often, however (and this is the type encountered most frequently by physicians), he absorbs negative feelings or unhappy impressions. Because he has difficulty expressing anger, he retains it, allowing it to fester; or, like Lot's wife in the Bible, who was turned into a pillar of salt as punishment for looking back, he develops pathology from mourning the past. He too vividly remembers past offenses, sorrows, and disappointments; he mulls over and hangs on to resentments. He "never forgets an injury and never forgives a wrong." Where another constitutional type would long ago have dismissed from consciousness an unpleasant experience or irretrievable loss and gone on to other things, the inconsolable *Natrum muriaticum*, with his inability to relinquish a grievance, virtually *cultivates* painful memories: "melancholy mood . . . cannot forget injuries which have been inflicted on him, which depress him so much that he has no pleasure in anything" (Hahnemann).

This is also the individual who for the longest time cannot seem to recover from a loved one's death (*Ignatia* is the remedy for the immediate or acute sense of grief). This longing for a lost love, whether romantic or other, or suffering from an gnawing sense of the futility of life in the absence of the beloved, can be unappeasable, unchanging, and unending—even lasting a lifetime as exemplified by Queen Victoria: for fifty years she dressed in strictest black and resolutely grieved over Prince Albert's death, as if determined not to forgive the Almighty for her bereavement. At times the individual veritably wallows in unpleasant recollections: "constantly recalls former disagreeable occurrences so as to worry himself by thinking about them" (Hahnemann). He may become obsessed with or "haunted by some unpleasant subject" (Kent).

Miss Havisham, of Dickens' *Great Expectations*, jilted by her lover on her wedding day and left standing at the church door, who wore her wedding dress for the rest of her life while nursing her grievance in a dark, dusty, cobwebbed room, caricatures this aspect of *Natrum muriaticum*.

He also "cannot remove from his thoughts injuries he has inflicted on others" (Hahnemann), thereby laying the foundation for the chronic guilt peculiar to this type.

To *Natrum muriaticum* time is not the "Great Healer." On the contrary, it serves only to crystallize the past. The insult or guilt festers, becomes magnified out of proportion, and ultimately holds the individual captive. Like a miser who hoards his gold and periodically goes to his strongbox to count it, *Natrum muriaticum* hoards his memories of injury and self-condemnation, periodically retrieving them for reexamination. He may even grow attached to them by virtue of their familiarity; or he may become chronically melancholy and morbidly "introverted" (Hahnemann), to the point of resenting any attempt to extricate him from his incubus or relieve him of his unhappiness: "*likes to dwell* upon past unpleasant occurrences" (Hering).

Childhood and Family Relations

Natrum muriaticum's grievances often stem from family relations. More often and more graphically than any other type, he exhibits the consequences of a poor relationship with one or both parents which breeds resentment and/or guilt. The adult quite commonly bears the scars of the parents' inability to respond appropriately to his emotional needs. "My parents never even *tried* to understand me; they never really approved of me; if I did things differently from the way they wanted, it was wrong," is a frequent complaint — yet he was never able to communicate to them his own need for approval or support. Another classic situation is the child whose emotional problems started when the mother took a job outside the home. But when she is home, he is neither affectionate nor outwardly happy, and, in general, is not easy to have around. The other children of the family are not affected in the same way, accepting the situation and enjoying their mother when she *is* home. Only *Natrum muriaticum* so deeply resents her betrayal, and is so sensitive to her rejection or neglect, that he cannot demonstrate his need for her affection. Thus, although these grievances against the parents are sometimes legitimate, he can also be accused of making excessive demands.

Even as an adult, he may forever harp on his parents' inadequacies or offenses. A woman who is practically a grandmother, and knows how difficult it is to raise children correctly, or a man successful in both career and family life, will still be passionately resentful of the father's disapproval, the mother's persistent inability to sympathize, or merely of some unwanted advice the parents have proffered. It takes but little to bring back all the disappointments of childhood and their accompanying resentments. One unforgettably immature reaction was encountered in a forty-year-old bachelor suffering from chronic hypertension (the potentized salt is predictably one of the best remedies for high blood-pressure) and a host of neuroses in dealing with people. He explained in all seriousness that he lost faith in humanity when, as a child of seven, he discovered that there was no Santa Claus. "My parents *lied* to me," he exclaimed indignantly. "So how could I ever trust them, or anyone else, again?"

The polar opposite, however, is also true. *Natrum muriaticum* often has a superabundance of sympathy and devotion to his parents and an extra-close relationship with them. He is likely to be the child who never leaves home (*Calcarea*) or the adult who insists on living next door to his parents to care for them in their old age.

Some of these children feel ill at ease when touched. They do not reach out for physical closeness and have trouble expressing affection. In contrast to *Phosphorus* or *Pulsatilla*, they have to learn to hug and kiss and generally to relate on the physical plane. This "don't touch me" syndrome contributes to the young *Natrum muriaticum*'s difficult relationship with his parents. The testily independent child pushes away not only any show of affection but also guidance. He rejects help when it is proffered and (like the *Natrum muriaticum* adult) is angry when consoled: "the more he is consoled, the more he is affected" (Allen). The parent then naturally turns to another child who is more receptive and cuddly, seemingly more appreciative. Thus the lessening of emotional rapport between parent and child that frequently occurs in adolescence with reduced physical contact may commence earlier in *Natrum muriaticum*. He projects a "leave me alone" attitude, and the parents leave him alone.

Yet, it is part of the nature's complexity and perversity to suffer inordinately from deprival of parental affection even when rejecting it. He thereby creates a "no win" situation for his parents and himself.

The "difficult" *Natrum muriaticum* child—or, more precisely, the one who finds life difficult—may originally have been well-behaved and affectionate but has turned moody, unhappy, even rebellious, because of real or imagined parental inattention to his needs or inappropriate reactions to his views and accomplishments (this type is always trying to dictate others' responses). His "heavy" relationship with parents can be seen in the abrupt and irritable manner that surfaces in sudden bursts despite an effort at self-control (his disproportionate anger at trifles will be discussed below). The physician can often recognize him by his determined avoidance of eye contact, reluctance to answer questions, and resentful expression as he looks down at the floor. A prescription of the medicine in high potency, however, can cause extraordinary changes: the child is now willing to look the physician in the eye, has an open instead of a forced smile, and is described by the parents as having a "lighter" nature generally.

At times *Natrum muriaticum*'s pathology stems from early sibling rivalry. The previously bright and happy child starts behaving badly or slackens in speech and intellectual development when he senses that the younger siblings are nipping competitively at his heels or receiving parental preference. In fact, "slow learning to talk" (Kent) is a strong indication for this remedy and a concrete reflection of the type's general inability to express emotion easily.

Other constitutional types in similar circumstances may feel equally jealous and resentful. They will fight for attention, argue, or intrigue; or they will learn to share or to yield; but ultimately they succeed in dealing with the situation. Not so *Natrum muriaticum*. He may confront it by being ultracooperative, obedient and responsible. The child is so sensitive to disapproval, so longing for approbation, so fearful of parental rejection if he does not please, that he will not even tell his parents that he is afraid of the dark and would like a night light, or that he wet his pants in school and would like to change them; and a mere glance from an adult will elicit the desired behavior. Indeed, when a parent or teacher describes a child as overconscientious, extremely anxious to avoid giving trouble, and "extra" or "unnaturally" good, the first remedy to consider is the potentized salt.

Even if this tactic is successful, however, he may still harbor resentment over having had to make the effort. If unsuccessful, if he still fails to elicit his parents' approval, the resentment is retained and thereafter sublimated into a kind of cosmic hurt.

Natrum muriaticum is prominent in the oldest and most vulnerable child of the family: the one upon whom parents learn by their mistakes, who has had to hew his own path and that of his siblings in the family structure, and who thus carries the most responsibility, whether seeking it or not. He often has a mature social understanding and feel for the relationships among family members but cannot easily handle stressful family situations. He is deeply affected by quarrels and subliminal hostilities and, like *Phosphorus*, can become actively ill as a result: "headache from excitement of the emotions" (Kent). For this reason *Natrum muriaticum* is the remedy most frequently administered to children and adolescents undergoing or who have undergone the trauma of parental divorce.

When *Natrum muriaticum* finds no excuse for injury in the parental or sibling relationship, he may seize on some other circumstance from childhood at which to take offense. Perhaps he was thwarted in some enterprise upon which his heart was set or was disappointed in not receiving some school honor. Down through the years he nurses the insults of childhood friends or the injustices perpetrated by his elementary-school teacher; or he retains some deep-seated disapproval of a family member who consistently shirked his share of responsibilities.

He does not always display his grudge at the time of the injury, nor does he necessarily withdraw into himself then and there (like *Calcarea*). But years later he will remember this grievance with passion: "recalls injuries long since suffered" (Hering). Thereafter, projecting his childhood experience onto the world at large, he will be quick to sense others' repressions, rejections, thwarted longings, and victimizations.

Much of this relates to the routine hurts and disappointments of everyday life which, in *Natrum muriaticum*, solidify into profound emotional traumas. This remedy is probably indicated if the physician is tempted to tell a "forever remembering" patient belaboring past slights and offenses, "Put that sorrow behind you. Don't look back! Forget it! Relinquish these grudges, and forgive those who trespass against you!" Elephant that he is, *Natrum muriaticum* will never forget, but the remedy's liberating and healing influence may induce him to forgive.

Thus, something in his nature—the inability to overcome life's normal hardships, the propensity to dwell on past sorrows or humiliations, and the rejection of consolation—leads one to suspect *Natrum muriaticum* of *seeking injury*, even if unconsciously, or at least of placing himself in a situation where injury can occur. This is reminiscent of a classic scene from the *Pogo* comic strip: the animals of the Okefenokee swamp are following the tracks of their supposed enemies when the endearing recluse Porkypine (with his typically *Natrum muriaticum* prickliness and benign moroseness), finally realizing that they have been walking in a circle and following their own footsteps, exclaims, "We have met the enemy and he is us!"

It should be noted, however, that the remedy not only suits imagined or exaggerated grievances but is *invaluable* in cases of legitimate tragedy and profound "grief" (Kent): sorrow and loneliness from the loss of (or rejection by) a loved one; a history of broken relationships; patients undergoing traumatic divorces; the effects of some deep humiliation or unbearable insult; alcoholism in a parent (resulting, for instance, in the classic problem of relating to a person of the same sex as the alcoholic parent); parental neglect, and sexual or other abuse. It is one of the most commonly used remedies for emotionally disturbed children (or for the parents of a brain-damaged or severely handicapped child) and for persons who appear to have been given so little in life; for loving conscientious parents devastated by ungrateful or disappointing children; for those who feel betrayed by someone especially loved and cherished; or for persons trapped in no-way-out marriages and other family situations who must bear the burden of others' selfishness and irresponsibility (see, also, *Staphysagria*). For this reason, while other constitutional types may come to the physician with equally serious physical or mental problems, they will not depress or affect him on as visceral a level as *Natrum muriaticum*, whose very person and emotional cast suggest the unalterably tragic make-up of the world.

These two parallel cases, the first *Natrum muriaticum* and the second *Lycopodium*, are vivid illustrations of their types.

A rather pathetic, middle-aged gentleman, exhibiting distinctly neurotic tendencies, was seeking homoeopathic aid for recurring migraines which required massive doses of aspirin. The source of his problem was not difficult to trace. He had grown up in France during the Second

World War, separated from his parents who were in the Resistance. For his own safety they had left him as a hired hand in a peasant household, and his headaches started during those trying years. He was never entirely free of them thereafter, and thirty years later the accumulated anger at his unjust fate and feeling of rejection by his parents were still close to the surface. He could not talk of his childhood experience without resentful passion. It took many months of homoeopathic treatment, primarily with *Natrum muriaticum*, for the emotional wounds and the headaches to heal. Even so, something in him remained traumatized for life.

The second patient, also a child of parents active in the French Resistance who had experienced even greater hardships during the War (having been left for long periods of time to roam the countryside and fend for himself, sometimes sleeping in barns and stealing food from the fields), was well-balanced and functioned effectively. He suffered from digestive troubles but otherwise appeared to be indestructible. Possibly because of his cooler affections, he was able to view his childhood and his parents' behavior with calm objectivity and equanimity. "They were true idealists who considered their cause more important than their only child. Perhaps they were right. Their work did save many lives and helped win the War, while I have survived just fine— at least I think I have, so please don't disillusion me. My wife [who complained of her husband's unfeeling aloofness] tries to do so enough already."

Bleakness

On the other hand, *Natrum muriaticum* can be his own worst enemy by allowing some specific emotional injury, or the cloud of depression constantly hanging over him, to be the lens through which he views reality. An apposite term for this distorting lens is "bleakness," implying, as it does, not only isolation, barrenness, and desolation, but also cheerlessness and discouragement ("sad and dejected": Hahnemann). It is less a question of his being negative or pessimistic than of an extra sensitivity to the minor-key forces at work in the world. The following are typical of his "bleak" physical and emotional responses to conventional symbols of life and joy.

1) Colorful, cheering, exhilarating *spring*, when all nature undergoes rejuvenation or rebirth, brings to *Natrum muriaticum* not only

an aggravation of various physical symptoms (*Lachesis, Sulphur*), but also depression of spirits (the remedy should be raised to a higher degree in the Kent *Repertory*). Contrary to custom and tradition, he is dejected and cannot feel a part of the regeneration and elation brought by spring. Whether it was a decadent pose or sincere conviction, the symbolist poets at the turn of the century were voicing a *Natrum muriaticum* sentiment when they lamented that spring's short-lived brightness and vitality are "deceitful" in holding out false hope and serve only to remind man of the brevity of life and the dissolving force of nature.

2) The warming *sun*, the quintessential symbol of life and growth, is frequently a source of physical pain to *Natrum muriaticum*, who is either enervated or drained by it. Its glaring rays, endowing our universe with heat and energy, are poorly tolerated by him (aggravation from "exposure to sun": Kent); the sun's light hurts his eyes, he is sensitive to its heat (feels "faint and weak": Hering), his skin may break out in various ways, or he develops headaches (*Lachesis, Pulsatilla*). In mythical and symbolic tradition the sun is associated with the heart and the affections, and predictably its throbbing energy threatens *Natrum muriaticum*'s most vulnerable side. Thus it comes to be associated with fatigue, burning, and depletion: "It is as though the sun, representing the supreme stimulus of life activity, would impose too much demand on [the] organism given to seclusion" (Whitmont). The type claims to function best on days that are not too bright. Some even prefer overcast to clear weather, especially for mental work (this trait should not be confused, however, with the *Nux vomica* and *Causticum* amelioration of symptoms in damp weather), and a number of symptoms as well his sense of well-being are ameliorated by "cold" (Boger—where *Natrum muriaticum* is listed in the highest degree with only *Lachesis* and *Gelsemium*) and "cold water" (Boericke).

3) Instead of being braced by the cool freshness of the *morning*, *Natrum muriaticum*, upon awakening, feels moody, despondent, or reluctant to face the day ("very ill-humored in morning": Hering; "the challenge of every sunrise to master life anew cannot be met": Whitmont). He is tired and slow to get started: the child does not want to go to school, or the adult to work, although both are perfectly happy once there. Or he may have morning headaches which increase in intensity between 10:00 a.m. and 2:00 p.m., as the sun climbs toward the zenith, and subside only at sunset. The spirits lift in the evening, and

there is a relieved feeling of "Whew! I managed to survive another day! Now I can rest until tomorrow." "Worse sunrise to sunset," in headaches and the emotional sphere is a key *Natrum muriaticum* symptom (*Medorrhinum*). However, the reverse: increased "apprehensiveness in the evening" (Hahnemann), is also encountered, particularly in more severely traumatized patients.

4) The *natural environment* can be as much an irritant as a source of joy to *Natrum muriaticum*. Such, at times, is his sensitivity to the environment that even exposure to a gentle wind or drizzling rain, not to mention a quick dip in fresh or salt water, can cause him to break out in skin eruptions such as welts or itching hives. The scent of flowers and other vegetation may bring on allergy symptoms (*Phosphorus, Nux vomica, Arsenicum*). At the same time, if the patient is a gardener with a passion for flowers, either *Natrum muriaticum* or *Arsenicum* (or both) will probably be prominent in the constitution.

He may also feel oppressed by the grandeurs of nature. High mountains give him vertigo: his sense of balance is shaky, and heights evoke a fear of falling or, even worse, an uncontrollable urge to fling himself down. In the valleys he feels claustrophobic and hemmed in: *Natrum muriaticum* is already too confined emotionally to tolerate further external enclosure without feeling suffocated and panicky (this claustrophobia in elevators and small rooms is listed in the Kent *Repertory* under the rubric, "fear of narrow places"). A beautiful lake may make him wonder how many persons, in their unhappiness, have felt the impulse to drown themselves (!) And the ocean, the matrix of life with all its symbolic association with the past, is bound to provoke a complex set of reactions. While some feel frankly miserable near the ocean, more often a patient will say that he loves it—that it is his favorite place, even while manifesting the key *Natrum muriaticum* symptom, "Worse from sea air, sea bathing" (Hahnemann). A host of complaints are aggravated at the seaside: allergies, asthma, headaches, constipation, skin eruptions after bathing ("herpes on tongue after sea bathing": Hering), cessation of menses, hair falling out or itching of the eyes, ears, scrotum, vagina (also *Arsenicum* and *Sepia*, all three contrasting with *Medorrhinum*'s "amelioration at the seashore" [Kent]). This same individual may add, "I don't know why I keep going back to the ocean for summer holidays. I never feel well there, but for some reason I can hardly admit it, even to myself. I have this pull to be by the ocean, no matter how poorly

I feel.''

This exemplifies an important *Natrum muriaticum* trait: *to be hurt by that which he loves best.* He is allergic to chocolate or cherries or to some other food he particularly enjoys. Animal lovers become allergic to their pets and must give away the dog or stop riding the horse. One patient who loved and read nothing else but the daily paper, developed an allergy to printer's ink, with streaming eyes, itching ears, and numbness around the mouth if he so much as picked up a newspaper. It took many doses of the remedy to overcome this sensitivity. And patients have been treated with this medicine for a tendency to embarrassing asthma attacks or other allergic reactions in the presence of persons whom they truly loved.

5) Beauty in *artistic form* can also be a source of pain to *Natrum muriaticum*. Poetry, literature, the cinema, all cause him to reverberate in a painful as well as a pleasurable response; he is saddened by music's capacity to evoke unhappy memories and unsatisfied longings or emotions he would prefer to leave untapped (*Natrum carbonicum*). But the heartache is not unmixed with pleasure, as at times he will turn to affecting music to indulge his bittersweet sorrow or voluptuously to reinforce some ancient (or recent) hurt (''worse music'': Boericke).

6) To experience *fun* can be foreign to *Natrum muriaticum*, whose nature is essentially serious. He becomes dejected at happy social gatherings or family celebrations, and holidays, especially the Christmas season, can be the worst time of the year for him. When everyone is supposed to be full of the holiday spirit, and many are truly enjoying themselves, he is more aware than ever of man's intrinsic loneliness. Even when participating pleasantly in a group, he may still feel an outsider and act left out: listening to others and observing their feelings, experiencing the warmth and fun vicariously rather than participating directly in the comradeship. In any gathering larger than a few, close, like-minded friends, *Natrum muriaticum* easily feels *de trop* (''avoids company, because he foresees that he might easily annoy others'': Hahnemann). This is due partly to insecurity, partly also to an egotism that makes him unwilling to remain an insignificant member of a group. Thus the reverse side of his sincere preference for remaining unnoticed in the background is a subliminal demand for special attention and an aggrieved feeling when others do not respond. He cannot grasp that being overlooked is not synonymous with being attacked and may in-

terpret inattention as dislike or even magnify it into condemnation. Traces of paranoia are detectable in this type.

7) More abstractly, *happiness* to *Natrum muriaticum* is only a "transient" (Allen) ephemeral feeling. How can anyone feel lasting happiness when loss awaits just around the corner, and suffering is encountered at every turn? Happiness is, at best, a temporary haven of rest, a momentary break from the true tenor of the world. He can feel fulfilled and useful, be content and full of enthusiasm for his work or the people he loves, yet remain unhappy. Patients admit to a *Weltschmerz* that prevents them from knowing the meaning of spontaneous, unalloyed happiness: "I have to work constantly at being happy," they say. This is due, in part, to the type's ever-present and unrelenting thoughts of duty and obligation that temper his ability to experience happiness.

8) Another facet of *Natrum muriaticum*'s bleakness is a *tendency to look at the dark side of things* (*Sepia*). On a day full of happy events, but with one untoward incident, he will focus on the latter. If he hears a dozen compliments and one mildly critical remark, he will be offended ("offended at every word": Hering). If things are going tolerably well, he wishes they were better, or he sorrowfully dwells on missed opportunities. He is so busy suffering that he overlooks the other dimensions to life. Also he anticipates the worst. If he has been looking forward to an outing and wakes up to a lovely morning, he will remark, "What a pity that the weather probably won't last; it will probably cloud over later in the afternoon." In a satisfying relationship, with no sign of rupture, he will think, "I know she will eventually drop me. But, anyway, I'm not sure she's the person for me, so maybe it's just as well . . ." This attitude is not simply pessimism but rather a precaution against being caught emotionally off guard. He wants to build up his defenses, the better to be forearmed if, or when, any disappointment comes his way. There is also an element of superstition here, a warding off of perverse fate that appears resolved to undermine his happiness, complacency, or security. Patients under treatment will be reluctant to admit improvement out of fear that the remedy will stop acting (not out of *Lycopodium*'s critical scepticism or *Arsenicum*'s demand for perfection).

9) *Natrum muriaticum* may even regard a *smile* as but "a brave effort to cover up tears," as more than one patient has put it. Yet they

themselves can possess the loveliest of smiles which literally transform their faces, making a plain woman pretty and a homely man charming. Almost any smile is an attractive phenomenon, but this "face transforming" quality is peculiar to the type. Sometimes the physician feels his heart sink, sensing another long and complicated case, when observing yet another dejected patient in the waiting room, the very lines of his face projecting misery and a low self-image. Then the individual looks up with that vulnerable but beautiful *Natrum muriaticum* smile, and suddenly the doctor feels reassured; everything will be all right, after all.

10) Over and above everything else, there is *romantic love*! With its enormous potential for pain, disappointment, and sorrow, it is fated to catch *Natrum muriaticum* at his most vulnerable. Being so easily hurt in friendship and family relationships, he can extract that much more suffering from romantic love. Here again, much of the grief he brings on himself, time and again misplacing his affections or tenaciously hanging on to an unrequited passion. He may seek out the company of those in whose presence he suffers, like a hovering moth repeatedly burning itself on a candle but unable to tear itself away. Young and attractive patients, with their lives and futures before them, confess that they do not know why they are sustaining a relationship which from the beginning has brought little happiness in proportion to the sorrow. "During the five years I have known her the deepest bond between us has been that she makes me consistently unhappy," is a typical remark. And many doses of the remedy may be needed before the person will finally let go of the painful relationship or equally painful memory. A common refrain of this type, when forsaken by another, is, "You don't stop loving a person just because she's hurt you"; or "You can't forget a person just because she's left you"; or the woman asks, "How can I *stop* loving him? He's still a part of me — and will never cease being a part of me — even though he's no longer around." Adamantly reinforcing the wound of rejection and holding on tenaciously to the memory of an injury, *Natrum muriaticum* has an unsurpassed ability to beat an unhappy emotion into the ground (in the Kent *Repertory*, this remedy is listed highest under the rubric "persistent, tormenting thoughts").

Even if the love is requited, he may put himself into insoluble difficulties, courting relationships that will inevitably lead to grief. He falls in love with a married woman or with someone so unsuitable as to be

unattainable. Kent has encapsulated this tendency in the portrait of the
great lady who falls in love with her coachman. Perhaps the unconscious
fear of love is behind his choice of object. A love that cannot be realized or fulfilled is ultimately safe, even if it does lead to suffering and
decline. Other constitutional types also become enamored unsuitably,
without hope of fulfillment, but *Natrum muriaticum* hangs on the
longest to empty yearnings and defunct memories, allowing them to
become obsessive, or clinging (it sometimes seems) less to the feeling
of love than to the remembered pain of rejection.

How different all this is from the love patterns of other types: from
the spontaneous, unselfconscious *Phosphorus* who can enjoy many
partners and relationships; or *Pulsatilla* who responds more simply to
her sexual needs and easily enters into tender and affectionate relationships; or from the strong even while equivocal passion of a *Lachesis*;
different too from *Arsenicum*, who generally does not allow himself
to be placed at an emotional disadvantage; also from *Lycopodium*, who
can remain detached and unperturbed even in love; or from *Sulphur*,
who rebounds easily, attaching himself to another if one love has failed.
To *Natrum muriaticum* love is a tortured, complex feeling, all too often
the source of profound sadness, unfulfillment, longing—and ill-health.

Loneliness and Isolation

All of this leads up to that special loneliness, that feeling of not
truly belonging anywhere in the world, which is often experienced by
Natrum muriaticum.

Whitmont offers an interesting thesis: this constitutional type represents man "in search of his Ego," in that period of mental or spiritual
development when he is breaking away from the "collective unconscious" (Jung's term), from family, heredity, traditional religious beliefs
or cultural values, and is seeking to find his own true nature. The remedy's "worse at the seaside" modality could thus arise from a subliminal
fear of being drawn back into the collective unconscious, symbolized
by the sea from which all life emerged. But between breaking with the
past and attaining the higher synthesis or integration represented by
discovery of the ego there lies a "transitional stage" which is of necessity
lonely, and "whenever the demands of the transition prove greater than
the strength of the personality, a state of pathology [ensues] which has

its remedy in *Natrum muriaticum.'**

This may be one reason for the key *Natrum muriaticum* symptom variously described as: "consolation aggravates" (Kent), "gets more agitated when consoled" (Hahnemann), "violent rage on being comforted" (Hering), "rejection of sympathy." The individual instinctively senses that no one *can* help him and that he must go through his difficulties alone. At the same time, concludes Whitmont, "his state of isolation is accentuated by the fact that love, sympathy, and communion with others are longed for; yet an inner command forbids their acceptance . . . and urges him to find the source of strength within himself."

This insistence on self-reliance, together with the patient's "joyless" (Hering) attitude, makes the typical *Natrum muriaticum* case long and difficult to treat. To be sure, it may happen that a dose of the remedy will bring about a lasting change of attitude, together with amelioration of physical symptoms (for an instance of this, see below, p. 375). But usually it is a long-term process, requiring abandonment of the acquired, and now firmly ingrained, lens of bleakness. For this patient, unconsciously clings to his despondency even while, on the conscious level, professing eagerness to cooperate in the cure.**

Thus, while *Natrum muriaticum* wants to withdraw from people ("aversion to company": Kent), he is also strongly attracted to them. He is the loner whose life is complicated by the need for company. Constantly vacillating between the desire for both isolation *and* companionship, he is never completely satisfied either with people or

---

* Many homoeopaths today find that *Natrum muriaticum* is the most commonly prescribed constitutional remedy—possibly because in our era traditional values are being more rapidly overthrown and superseded by new ones than at any other time in history. Consequently, more people are finding themselves alone, searching for new values and life-styles. *Sulphur*, however, remains the constitutional "common denominator" of mankind, being required not only by the *Sulphur* constitutional type but—at various stages of treatment—by all others.

** What Whitmont remarks of *Lachesis* (see that chapter) is equally true of *Natrum muriaticum*: its picture is found at the basis of many cancer cases where retained sorrow and repressed emotions crystallize over time into hard knots of malignancy.

without. At times, like *Lycopodium*, he wants others around but not too close: in the same house but not in the same room. People "drain" him. Unlike *Phosphorus, Pulsatilla,* or *Sulphur,* who are energized by human contact, *Natrum muriaticum*'s encounters with humanity are all too often traumatic, or at least depleting, experiences.

Being highly susceptible to hurt, he invariably seeks to avoid being emotionally injured by others. For protection, the more sensitive individual surrounds himself with a thick wall ("an impenetrable wall of scar tissue," as one *Natrum muriaticum* expressed it) and thus becomes even more introverted, even less capable of expressing emotion or affection. He is careful never again to be placed in a position to be wounded or humiliated and forearms himself against future injury by keeping others at a distance. In extreme cases he may never venture to love deeply again, to avoid the risk both of rejection and of hurting another. In fact, some of his reclusive tendencies stem precisely from a refusal "to go into society for fear of giving offense" (Allen). Here the picture of emotional exhaustion or numbness, of unresponsiveness following disappointment in some strong feeling ("deliberately repelling companionship": Whitmont) overlaps with *Sepia.* An *overdemonstrative* affectionateness (i.e., the insecure individual's "Please love me! I do *so* need to feel accepted!" demeanor) is, however, another facet of *Natrum muriaticum*

The blocking-off mechanism can even carry over into sleep, and the individual claims that he does not dream or, at least, does not remember his dreams, feeling only a vague depression or unpleasant sensation upon awakening. The reverse, "annoying, anxious, loathsome, horrible, and sad dreams, or vivid dreams of fire, murder fighting," etc. (Hahnemann), are also characteristic of the *Natrum muriaticum* picture. But, as noted in the *Sulphur* chapter, these are common to other types as well, and are thus less indicative of the remedy than absence of dreams. Finally, "walking, talking" (Hahnemann) and gesticulating during sleep, or sleeping an inordinately long time—a classic way of "escaping" from life—are indications for this remedy.

Natrum muriaticum may retain his distance by withdrawing into the reflective world of art or scholarship—an emotionally nonthreatening environment. One way or another, with "spirits subdued" (Hahnemann), he succeeds in turning inward to the introspective, often intellectual, life. He may enjoy spending hours alone in his room or retiring to work in some secluded place. The more reclusive type talks of wanting to live in a cabin in the woods, by the ocean, or high in the mountains, far away from people and from the glare of the world ("anthropophobia": Hering). Yet, if he does escape thither, bitterly resenting any intrusion, he generally returns again unless there is also much of the *Sulphur* hermit in him. The *Natrum muriaticum* exile from society becomes lonely living in glorious isolation. He even tires of solitary artistic or scholastic pursuits (some artistic *Sepias* and *Arsenicums* or scholarly *Sulphurs* are more true loners) and eventually returns to where he can interrelate with people even at the risk of emotional injury.

In more severe cases solitude becomes actively unbearable, since "when alone, he calls up disagreeable thoughts and has to weep" (Hahnemann). His grief wells up, especially when alone at night, when his emotions and "thoughts are not under his control" (Hahnemann), in the form of inconsolable sobbing. His heart begins to race or pound, and he suffers from total or partial ("on once awakening": Boger) insomnia. He desperately needs someone to call on for help but, in contrast to *Pulsatilla*, who always has a series of supporters lined up, finds himself isolated and begins a frantic search for human contact.

The fear of loneliness that strikingly underlies much of the *Natrum muriaticum* pathology differs, for example, from the *Phosphorus* need for immediate reassurance or the *Pulsatilla* desire for continuous support. He can stand long periods of time alone provided he knows that somewhere there is a person to whom he is meaningful. His is rather a fear of long-term loneliness. The type's prominent symptom, described as "solicitous about the future . . . anxiety as to what will become of her" (Hahnemann), usually reflects a fear of being left without some close meaningful relationship.

The lonely stage of adolescence can be helped significantly by this remedy. Usually these teenagers are difficult because they are uncommunicative and project unhappiness, not because they are unruly or disobedient. They may suffer from a self-imposed loneliness due to expressed or implied disapproval of the behavior of others and a general refusal to go along with the crowd. By standing for higher principles and stricter behavior (not only in sexual matters but also in reaction to the lack of consideration often shown by children to one another) they become somewhat estranged from their peers. *Natrum muriati-*

cum's loneliness, at whatever age, stems in part from an excessively critical attitude toward others. He feels both judged and judgmental—inadequate yet disappoving. Like *Arsenicum*, he harbors high expectations of people. But, whereas *Arsenicum* becomes angry at, then disdains, those who do not meet these expectations and, after frankly expressing his feelings, proceeds to ignore the unworthy, the disappointed *Natrum muriaticum* bottles up his displeasure and consequently feels more isolated and wounded.

The tomboy who is adamant in retaining her tomboyishness is frequently *Natrum muriaticum*. Typical here are Jo March and Naughty Nan (who grows up to become a homoeopathic doctor) in the works of Louisa May Alcott, and especially Peppermint Patty in the *Peanuts* cartoon strip.* Even those girls who try hard to fit the common mold may remain square pegs in round holes. However, for all their angularities and, at times, peculiarities, they are appealing and interesting individuals because of their good hearts, sound values and originality.

Natrum muriaticum is well aware of being different from others. Sometimes, embarrassed at standing out in the crowd and sensitive to others' comments, he will make a successful effort to adapt to the prevailing mode. Alternately, he is determined to preserve this difference and manifests a real dread of altering anything in himself. Even young patients panic at the very idea of homoeopathic remedies: "You aren't going to *change* me with the remedies are you?" is the anxious inquiry. They cling to their familiar quirks and neuroses as if fearing, with change, to lose their very identity. Adults also become heated, angry, and defensive if they feel the threat of possible change. They clutch their hangups and emotional knots as if these were their *one* source of security in an insecure world. As one patient expressed it, "Depressions and neuroses are like a blanket; they can be protective as well as terribly smothering. So that when I seemed to be losing them after the remedy,

---

* Peppermint Patty, the eternal misfit in school and an outsider even in her children's world, with her tomboy clothes, manner and tastes (her passion for, and skill at, baseball), her inability to conform socially despite sporadic efforts to this end, her touching but futile attempts to engage others in serious conversations about friendship, love and suffering—and who, growing up motherless, is always searching for closer and more meaningful relationships with her peers—is classic *Natrum muriaticum*.

I felt not only lighter but also more exposed."

Possibly *Natrum muriaticum* senses that neurosis, as Jung observed, represents the individual's protective adaptation to an inimical environment, or, in homoeopathic terms, a manifestation of the body's capacity for self-defense. In the *Natrum muriaticum* constitutional economy this defensive function of the neurosis may be vitally important (after all, salt *preserves*). Hence there may be genuine risk in tearing down these protective walls and exposing the vulnerable psyche to itself and to the world unless some better protection is offered instead. At times the remedy should *not* be prescribed, however much the patient's picture calls for it, so as not to disturb the defense mechanism at work. Remedies such as *Ignatia* or *Staphysagria* should be used until the patient is strong enough for an encounter with *Natrum muriaticum*.

To be sure, while preserving his dissimilarity, the individual may still feel guilty about it. Fearing society's rejection, as he formerly feared that of his parents, he wants assurance that his reactions and symptoms are just like those of everyone else and not distinguished from the norm. When asked by the physician what is his favorite temperature, season, or time of day, he may reply, "Doesn't everybody prefer the moderate seasons to heat or cold; or the evening when the day's work is over?"; if asked whether he is habitually thirsty, he may reply, "Yes, I drink a lot of water, but I'm not diabetic or anything like that, if that's what you mean." Asked about his cravings, a teenage boy will reply, "I'm like other boys. I have the normal craving for chocolate and potato chips" (among *Natrum muriaticum*'s most prominent cravings are salt and chocolate).

Thus, although most people like to feel they are somehow unique, *Natrum muriaticum* already sensing his difference, needs to know that he is not alone in his problems and neuroses. One of the greatest comforts the physician can accord him is reassurance that he does indeed belong to the great human family ("Many people feel exactly the same way you do. I have treated a number of patients with similar troubles. Yours is a normal reaction for persons in your situation . . . ").

Frequently *Natrum muriaticum* projects an aura of *heaviness.* During consultation the physician almost physically senses the weight of the patient's problems, and it can even be discerned in his facial features and carriage. There is a heaviness in the lines running from the nose to the corners of the mouth, and especially in the downcast or hang-dog look of the eyes. Or he sits there with crossed hands clasped tightly to the chest, holding in his anger, resentment or unhappiness. Some-times the legs (from the knees down) feel too tired to support the body: he walks wearily and toilsomely—trudges—and the ankles sprain easily (*Calcarea*); or the scrawny "chicken neck" cannot support the head, and the individual constantly rests his head on his hand when sitting.

The patient's aura of being burdened by grief or weighed down by the cares of the world is also projected psychologically. Whatever he may state explicitly, if he touches upon such perennially unanswer-able questions as—"Why is man subjected to so much suffering, in-justice, and loneliness? Why is he placed in intolerable situations with no way out?"—the chances are good that he will require *Natrum mur-iaticum*. Indeed, children needing this remedy from the earliest age are already sensitive to the existential dilemma and may begin to inquire into the meaning of life, even asking adults whether they have found happiness, believe that life is worth living, have ever wanted to die, and so on. These same questions, of course, continue to plague them throughout life.

It is thus hardly surprising that such patients often admit not only to the classic forms of depression "melancholic sadness with aversion to exertion": Boenninghausen) but even to a *chronic longing for death*, sometimes low-grade, at times stronger. This "tiredness of life" (Her-ing) or "wishing for life's termination" (Whitmont) contrasts with the sudden loathing of life, or acute suicidal impulse due to some specific misfortune, of other constitutional types. A history of repeated emo-tional injuries, overcome on the surface but never truly resolved, may lie at its source, but sometimes no specific motive is needed ("melan-cholic dejection . . . without any known cause": Hahnemann). The cul-prit is, once again, the ingrained bleak *Natrum muriaticum* outlook, "a centrally rooted attitude of dejection . . . [which] disintegrates the vitality at its very beginnings" (Whitmont), inherited from the past or from childhood. "My whole adolescent and adult life has been one con-stant battle, sometimes successful, sometimes less so, against this longing for death," will be the unexpected admission of a patient who seems to have everything going for him. Another will state, "Life is such a struggle. I work hard on myself, doing what I should be doing and trying to cultivate a cheerful outlook, but there seems to be no progress. I am far more often depressed than not. For no particular reason I feel exhausted and want to give up—just throw in the towel and die."

When the suicidal urge becomes pressing, the *Natrum muriaticum* patient may require *Natrum sulphuricum.*

At the same time *Natrum muriaticum* feels profoundly that these burdens are his destiny and that he may as well endure them now ("he is tired of the load he has to carry without hope of deliverance . . . yet he knows he must go on": Whitmont). He is good at stoically bearing difficult situations: "I must have done something to deserve it," he will think guiltily, or, trying to find meaning to his suffering, "I, obviously, have some important lesson to learn." Occasionally, however, the remedy has the most unexpected effect on this enduring individual, and he becomes better attuned to the happy and uplifting elements in his situation. What was formerly all duty, sacrifice, and responsibility now takes on a dimension of joy: "internal contentment, hopefulness, as a result of curative effect" (Hahnemann).

Hope and Laughter

Every constitutional type is sustained through trials and tribulations by hope, and *Natrum muriaticum*, who is subject to the most profound "despair, hopeless feelings about the future" (Hering), is, curiously, also distinguished by the intensity, persistence, and even utter groundlessness of his hopes and dreams—upon which he may live as if they were realities. A city child will spend countless hours dreaming of owning a pony. He knows that he cannot have a pony in an urban environment but will concentrate day and night on this unrealistic vision, meanwhile missing out on the actual happiness available to him. But then, he may derive more satisfaction from hopes and dreams than from their actual fulfillment. One young patient (with recurrent fever blisters) hoped every year to be elected class president.* He finally attained this

---

* *Natrum muriaticum* has many mouth and lip symptoms (Hahnemann lists over 80), including: fever blisters, cold sores, herpes around the lips, canker sores, vesicles and ulcers of the mouth and tongue, the characteristic "mapped tongue" with red patches, dry and cracked lips, cracks in the corners of the mouth or on the lower lip, blood blisters on the insides of the lips, numbness of the lips, and so on.

wish in the seventh grade and was an excellent officer. Yet the following year he refused reelection, as the distinction proved not so interesting after all, and went on to dream happily of becoming president of the United States.

This could explain why *Natrum muriaticum* hopes for the impossible or refuses to take the necessary steps to realize his desires. Having been burnt by his previous idealism and learning a lesson from this, he now senses or fears that the reality will fall below his expectations. The adult, we saw, falls in love with an inaccessible person or with someone who is hardly aware of his existence, and would rather worship from a distance or on a platonic level than risk the disillusionment that may follow love attained. Furthermore, he is so sensitive to rejection or humiliation, so fearful of appearing ridiculous or annoying with unwanted attentions that, like *Calcarea* , he may refuse even to venture a move to attract attention or express his attachment. Instead he spends energy *hoping* that his love will be reciprocated. And yet, he also succeeds who only hopes and waits, and those nineteenth-century heroes and heroines of fiction who silently, faithfully, and uncomplainingly waited through several hundred pages for their love to be reciprocated are usually *Natrum muriaticum*. Parenthetically, the types's emotionalism often takes refuge in the romantic novels for which he or especially she, harbors a passion: they enable her to experience love vicariously and ideally, without danger of being wounded or disappointed.

On a broader scale, the socially concerned *Natrum muriaticum* is equally full of idealistic longings—for various never-to-be-realized utopias, for the dawn of some Aquarian Age which will resolve all the world's problems. He is always hoping for a magic breakthrough in consciousness that will guide humanity to happiness. Above all, he has faith in man's innate capacity for unlimited improvement, faith that the fabric of society can and will change once people understand their own best interests. Consequently, his disappointment is all the more severe when people do not live up to his expectations.

In contrast to the sceptical *Lachesis*, who sees institutions as corrupt by their very nature whoever may be involved in them, or to *Lycopodium*'s belief that people will not change until the laws and administrative procedures are themselves reformed, or to *Sulphur*'s confidence that humanity can be improved by one grand, cohesive, and all-inclusive ideology (his own, naturally!), *Natrum muriaticum* feels that institutions are, after all, only made up of people and are thus no better or worse than the individuals working in them. It follows that the world's problems would be resolved if only good, honest, and conscientious people could be put to the task.

In fact, his eyes light up, his complexion gains color, the lines of the face seem to disappear, and his whole person sparkles, when talking of some hope, some ideal, some Five-Year-Plan, that will *change* the world. At these moments he can resemble *Lachesis* in intensity and rush of words, *Arsenicum* in drive and energy, *Phosphorus* in liveliness and ability to project enthusiasm and establish rapport with his audience, or *Sulphur* in his contagious messianic spirit. He goes into high gear when waxing enthusiastic over some dream. *Natrum muriaticum*, in general, is future-oriented. Since the past is full of painful memories, and the present is burdensome, only the future promises happiness and fulfilment. Thus he may actually view the present from the perspective of a "better" future, talking of and living it, as if it were the past to come ("In ten years, when we look back on the present times, we will wonder how we were able to bear . . . "). Once the immediate enthusiasm subsides, however, these characteristics recede, the features droop, the spark is extinguished, and he returns to his brooding introspective self. In this way he can be distinguished from other constitutional types.

Another classic deterrent to melancholy is laughter. The heart of the most stubbornly gloomy or introverted *Natrum muriaticum* can be reached not by the display of affection, not by sympathy and understanding, but by laughter: "he is not cheerful at all, and yet readily moved to laughter" (Hahnemann). He does not necessarily possess a better sense of humor than other types. In fact, being of a serious nature, his sense of fun is not equal to that of the sparkling *Phosphorus* or the gregarious *Sulphur*; and, like *Calcarea*, his all too shaky ego can be devastated by ridicule ("offended at a joke": Hahnemann). Even when possessing the sharp tongue of a *Lachesis* or an *Arsenicum*, he might hesitate to use it out of reluctance to wound others. Yet, even though not generating humor himself, he greatly *appreciates* those who do, and laughs much and easily ("striking inclination to laugh": Hahnemann). However profound his despondency or impregnable his isolation, it cannot withstand the assault of humor. This alone disarms him, since laughter, which engenders self-forgetfulness and dissociation, unblocks his emotions and thereby opens up a line of communication between his secluded self and the outside world.

Natrum muriaticum displays various types of laughter. There is the uncontrolled schoolgirl giggle, with its subliminal note of hysteria, which can easily turn into tears (*Ignatia*). Characteristic, too, are his loud laughter (*Belladonna*), his explosive guffaw (*Sulphur*), or his "immoderate" (Allen) laughter (*Nux vomica*) where "the individual laughs too much for the occasion" (Kent); and Hahnemann describes the woman who "laughs so violently about things in no wise ludicrous, that . . . tears come into her eyes, and she looks afterwards as if she had been weeping."* Then there is the nervous little laugh at something not at all funny; or the patient smiles inappropriately and too much when recounting his symptoms, as well as when describing some sad event. This inappropriate smile (or "laughter over serious matters": Kent) reflects the patient's unease, or is an unsuccessful attempt to lighten the burdensome recital, and does not arise from lack of feeling. The uneasy smile is distinguished from the sincere, face-transforming one; only the mouth smiles in a rather forced manner, instead of illuminating the whole face. There is also the loud cackle, betraying an element of discomfort, when some sensitive point has been dealt with humorously; and the remedy's "spasmodic" or "involuntary" laughter (Kent) is, of course, a release of pent-up emotions in a heavily repressed type (hence the uncontrolled nature of the laughter or its underlying hysterical tone). Last but not least is the classic *Natrum muriaticum* striking alternation between "sad and excessively merry" (Hering).

Thus laughter is the reverse side of his heaviness or bleakness, and

---

* One memorable case comes to mind in this connection, a patient who was being treated for severe and long-standing food allergies. He also evinced a particular phobia to spaghetti, less to the taste than to the sight of those white worm-like strands that seemed to wriggle and squirm on the plate. A prominent symptom was his laughter; the mildest humorous remark provoked shrieks of loud laughter and streaming tears. While it was gratifying to have such an appreciative audience, the explosions of mirth were out of proportion. This trait guided the prescriber to *Natrum muriaticum*. And as the allergies disappeared with treatment, so did the aversion to spaghetti.

the remedy should not be overlooked in the individual who is full of humor and good cheer: "cheerful, merry and in good humor" (Hahnemann). To be sure, the excessive heartiness may be only a mask—putting on a good face in difficult circumstances—and the patient laughs so as not to despair. The physician learns to sense the tense surface of *Natrum muriaticum*'s mirth which is underlain by an ineffable sadness and, still deeper, by an indomitable valor.*

. Finally, *Natrum muriaticum*'s essentially sober, earnest nature is apt to take even humor seriously, treating it as a kind of therapy. Patients aver that viewing a funny movie or reading humorous literature will cure them of their various pains; some call this the best form of psychotherapy: "Cheaper and far more agreeable than the other." Any patient who speaks overenthusiastically of some humorous work, or insistently recommends a book about laughter as a healing agent, will probably require this remedy.

Stoicism

Classically, *Natrum muriaticum* manifests reticence and reserve. He may appear open and confiding, but this is deceptive. One knows his opinions about religion, politics, education, and his vocation, but little about him personally or about the emotions that affect him most. Even the individual who constantly analyzes himself does not want

---

* The works of Anton Chekhov, whose short stories and plays portray that specific edgy humor known as "laughter through tears," are among the purest examples of the *Natrum muriaticum* mode. They capture all the shades and varieties of the remedy's bleakness: the unhappiness of people caught in ineluctable circumstances, their thwarted longings and ideals, their ultimate loneliness and inability to communicate despite their love for one another; where the only glimmerings of hope reside in finding, in some shared human experience, a universal meaning to man's inescapable and burdensome lot.

Chekhov, interestingly, was a physician who became disillusioned with medicine's power to help the real ills, and deep psychological maladies that affect humanity. In his frustration he turned to writing. He even occasionally ridiculed homoeopathy in his fiction; but this is one instance where we can be grateful for a physician's non-appreciation of the science. Had he practiced homoeopathic medicine, he would perhaps not have written at all.

others to intrude; any relinquishing of the protective blanket of reserve makes him feel exposed and even more vulnerable.

The ramifications of this inherent reserve are an uncomplaining stoicism and lack of demonstrativeness—the quality inculcated in the British of maintaining a "stiff upper lip" and presenting a strong front to adversity. In an interesting physical parallel, speaking through clenched teeth or moving the lips minimally when talking, i.e., literally preserving a stiff upper lip, often point to this remedy. This reserve may prevent the patient from communicating with the physician. To all inquiries, "Tell me what happened before your symptoms began three years ago," "How do you *really* feel about his desertion?" "Tell me what's bothering you," the depressed patient sits silent and unresponsive. Sometimes his "emotional constipation" is only unblocked upon reception of the remedy.*

He does not cry easily. He is so constricted inside that the choked-back tears will not flow. When he does cry, it is alone in his room, in broken sobs which cause an aching or constricting pain in his throat and upper chest, as well as in his eyes and head. He may even burrow his head into the pillow to stifle his sobs so that others will not hear him and proffer sympathy. His grief is too fundamental, too all-pervasive for expression, and too deep for consolation. Unlike *Pulsatilla*'s tears that clear the air like an April shower, *Natrum muriaticum*'s tears are a tropical rain which leaves the atmosphere heavier than before. Yet this type may react to sentiment in the same way as *Pulsatilla*. All that is noble, beautiful, or touching readily brings tears to his eyes. When moved, or even at the remembrance of being moved, his voice will break, there is a catch in this throat, and his eyes begin to water. But *Natrum muriaticum* is ashamed of his tears and tries to hold them back, while *Pulsatilla* lets them flow freely.

Thus, although *Natrum muriaticum*, like *Pulsatilla*, may cry for others or from sympathy or, like *Arsenicum*, from anger and frustration, he finds it difficult to cry when grieving for himself ("I am *just*

---

* Many homoeopaths feel that *Natrum muriaticum* is the national remedy of the British, with their high sense of duty, reserved and understated manner, and inability or refusal to display emotion. Could their personality development have been shaped by the salty ocean surrounding their island?

beginning to learn how to cry," is an often-encountered phrase in the physician's office). This trait reflects his general tendency to be harder on himself than on others—at least with respect to displaying emotion.

This basic inability to cry easily is not contradicted by the numerous "weepy" symptoms found in the homoeopathic texts: "weeps involuntarily . . . as soon as anyone merely looks at him," "lachrymose depression," "anxious disposition . . . much inclined to weep," (Hahnemann). All this usually emerges only after long restraint and a brave effort to hold back the tears and carry on alone. Indeed, *Natrum muriaticum* is one of the major remedies used for the profound weakness and emotional breakdown that arise from *too much* or *too prolonged* stress.

A woman in her mid-thirties was constantly tired and constipated, weepy and low-spirited, and regularly missed her periods, all for no apparent reason. Physically, she exhibited the characteristic *Natrum muriaticum* adult acne, oily hair requiring daily washing (hair that goes limp within twenty-four hours after washing is a guiding symptom), and waxy, greasy skin on the face. She received the remedy in the 10M potency and for two days thereafter experienced moderately severe headaches. After that came inexplicable crying fits, then two days of diarrhea. Following these aggravations everything started to improve. It turned out that she was homesick for her family in the Midwest but, trying to be brave, had not admitted it even to herself. This fact emerged only when the homoeopathic medicine had released her reserve and for the first first time made her fully aware of this feeling. She then planned regular visits home with her children, and her physical and psychological problems disappeared.

Natrum muriaticum's reserve sometimes makes him appear distant or unresponsive. He seems standoffish, as if uninterested in another's problems. But underneath (or behind the "impenetrable wall") he *does* care and takes to heart what others tell him ("his mind is much affected by a conversation": Hahnemann). And every chord in him responds to the misery of others; in fact, he may suffer more than they do themselves. They eventually get over it, while he continues to brood.

This sympathy and compassion, however, are at times incapable of expression otherwise than in some professional capacity (physician, nurse, counselor, etc.). He lacks the suitable manner and gestures, or even the right words. Contrary to *Phosphorus* and *Pulsatilla*, it is difficult for him to "open up" to others. Their suffering makes him shy and awkward, or else indignant at a world that permits such things to happen. Happy emotions as well as sad can rob him of the power of speech, sometimes prompting him to inappropriate remarks. He feels so tongue-tied in displaying emotion, even with those who are close, that he may ponder for hours over a short letter to his spouse, child or loved one, and even then it comes out wrong. And it can be sheer agony for *Natrum muriaticum* to articulate his love in a romantic relationship.

In his reserve, self-consciousness, and sense of his own awkwardness the individual can also develop an ultrapuritanical sexual attitude. Some minor childhood sexual experience, or adult sexuality observed too early in life, can breed in him a distrust of the physical expression of love. Although he feels strong affection, there may be an aversion to the sexual relation (*Lachesis, Sepia*), inability to demonstrate love, or homosexuality. Even in the absence of such early experiences, he can be extremely delicate in all sexual matters, abhorring suggestive language and innuendo. The adult refuses to see films which portray sexual matters too explicitly, while the child will cover the word, "love," with his fingers when reading a book or close his eyes at every kiss on the screen. Possibly the *Natrum muriaticum* guiding symptom, "inability to pass urine when others are present" (Hering)—certainly the amenorrhoea of the teen-age girl who resents her periods and wants to deny her femininity—arise, in part, from the same sensitivity to sexual implications.* At the same time, in a characteristic homoeopathic polarity, patients who suffer physical or mental problems from lack of sexual activity will most frequently require this remedy (and secondarily *Lachesis* or *Staphysagria*).

The reserved *Natrum muriaticum* gives an impression of strength. Like Atlas, he seems capable of bearing the whole world on his frequently broad shoulders and back. But he is less strong than he appears, as can be seen in the physician's office. On entering, he looks bright and hearty, with a flushed appearance and good coloring; he may even have the lively outgoing manner and sparkle of *Phosphorus* or the vitality of *Lachesis*. But as the hour advances, the spirits flag, the visage droops, and the features hang heavier. Lines of tiredness emerge, especially

* As if to intensify the individual's already painful feelings of guilt and retribution in matters sexual, *Natrum muriaticum* is the remedy most often used in the successful treatment of genital herpes.

around the mouth, and the skin takes on a duskier or paler hue (Borland observes that the type is often relatively anemic: "It may not be obvious because they tend to flush up quite easily, but when the flush settles, there is a definite pallor, and they usually have a lowish blood count. Most of them have rather pale mucous membranes"). It is as if the patient cannot sustain the impression he is trying to project. But he hides his vulnerability under a facade of strength less from a desire to impress than out of an instinct of self-defense and a concern not to burden others. In contrast to *Lycopodium*, he himself is not deceived.

This front even vis-a-vis the physician is often expressed by the characteristically *Natrum muriaticum* "doorknob symptom." The patient smiles and insists that he is doing very well emotionally, thank you; that nothing in the present or the past is disturbing him, that he (Thank God) has always been able to deal with the hardships and sorrows that have befallen him. And indeed he has. Yet, just as he is leaving, with his hand practically on the doorknob, he turns around, the tears well up in his eyes, and, unable to bear his burdens alone any longer, he breaks down. With a red nose and a blotched and swollen face from the effort of holding in his emotions, and with tears whose violence (from long restraint) can no more be arrested than water bursting through a dam, he pours out his troubles—and the most important features of his case.*

Or, when asked on the return visit how he has felt since the remedy, *Natrum muriaticum* replies, "Well, thank you," or "Much better, really," then hesitates and gives a tenuous smile. But closer questioning reveals that this is not so at all. Some physical aggravation or the surfacing of suppressed and painful emotions have made him miserable.

Such behavior is motivated first by his instinctive rejection of consolation, even from the physician. The ailing patient is not seeking sympathy (*Pulsatilla*) or reassurance (*Phosphorus*) but *answers:* practical ways to help himself. There is much convoluted politeness here also. He does not want to offend the physician who, after all, *is* trying his best to help. In the third place, the type's pervasive guilt also comes into play. He feels that *he* has not responded to the remedy as he should; in some way he has let the physician down. He must be reminded that

---

* All this takes place when the homoeopath no longer requires the information; from the "doorknob symptom" alone he will have established that the patient needs *Natrum muriaticum*.

he need not spare the physician, who is seeking the truth not politeness, and is quite prepared to shoulder responsibility for lack of improvement. An additional reason might be his subliminal fear that if he does not do his share and improve, the physician may give up on him, and he will be left alone again, without hope.

Natrum muriaticum also retains a superstitious belief that verbalization influences reality. As long as something is not admitted in words, it does not exist, while if he says he is better, he may become so. This may explain in part why he is aggravated by discussing his symptoms: it makes them more *real*. His stoicism and reserve is thus a defense mechanism: certain depths of emotion should remain, not unexamined, but *unarticulated*. It is often best and easiest to let lie the sleeping dogs of the psyche.*

Yet, once the reticent individual does unbend, and the long-repressed emotions finally surface, the patient tells all, often to the accompaniment of uncontrollable sobs that rack the whole body. This remedy should thus be added in bold type to Kent's *Repertory* under the rubric: "weeping when telling of her sickness [problems]."

Natrum muriaticum patients who came of age in the '60s and '70s (the "me" decades) may present a somewhat different picture from that of their elders. Encouraged to express their emotions on all occasions, and prompted by innumerable self-help books, group therapy, and individual counselling sessions not to keep silent about anything, this younger generation has emancipated itself with a vengeance from the prototype of reticence. The individual is now as ready as anyone (or more so) to talk at length about his body, soul, and sorrows. He will recount to any listener the dark workings of his mind and his innermost feelings, as well as the defects or malfunctionings of each organ. Conceivably, with age the basic character will reassert itself, and the young *Natrum muriaticum* will grow more reserved.

Thus, where the older person must be encouraged to express his feelings more, the younger may have to be discouraged from doing so. Unlike *Pulsatilla*, for whom the mere talking out of her problems is

---

* One of Snoopy's short stories humorously depicts this attitude: " 'Do you love me?' she asked him. 'Yes,' he said. 'Do you really love me?' 'Yes,' he said. 'Do you really *really* love me?' 'No,' he said. She then asked, 'Do you love me?' 'Yes,' he said. So she asked no more."

a healthy catharsis; or *Phosphorus*, who derives emotional support from an audience; or *Arsenicum*, whose pains and anxieties are greatly ameliorated by speaking about them, *Natrum muriaticum* is not intrinsically *helped* by talking excessively of self. Verbal self-expression only becomes an addiction, an overindulgence that aggravates rather than heals. The patient can work himself into such a passionate state that pouring out his troubles only makes him feel worse. We recall that whereas *Lachesis* defuses his negative feelings by expressing them, *Natrum muriaticum* brings negative emotions into being by articulating them.

This is due in part to the emotional inflexibility of persons with the salt diathesis. Their tendency to become stuck in grooves encourages a fixed and polarized understanding. Thus, if the *Natrum muriaticum* idealism is shattered, if he admits to not truly loving some person, all suddenly turns into bitterness. Articulating his frustrations and disappointments can precipitate a regular avalanche of anger, hatred, and resentment, and a desire immediately to break all ties. Many months of homoeopathic treatment may pass before he realizes that complex feelings for close ones need not be absolutes; that, despite intellectual and emotional differences, they can incorporate devotion, dedication, and respect, making the relationship worth preserving.

Especially the *Natrum muriaticum* woman of the "me generation" may resemble *Arsenicum* in the physician's office: a "hypochondriac" (Hahnemann), overconcerned about her health, excessively frustrated, impatient and even resentful about every symptom, overindustriously striving for self-improvement, or overmeticulously applying some chosen dietary regime. The two have in common many fears and apprehensions (see the chapter on *Arsenicum*). Like *Arsenicum*, too, her behavior may initially require the physician to manifest the patience of a saint. If *Arsenicum* is sent to *try* the true homoeopath, *Natrum muriaticum*—with her traumatic emotional history—is sent to *test* him. Yet, by the same token, these last eventually become most satisfying patients. The physician can count on them carrying out his instructions to the letter and adhering religiously to his advice. They will be the homoeopathic "purists" who are willing to suffer any torment rather than take an aspirin. This contrasts with *Phosphorus* who, after the initial love-feast with the physician, does not always wear well, often failing to adhere long enough to the treatment to obtain the profoundly satisfying results that homoeopathy can attain.

There are, however, several significant differences between *Arsenicum* and *Natrum muriaticum*. The latter gives off an aura of heaviness and dejection, while the former projects frantic anxiety and despair. Whereas *Arsenicum* is critical of the physician and belligerent when results are not up to expectation, *Natrum muriaticum* burdens him with *guilt*. She herself assumes guilt so easily that, in unconscious retaliation, she also attributes it to others. Mild enough during the first visit, in the following one she may express disappointment at the physician's lack of *true* concern with her case. Especially on the telephone she may complain of insufficient interest when not allowed to talk out her interminable problems in all their detail. She is the type that must be reminded that, while homoeopathy always incorporates the individual's mental and emotional symptoms, it is not psychoanalysis. Moreover, she does not *enjoy* visits to the doctor as much as *Arsenicum*; nor does she seek to dominate the case or take over the prescribing. She does not know better than the physician or try to score points over him but defers to his opinion. Finally, *Arsenicum* usually appears tolerably well-balanced except on the subject of health, while *Natrum muriaticum* seems more neurotic overall—this, indeed, often being the cause of her health problems.*

High-mindedness

For all his heaviness, *Natrum muriaticum* is a likeable type. He has a definite character, solid virtues, and an undeniable high-mindedness. He is prepared to stick tenaciously to his ideals and, wary of inflicting pain on others, is usually motivated by kindness. Borland claims that the type is pleasant to meet but difficult to get along with, and on one level this is so. On first acquaintance he cheerfully and willingly

---

* The following quote from Margery Blackie is relevant: "In writing about homoeopathy, one must also mention the neurotic patients . . . [who] have no actual disease, and are not really ill, but find it very difficult to lead a normal life and are afraid of tackling a job. They come to the doctor with a great many symptoms which they like to describe fully but which quite often mean very little . . . In these cases one likes to use a high potency and see how much it will do, but there are often so many complaints that it is justifiable to give a low potency [over a period of time] of a remedy like . . . *Natrum muriaticum*, [especially] if they feel rather resentful that life has not treated them better."

puts himself out but later shows his unyielding side.

He may have peculiarities of personal behavior which he asserts with tenacity, even insistence, while demanding acceptance on his own terms and ignoring the fact that in society one cannot always afford to be completely true to oneself. If absorbed in his own broodings, he is "apt to be peevish and abrupt" (Hahnemann) and can display the gruffness of an unhappy person. Or when in one of his egoistical moods, he "wants to talk . . . but does not want to be talked to; when he has nothing to say he becomes depressed and melancholy" (Allen). He can also be surprisingly vengeful against those who have injured him ("hateful and vindictive nature": Hering)—although usually he confines this characteristic to a fervent wishing that some "Hand of Destiny" might severely chastise his offender. But then he takes everything in life so hard—on the chin, as it were. He fights desperately on every front and to the last breath, even when little or nothing is to be gained, and can be needlessly intransigent, refusing to submit on the smallest points. He would accomplish so much more, and would find life so much easier, if he did not perceive compromise or flexibility as a threat to his very identity.

He is a good person but, as with salt, a little goes a long way, and sometimes others can take only so much of his distinctive flavor (i.e., heavy presence).

He suffers, furthermore, from oversensitive pride. To admit error is a humiliation, and to apologize is extremely difficult (*Sepia*). Thus a child who has shirked his household chores and been criticized for not laying the breakfast table becomes indignant, angry, and defensive, insisting that it was not his turn. But for the next few days his guilt feelings make him not only lay the table without being told but also clear and clean; he admits his error by his actions, even though he cannot say it in words. "I would rather die than say 'I'm sorry'" is the typical refrain of the *Natrum muriaticum*, both young and old.

Finally, he can be highly argumentative. Other constitutional types also argue, to be sure, but are not as deeply upset by it. Like *Phosphorus* and *Staphysagria*, *Natrum muriaticum* may start to tremble and have to lie down after an angry confrontation, or he may develop headaches and heart palpitations ("bad effects of anger": Hering), but he still cannot learn to avoid arguments. He must prove that he is, always has been, and always will be right on this issue and, in contrast to *Lycopodium*, *Pulsatilla*, or *Phosphorus*, seldom knows when to stop or retire from the scene of conflict. Even when victorious, he will continue to pile

Ossa upon Pelion in further demonstration of his rightness.

Thus, while *Natrum muriaticum* may be insecure in his social behavior, as exhibited by an exaggerated concern with what people think and whether they approve of him (an important factor in all his actions), he is not insecure in his understanding. He knows, or thinks he knows, what is right. This contrasts with *Lycopodium* who on the surface appears secure and self-possessed but is still a sceptic underneath; if he avoids argument, it is because he is uncertain of the strength of his position.

When *Natrum muriaticum* is accepted on his own terms, however, he "grows on you." He is a true and thoughtful friend who can be relied on implicitly, a Dr. Watson to another's Sherlock Holmes who is always willing to give aid and relinquish the limelight. He is steady and comforting in times of stress and easy to talk to, ever prepared to engage in long serious or lively conversation. Having been burnt emotionally (maybe more than once), he may be undemonstrative or tend (like *Sulphur*) to relate more on the intellectual level, but (unlike *Sulphur*) his emotions remain close to the surface or even paramount. And where *Sulphur* will discuss theories and abstractions, *Natrum muriaticum* enjoys analyzing human nature, deciphering what people are *really* like inside and how they truly function in mind and spirit. He is an intelligent and compassionate listener, a good foil for those who enjoy talking. While he may need to be drawn out somewhat, once he feels secure in his surroundings and sure of himself intellectually, he can be as talkative and outgoing as anyone. In fact, on familiar subjects he may get carried away by the "pleasure of his own talking" (Kent). Sometimes (like *Arsenicum* and *Nux vomica*) his symptoms are "aggravated by the talk of others" (Kent), especially if the others are monopolizing *Sulphurs*.

Consideration of others underlies much of *Natrum muriaticum's* behavior. It is his intellectual credo, his "inalienable duty," not to hurt others, but to support them and, whenever possible, be sympathetic to their needs. Typically, a family member who has constantly effaced herself for the others, when prompted to assert her rights, will reply, "I've had my share of attention. I don't want to take it away from the others." Or a gruff and taciturn man turns out to be nobly putting up with an unbearable in-law situation without seeking praise or acknowledgment. Thus he can be an unsung martyr, a role which, although courted by himself ("I don't want thanks . . . I don't look for gratitude . . .

I don't expect praise . . . ''), he may then resent. Outwardly he scorns and spurns recognition but, as becomes apparent months or years later, was craving it all along.

Natrum muriaticum is also motivated by love of truth. For instance, he will not accept unearned praise. Where another would have been delighted to produce a good impression, he will disclaim the compliment or qualify it. Even when responding to legitimate commendation, he acts embarrassed or pretends he has not heard, attempts to pass the credit on to someone else, or ascribes his success to luck. He may even denigrate himself unnecessarily (*Sepia*). The mother who is complimented by the physician on her attractive and well-behaved children will reply, ''It isn't only me. The credit should go also to their grandmother who lives next door''; then, turning the compliment around, ''And also, of course, to your homoeopathic prescribing.''

The type is seldom boastful. He would rather understate his accomplishments than aggrandize them and will energetically promote some cause rather than himself personally. If ambitious, he is quietly so. Superstitiously, he will not tempt capricious fate by premature boasting. He accomplishes things first and talks about them later.

In his honesty, however, he can be outspoken to the point of ''tactless'' (Whitmont). When his hostess asks what he thinks of her homemade cake, he will hesitate on the verge of some empty politeness and then blurt out, ''As a matter of fact, I have never liked coconut, so I can't really tell.'' Even his white lies are simply not convincing. If he says he *likes* the cake, it will be clear from his mien that he is not telling the truth. A *Phosphorus* who hates coconut will say with utter conviction, ''It was the most delicious cake I've eaten in months. How *did* you make it?''*

---

* It is always enjoyable to receive a letter from a self-consciously honest *Natrum muriaticum*. He cannot begin with the conventional ''Dear John.'' It will be ''Hi!'' or ''Greetings'' or just the name, ''John!'' There is no ''Dear'' because the person addressed is not especially dear to the writer, and it would thus not be completely honest to address him as such. The same happens again at the end of the letter. *Natrum muriaticum* will not sign off with the conventional ''Love'' or ''Yours,'' since, here again, it would be insincere; the correspondent does not necessarily ''love'' the recipient of the letter nor feel that he is ''his.'' So he signs ''Peace'' or ''Take Care'' or simply his name; or, if dealing

This bluntness, sometimes amounting to "lack of discretion" (Hahnemann), is often involuntary, coming out despite himself, more like an occasional bark than a habit of biting. *Natrum muriaticum* is well aware that truth in social relations is a luxury that can be afforded only infrequently. *Arsenicum* or *Sepia* may tell you to your face what they think, regardless of the consequences, but *Natrum muriaticum* feels terrible about blurting out home truths (even after long restraint) because of the hard feelings or estrangement which may ensue, and consequently seldom indulges.

As a rule, this person learns the difficult way—not surprising, given his unbending, pillar-of-salt personality. *Phosphorus* can be headstrong, *Lycopodium* is thick-skulled, *Calcarea* is stubborn, but *Natrum muriaticum* is inflexible and rarely chooses the easy way out. In antithesis to *Pulsatilla*'s adaptability, he must receive a number of hard knocks from life before his crystallized patterns of behavior and thinking are shattered, and he can change. In further contrast, *Pulsatilla* externalizes problems while *Natrum muriaticum* internalizes them. The former reacts quickly and visibly to affecting circumstances, while the latter may take a long time to react or even to admit that he has been affected. *Pulsatilla* is yielding, *Natrum muriaticum* unyielding. *Pulsatilla*'s symptoms are fluctuating and always changing (with "here and there" [Boger] symptoms, and no two pains alike), reflecting the flexible nature of the meadow anemone, while *Natrum muriaticum*'s symptoms (such as headaches, constipation, or joint pains) are fixed and unbudging, reflecting the solidifying nature of salt.

Antimaterialism and Unconventionality

Natrum muriaticum possesses a prominent streak of *unconventionality*. If he can, he will buck the conventions. This is seen in his dress, behavior, manner, and way of thinking. He has difficulty adapting to established values, refuses to be impressed by what is popularly

---

with medical issues, might use some tortured phrase like "Yours in Health.". Others realize that the conventions of address are there merely to make letter-writing easier. *Natrum muriaticum*'s insistence on uncompromising honesty at all times complicates correspondence for the writer (this, in part, explains why he finds letter-writing so difficult) while providing entertainment for the recipient.

praised and, as we saw earlier, may find it personally hard to conform.* Thus it can be instinctive with him or a matter of principle. Either way, he may pass through life acting not in the generally accepted fashion: neither more "right" nor more "wrong" than others, simply in his own different way.

This trait can express itself in a proclivity for minority causes, the more unpopular, the better. He will do everything in his power to spread "the Word" to the masses; but when his cause is accepted, he may lose interest in it and turn to championing a less sucessful one. Something in his very bones attracts him to the underdog. To take an example close to home, *Natrum muriaticum* is probably the wavelength that binds together all unorthodox physicians; this type is drawn instinctively to the anti-establishment, even if it entails less prestige or financial remuneration.

His unconventionality is sometimes displayed as antimaterialism. Uninterested in money per se, he constantly loses or misplaces it. Dollar bills which have been left in the pockets of his clothes come out bleached or shredded from the washing machine, and he seldom actively enjoys prosperity. He is quite satisfied with enough money for his simple needs. The child of wealthy parents who are quite willing to help him financially decides to slum it on his own, living in a cold and depressing attic in a poor section of town, just to do his "own thing" (*Sulphur*).

Natrum muriaticum's lack of interest in the material can be seen in his dress. The president of a large company will wear a threadbare suit and neatly starched shirt with frayed collar and cuffs, not caring for an ostentatious display of wealth. At home he will don a favorite and well-worn jacket or bathrobe, remaining attached to it for years (*Sulphur*). A woman can be neatly dressed but is seldom stylish or elegant, preferring above all to be "comfortable." She cannot be bothered to keep up with fashion and dresses in the same article of clothing

---

* One of the *Doonesbury* cartoon strips shows *Sulphur/Natrum muriaticum* Mark Slackmeyer fishing with his well-to-do, "bourgeois" father. Mark is saying, "Here I am, fishing on the best lake in northern New Jersey . . . I have just caught my first pink-bellied trout." The father, beaming at his hitherto renegade son, whose main ambition in life is to be a disc-jockey, eagerly questions, "Yes?" Mark replies, "And I've never been so bored in my entire life!"

until it wears out. "As long as it fits, why stop wearing it?" is her philosophy.

Thus she rarely dresses quite correctly for the occasion, but is either over- or under-dressed or merely different from others. She does not possess the instinct for clothes of *Sepia*, *Lachesis*, or especially *Arsenicum*. Conversely, the young girl who spends half an hour putting a barrette in her hair or arranging her ponytail in some over-precise way is also *Natrum muriaticum*. She will be as fastidious as *Arsenicum* about some inconsequential aspect of her toilet that others hardly notice, while ignoring the rest of her outfit (*Arsenicum* is fastidious about everything).

Frequently she will wear muted or subdued colors—blues, grays, browns, and other "earth colors"—rather than bright ones. Yet she may have a strong affinity for purple ("It just seems the *only* right color to wear!"), and in any constitutional type a propensity for purple clothes may be a sign that the time to prescribe this remedy is at hand.

The *Natrum muriaticum* atmosphere can at once be sensed upon entering the individual's living quarters: Salvation Army furniture, modified odd pieces of lumber upon which to sit or place things, ("Why not give even the lowly orange crate a chance to be useful" he thinks charitably), and frayed upholstery, with nothing really matching. The whole gives evidence that little energy or care has been directed at furnishing or decorating the house. Even the well-to-do individual may choose to live in shabby gentility. With so many world problems to resolve (saving the whales or baby seals, universal disarmament, the propagation of homoeopathy), he has no time for superficialities.

Sulphur displays similar tendencies but differs from *Natrum muriaticum* in being less affected by his surroundings. He can be perfectly comfortable in his domestic pigsty ("The house is a mess, but I *love* it this way. It is my idea of comfort!"), whereas a bleak environment disturbs *Natrum muriaticum*'s serenity and contributes to his already low spirits. Appearances to the contrary, he does have a strong feeling for beauty. Responding to all that is noble and uplifting in art, he will habitually listen to classical music and read Milton or Shakespeare, but will do this in the grubbiest surroundings, for some reason refusing *even once* to devote a few hours to improving the physical environment.

However, just as depressed patients can put aside some ancient grief or other incubus after a course of *Natrum muriaticum*, so they can also discard their drab clothes and start wearing something more attractive. They will hang up some cheerful curtains or purchase a comfortable armchair, reflecting their improved self-image and a raising of spirits.

In the realm of food, the present popularity of granola and other mutually indistinguishable pre-cooked grain and seed mixes, to the exclusion of what has traditionally been regarded as good food, probably represents a *Natrum muriaticum* cultural influence. The type is content to subsist on simple and easy-to-prepare dishes such as boiled combinations of vegetables and legumes. There are several reasons for this. Wholesome food that requires little cooking and can be eaten at any time appeals to the individual who likes to eat irregularly or skip meals; who, in fact, feels better from "irregular meals" (Hering). "I feel wonderful as long as I don't have to eat," is a common *Natrum muriaticum* refrain (and, at times, becomes a basis for anorexia in an emotionally disturbed individual). Complicating this picture, however, are the headaches caused by irregular or late meals (*Sulphur*); if he does not eat at his accustomed time, he develops a headache that may last the whole day and resolve only with a good night's sleep (Borland). Then, also, on the ideological level, grain mixes or stirred-up brownish-green mushes make *Natrum muriaticum* feel virtuously in tune with the universe. This is important to him. Duty as much as taste determines his choice of food. If convinced that a substance such as wheat germ or tofu is good for his health and that eating it manifests responsibility toward the environment (or meets some other ideological stricture), he will conscientiously set about eating it three times a day, insisting all the while that he loves nothing better. Admirable though this may be, he sometimes seems to promote a given victual the more strongly, the less palatable it actually is.

His diet thus reflects an important aspect of his character, specifically, his strong sense of principle and moral obligation and a conscious or unconscious streak of self-denial. These induce him to impose the strictest regimens on himself and his family, whether relating to food, clothing, surroundings, certain forms of abstention, or self-imposed obligations: "I'm a specialist at *forcing* myself to do things" or "If I have a choice of several things to do, I always choose the hardest" or "I usually find myself doing that which I most dislike" are typical *Natrum muriaticum* comments. The self-denial, in turn, reaffirms his instinctive conviction that life is a serious business, that we are here on earth for duty, hard work, and no mean share of suffering.

Natrum muriaticum may be wanting in natural elegance and ease Even on the purely physical level the individual is deficient in these. The carriage and gait are characteristic. There is a certain gawkiness in his build, movements, and bearing. Either he treads heavily on his heels (clumps), or he shuffles or lurches as he walks, or he strides with determination, body straining forward, and with flailing arms—or, conversely, with arms held too stiffly by his side. In contrast to *Phosphorus* and *Arsenicum* he is "clumsy" (Borland), hasty in his movements, or "awkward" (Hahnemann) in his gestures. He knocks things over or spills them, stumbles over thresholds, trips over carpets, or nicks himself on the corners of tables. He cuts himself when peeling vegetables and is always dropping things (the other clumsy or accident-prone constitutional type is *Kali-carbonicum*). This contributes to his overall feeling that the whole world is against him, even animate and inanimate objects of nature. One patient stated in a seriously aggrieved tone, "Not a single mosquito flies by without first biting me" (interestingly, *Staphysagria*, the foremost remedy for persons who uncannily attract mosquitoes, is more closely related to *Natrum muriaticum* in its mental picture than to any other remedy).

He may lack delicacy in his finer movements. His handwriting can be atrocious, with a general air of imbalance: no two paragraphs look alike, the letters slant in different directions or alternate in size. The poor speller or one who "readily makes mistakes in writing" (Hahnemann) is frequently *Natrum muriaticum*, but whether from a *Sulphur*-like inattention to detail or a trace of dyslexia is difficult to ascertain.

Even the articulate individual may have difficulty expressing himself verbally ("difficulty in articulation": Borland; "speech is thick": Kent). His delivery is not smooth, and his enunciation is poor. Thus *Natrum muriaticum* is one of the best remedies in cases of multiple sclerosis, where loss of balance or control of the fingers, impaired spatial judgment, tripping, a lurching gait, stumbling ("instability": Boenninghausen), and slurred speech are among the earliest symptoms.*

Natrum muriaticum at times lacks the social graces as well and is, like *Sulphur*, a bull in a china shop. In unfamiliar situations or when not completely at ease, he is all angles and abruptness. Aware of his

---

* Interestingly, an increasing number of homoeopaths are discovering in their multiple sclerosis cases, that the above symptoms commenced fairly soon after a severe emotional trauma. If these patients could be

social awkwardness and fearing ridicule, he wishes he were inconspicuous but does not want to offend by standoffishness. Thus he will be taciturn or loquacious in spurts, first sitting in uncomfortable silence and then, to cover up his shyness, suddenly bursting out on a subject that interests him and talking at too great length. Then just as suddenly ashamed of his outburst, he relapses again into silence.

It is especially difficult for him to express thanks (in contrast to *Lycopodium*). He feels gratitude but cannot articulate it suitably. He may not know how to say "Hello" or "Goodbye" properly. He is either embarrassed or curt or, to cover up his embarrassment, draws out the civilities excessively. This is apparent even on the telephone. For fear of offending the person at the end of the line he does not know when or how to hang up.

This all happens because, unless he is sophisticated or among close friends, *Natrum muriaticum* is excessively *self-conscious*, suffering from the conviction (sometimes groundless, sometimes justified) that everyone is looking at or judging him. In unfamiliar situations he may try to disguise his shyness with humor that is too heavy, his unease with a casualness that is too studied, his dislike with a politeness that is forced. This makes him act without spontaneity and therefore falsely, so that, even if he says and does the right thing, others will still feel uncomfortable. At times, too, he is *overanxious* to accommodate, compliment, please—in a way that makes others wish he would desist (with the ingratiating *Phosphorus* one always wishes for *more*). His unease is most readily betrayed by his *unsteady* eyes. Unless completely at ease with another, he will not look him straight in the eye when talking. Reluctant to betray his true feelings—which are written plainly in his eyes—he averts them to prevent the other from peering into his soul. Thus the patient's glance will shift ever so slightly to the side, or he looks over the doctor's shoulder, or down at the floor, or just enough above or below to avoid eye contact. In addition, the patient requiring this remedy sometimes has eyes of different sizes or shapes, or which slant at different angles.

Diplomatic polish is clearly not *Natrum muriaticum*'s strong suit.

---

identified, and their symptoms treated with the classic remedies for trauma during the premonitory stages of this tragic disease, homoeopathy's preventive powers could really come into their own!

Despite attempts at politeness, at trying to hide his feelings, these last are easily discerned by others. Just as he is bound to display pleasure and enthusiasm by the way his whole face and eyes light up, so he cannot hide displeasure, critical feelings, or disgust. He may not say anything outright, but the silent disapproval is nonetheless apparent, as his face is always easy to read. This inability to pretend what he does not feel may land the *Natrum muriaticum* child in trouble. If it involves the teacher, for instance, his grades may suffer. He then considers this highly unfair, since he has *tried* to disguise his true feelings and has *done* nothing wrong.

At times the type's social awkwardness is revealed in a tendency to verbal blunders ("readily makes slips of the tongue": Hahnemann) from which he later suffers grievously. One such incident was recounted by a patient with plantar warts (*Natrum muriaticum* is the principal remedy for this complaint and, secondarily, *Thuja* or *Sepia*), who, greeting an acquaintance whom he had not seen for some time, asked, "And how is your wife?" Then, remembering that she had passed away, he added in confusion, "Still dead?" The patient said that, twenty years later, he still writhed in mortification every time he recalled the incident (*Staphysagria*). Or a *Natrum muriaticum* university department chairman will ask one of the younger professors, "Would you like to teach a course next semester? We are really scraping the bottom of the barrel. Our best teachers don't want to remain in the city during the summer, so I thought of you—" Then, recollecting himself and with a look of dismay, he compounds the gaucherie by trying to right it: "Of course, you are not the scrapings—What I meant was. . . . " and continues in this fashion until his interlocutor feels like crying out, "Just drop it! Forget it! It's all right, I am not offended."

In general, this person justifies, excuses himself, and explains too much, thereby placing himself further in the wrong. He is aware of this but cannot help himself.

Reliability and Unpredictability

Natrum muriaticum is the antithesis of the smugness which arises from a sense of stability and security. Even if everything is going well in his life, he is seldom complacent. Fearing a reversal of fortune, he will begin to think superstitiously, "This is too good to last," or, in a fit of unworthiness, "I don't deserve such happiness"; or, immediately relating to any grief he hears about, he thinks, "There, but for the grace of God, go I!" ("he absorbs the pain of others . . . particularly wondering 'How would I react in such a situation? Would I be able to take it?'": Vithoulkas).

He is not cowardly, although he does display specific fears and phobias, such as of heights and closed-in spaces (*Argentum nitricum*) or of robbers ("awakes at night from fear, believing that there are thieves in the room": Hahnemann), against whom he takes elaborate precautions (*Arsenicum*), double checking the door locks at night, even to looking under the bed or into closets before going to sleep (he also "dreams of robbers": Kent). When confronted with a real difficulty, he rises to the occasion and grapples with it courageously. He is more self-reliant than *Pulsatilla*, faces unpleasant situations more squarely than *Lycopodium*, and withstands stress better than *Phosphorus*. He may almost welcome a tangible problem as a relief from his brooding self-absorption—finally confronting the enemy in the open after having long fought him in a fog. Also, a concrete difficulty assuages his subliminal superstition. He hopes that the fates which seem hostile to him will now be appeased. Some deep-seated apprehension of the wrath of God renders *Natrum muriaticum* insecure. His God is not *Lycopodium*'s compassionate and forgiving Savior, nor yet the comfortable bourgeois God who always rewards the righteous, but the stern, *unpredictable* and demanding Jehovah of the Book of Job, who tries his subjects' strength and loyalty.

Natrum muriaticum here projects onto life one side of his own temperament. As a rule he is ultrareliable, sometimes even too predictable (i.e., rigid) in everything he says and does. In any situation his dogged determination compels him to hang on at all costs, and, like an English bulldog, he never lets go when he has his teeth into something—an attachment, an emotion, an idea. This tenacity is not *Calcarea*'s stubbornness (the unbudging oyster embedded on a rock), and it differs somewhat from *Arsenicum*'s terrier-like worrying persistence. It is a focussed, single-minded approach to every issue, a refusal to be distracted, which permits him, slowly but relentlessly, to attain his goal.

Stability and dependability are exhibited in *Natrum muriaticum*'s love relationships. These men are the most uxorious of husbands, mo-

nogamously devoted and unshakably loyal to their wives. Patients repeatedly volunteer such remarks as, "I can never get over how capable
my wife is" or "As far as I can see, she has practically no defects." The
woman is also capable of the deepest and longest-lasting attachments
and barely notices (in a sexual way) any man other than her husband;
even after twenty or more years of marriage, she will say, "My life would
be meaningless without him. If anything happened to him or to our
marriage, I don't think I could ever love anyone again." Thus, in a successful longstanding marriage there is usually much *Natrum muriaticum*
in at least one of the partners.

The type is monogamous for several reasons. Aware of the power
of passion as a source of injury, he shies away from playing with fire.*
Also, he is dutiful, willing to put up with the hardships and difficulties
inherent in any longstanding relationship. These are still preferable to
being left without someone close. In a highly stressful marriage he is
prepared to make sacrifices and stick it out for the sake of a *steady* relationship. Then, too, his fixed nature makes it difficult for him to *cease*
loving someone ("I don't separate easily from anyone I've once loved").
Or he simply loves his home (*Calcarea*), feels miserable when away,
and endures much to avoid breaking it up.

But, despite the solidity and reliability emanating from *Natrum muriaticum*, the underlying emotional state can be surprisingly unstable.
The individual is more strongly governed by emotions and moods than
would at first appear. Behind his outward reserve or intellectual approach his "cheerfulness alternates with sadness" (Kent), or he oscillates
between excitement and despondency (*Phosphorus*), an overconscientious devotion to work and total lack of concern ("in the midst of work

---

* It is worth stressing that often it is *only* the grief of a broken romantic
relationship or thwarted sexual passion that can finally break down
the stoicism and fortitude of a strong *Natrum muriaticum*—not financial ruin, loss of professional prestige or a job, illness, nor even the
loss of a beloved family member or friend. This type simply cannot
handle the emotions accompanying romantic loss and may display the
Ignatia picture of hysteria, despair, and complete breakdown of the
ego. The patient will then require the latter remedy for his acute condition prior to being able to respond to, and be helped by, *Natrum
muriaticum*.

he suddenly loses all pleasure and interest in it": Hahnemann), the craving for companionship and rejection of it, an overassertiveness and a *Calcarea*-like diffidence and insecurity. Even his affections can be unpredictable. He is subject to ardent and overwhelming attachments of long duration. Nor does it take much to trigger this transport of emotion. An affectionate glance, a few kind words, can spark his romantic feelings and launch them into completely unrealistic realms. Then, seemingly overnight, he becomes indifferent. The feeling disappears, the longstanding rapport is gone. The candle goes out for want of anything to burn.

A child will be passionately attached to his pet, lavishing on it all the affection he cannot give to humans. In fact, excessive attachment to a pet, especially a horse or a dog, is often a sign of *Natrum muriaticum* (cat lovers are more often *Arsenicum*). This is because a pet is a "safe" object of affection: animals do not turn on their masters, letting them down and disappointing them. But, just as in human relationships, he may suddenly lose all interest (*Calcarea*, who also likes animals, does not display this change of heart). Having extracted all that is needful for his own development, he is ready to move on to the next stage in his process of self-discovery. Strong attachments, he feels, will only hold him back.

Thus, although no one values consistency and predictability more than *Natrum muriaticum*, who always cultivates these qualities in himself, he is prone to sudden and strange reversals that astound him almost as much as others. Sometimes he takes the most important and irrevocable decisions purely on impulse. A promising student on a much-needed scholarship suddenly abandons college and sets off to rough it in Alaska, or switches fields entirely and starts from the beginning again. A forty-year-old with a successful career will enter a completely different occupation or retire to the country. Or he walks out on his spouse after twenty-five years of seemingly happy marriage. There had been few harsh words between them, but one day he packs two suitcases and disappears without a word of explanation, never to return home again. All he says is, "It seemed like the right thing to do." Alternately, he decides to marry someone he has known for years as a friend and whom he had never considered marrying until that moment. He may undergo equally dramatic changes in artistic taste. Giving away his enormous collection of folk music, he now listens only to jazz—or Bach.

All of these reversals convey a subliminal determination to *obliterate* the past, which is the shadow side of the constitutional type's tenacious unwillingness to relinquish it. Once he has decided to put the past behind him, he will refuse to see people or visit places even remotely connected with these unpleasant events. The break with a person, an institution, a hobby, a job, an intellectual discipline, or an ideology is final and complete; in contrast to the conciliatory *Pulsatilla*, the "mending" *Lycopodium*, or the ready-to-make-up *Phosphorus*, *Natrum muriaticum* will sever the relationship irreparably and deliberately burn his bridges to eliminate the possibility of reconciliation except on a superficial level. This individual can be an "excellent hater," as Borland puts it. Overflowing with rancor, his hate ("against persons who have formerly offended him": Hahnemann) is more lasting than that of *Lachesis*, whose feelings, while stronger at the moment, can easily switch back to love. *Natrum muriaticum* is unbending and keeps on hating.

He has only one justification for such reversals: some inner process or intuition of which he himself is barely aware has suddenly crystallized into an unshakable resolution, out of which he can be neither reasoned nor argued. Unable to predict in which sphere such an overwhelming reversal might take place, even the steady reliable type who never *acts* in this way senses in himself an underlying unpredictability which renders him insecure.

Another facet of *Natrum muriaticum*'s unpredictable behavior is seen in the unexpected rages—instigated by disputes over relatively minor issues—to which this normally even-tempered and considerate individual may be subject: "becomes vehement without any particular cause" (Hahnemann) and "flies into a passion over trifles" (Hering). The obedient and responsible child, told that his clothes are inappropriate and asked to change them, or who is requested to cooperate with his parents in some small way, flies into a temper which no amount of reasoning or soothing can assuage. When consoled, he responds vehemently, "Go away! I hate you! I am ugly; no clothes suit me; and I wish I could die!" The adult becomes violently angry over a minor change of plans or through recalling some past vexation, insult, or humiliation (also *Sepia*, *Staphysagria*, and, surprisingly, *Calcarea*: Kent).

Serious cases of legitimate rage, however, also call for *Natrum muriaticum*. A classic picture is the elderly man who suffers from stroke and ensuing senile behavior, from anger at having been defrauded by his business partners and possibly facing financial ruin. *Arnica*, administered at regular intervals for impaired speech and voluntary motion, is usually the best remedy to give first ("Apoplexy: . . . from traumatism of grief, remorse, or sudden realization of financial loss": Boericke). But if the speech remains rambling or slurred and the patient continues to rage against, or dwell on, the wrongs inflicted on him, *Natrum muriaticum* 30x, prescribed twice daily, may restore him to his former self.

A more unusual case was a formerly healthy woman of seventy-five who, seemingly overnight, turned senile and developed concomitant symptoms. She was treated with *Arsenicum* for her anorexia and suspicion of doctors, *Causticum* for incontinence, and *Helleborus* for the tendency to pick at her clothes and bedcovers. These all helped the particular symptoms but left her mental state untouched. *Calcarea* and *Lycopodium* were also unavailing. After much probing it became clear that the problem was rooted in an incident occurring a year earlier: the synagogue where she used to arrange flowers had been badly vandalized, and such was her anger at this outrage, and shock at being deprived of her one emotional outlet in an otherwise lonely life, that senility set in a few weeks later. With *Natrum muriaticum* in high potency her mental condition improved substantially.

Natrum muriaticum can become disproportionately angry when interrupted in his work (*Nux vomica*: Kent). He is single-minded and drives himself to complete whatever he undertakes. His excessive irritability at noise and distraction when concentrating on some intellectual occupation may prompt him to push others away roughly, even bad-temperedly ("Get out, and leave me alone!"). But later he suffers remorse over such outbursts.

This characteristic stems, in part, from an inability to switch moods easily. When immersed in some activity, he wants to remain there and does not willingly respond to a new stimulus. He can be grumpy and bearish when aroused from sleep and at meals prefers to eat without distraction or interruption. He does not dawdle over food but eats rapidly and methodically and, when finished, pushes away the plate: only then is he ready to talk and be sociable. The typical singlemindedness can be seen in the way he walks. He does not saunter and look around, hoping to catch sight of someone familiar (*Lycopodium*, *Pulsatilla*) or of something interesting (*Phosphorus*). *Natrum muriaticum* walks rapidly, with neck stretched forward, looking neither to right nor to left as if blinkered and with the "deliberate stride" (Blackie) of a person who knows where he wants to go, is determined to get there as soon as possible, and is irritated at delays. In general, he can be "hasty and impatient" (Boenninghausen). If he wants something or is seeking assistance, he wants it immediately or would rather do without. To him, help delayed is help denied.

To an outsider *Natrum muriaticum*'s anger appears irrational and uncalled-for, a hysterical overreaction suggestive of imbalance. "He is carried away by anger; every trifle excites him to anger; vehemence without particular cause" (Hahnemann). But anyone who has worked as a counselor and recognizes depression as "anger turned inward" understands how well such behavior fits the nature's pattern of enduring a difficult situation while becoming increasingly depressed until the inevitable explosion of rage and resentment occurs. The individual puts up with frustrations and iniquities until some small incident "breaks the camel's back." Suddenly his stoicism founders, and he cannot bear the situation a minute longer.

Uneasy Relationships

Thus there is method in *Natrum muriaticum*'s rash acts and impulsive anger even as there is some madness in his method. The madness lies in a refusal to take constructive steps when he is still calm, instead of waiting until he is in a passion and then reacting in an extreme fashion. In an effort to avoid unpleasantness he will not coolly confront the person injuring him, but either hopes that the situation will improve of itself or attempts to convey his disapproval by indirect methods (this is either not perceived or conveniently ignored by the other). Thus he permits others to injure or exploit him and then bears a grudge.

This pattern is especially apparent in family relationships. For instance, a *Natrum muriaticum* woman might do more than her share in caring for her elderly and sick parents and will lament to the doctor that other family members are not pulling their weight. His obvious reaction is to ask, "Have you talked it over with them and divided the responsibility in a way that is satisfactory to all of you?" It then materializes that she has not done so because "It wouldn't work . . . No one will stick to the agreement," etc.

"Well, why don't you just try. Tell them how you feel, and see if it works?"

"What's the use? If after all these years they don't see for themselves that I am bearing the brunt of the responsibility, they will never understand."

"Still, you should *say* in so many words that you are being imposed on. Confront them directly, and see how they respond."

"I'm hoping they will understand without my having to tell them . . . "

So she continues, hoping for a change, without taking effective measures to lessen the burden of her grievance, unconsciously trying to make the mountain come to Mohammed. Her resentment grows when the mountain does not move, and one day some trifle sets her off in a rage which is incomprehensible to others.

Thus, although *Natrum muriaticum* may be morally in the right, politically he is not, and the deterioration of important relationships is partly his own fault. Similar patterns of behavior occur with colleagues at work, with friends, and even in relatively impersonal relationships such as dealings with salesmen or repairmen.

His uneasy relations and misunderstandings arise then from not being straightforward with people. A fear of offending them, and also of being offended by the wounding remarks they might utter in reply or maybe even rejected, induces him to take a convoluted approach. His feelings are definite and clearcut, but his manner is evasive. Instead of refusing outright to do a friend a favor (this would violate his idea of how friends should behave), he resorts to lengthy explanations, rationalizations, and justifications. To avoid offense, and in an attempt to please, he moves circuitously but ends by irritating even more.

The source of this behavior is, once again, his readiness to assume guilt. *Pulsatilla* waffles and cannot say "no" out of irresolution; *Phosphorus* will not say "no" out of eagerness to empathize; but *Natrum muriaticum*, with his ingrained or subliminal "anxiety of having done something wicked" (Hahnemann), cannot say "no" without feeling guilty. The individual then finds himself in the ungratifying situation of fearing he is not doing enough for people, while still doing more than he desires. Resentment builds up while his conscience remains unpacified. He also feels guilty asking for help. His sudden and severe breakdowns in health, the episodic hysteria in which he becomes excessively demanding, could actually be regarded as the subconscious revenge of the constantly giving and supportive individual who only through illness can receive the attention he needs.

Sometimes, in his convoluted fashion, *Natrum muriaticum* ascribes to others thoughts and motives they do not possess. He will not respond to the express words of another's question or statement, but rather to what he sees as their implication, hidden meaning, or unconscious motive. Thus an important link may disappear from the chain of communication, giving rise to misunderstanding. He also has a tendency to enact in his mind imaginary quarrels or distressing conversations with those who have offended him. "If X says so and so," he thinks to himself, "I will say such and such . . . Then he will reply with . . . but I will cut him down with . . . " and so on in these mental harangues, to interminable lengths (the other remedy that "quarrels in mind with absent persons" [Hahnemann], is, *Lycopodium*).

All this transpires only in his mind; *Natrum muriaticum* seldom finds the courage to come out with all these angry and harsh words (as *Arsenicum, Nux vomica,* or *Lachesis* would do). But he becomes just as upset as if the conversation had taken place. And when the anticipated confrontation does materialize, it is rarely as traumatic as he had apprehensively imagined.*

The Reformer

Natrum muriaticum displays prominent reformer instincts. He is convinced that he knows how people should think and what they

---

* An illustration of how convoluted relations can lead to desperate misunderstanding is found in *King Lear,* one of the most concentrated dissertations on *Natrum muriaticum* ever penned. Shakespeare seems to explore the various tragic aspects of this mode. The characters wander about on the heath, so close to each other and yet so distant, so unable to communicate and thus to unravel their differences, that all their true and noble feelings go to waste. Not only is Lear himself a true *Natrum muriaticum* in seizing on an imagined insult, exaggerating it beyond reason, and reaching the thoroughly erroneous conclusion that his daughter, Cordelia, has betrayed him. Not only does he go through circuitous and wrongheaded rationalizations to deny his love for her, but Cordelia herself is of the salt diathesis in her emotional self-consciousness, inability to express filial love in the correct words and gestures, and inflexible honesty and intransigent refusal

should do to make this a better world. More than any other type, he takes on the role of "his brother's keeper." Ironically, this individual who so fears being influenced and so adamantly fights guidance, is always trying to guide others and influence them: while not wanting to change himself, he is ever anxious to change humanity.

Even as a child, he finds it especially difficult to accept the injustices of the world. At school, during games or in the classroom, he is the one who reacts to small injustices most vigorously, even to the point of hysteria: "Hey, no fair! That's no fair! It was *my* turn to be at the head of the line!" he shouts *in fury*, his face scarlet with indignation at the miscarriage of justice. Nor is he anxious only about injustice directed at himself. He defends fairness in principle and will rush in to defend others, protesting vehemently, "That was John's ball. Make Tom give it back!" even if John is on the other team.

The child sometimes appears to be a prig or a tattle-tale, but he is seeking justice more than approval, and reparation for his offended sense of propriety. We recall how the *Lycopodium* boy shrugged his shoulders and went on to other things when treated unfairly by his teacher (see page 83). *Natrum muriaticum*'s sense of justice would have been outraged, and his anger could affect his whole future outlook.

Typically, also, the otherwise gentle adult lashes out in uncontrollable anger at a driver cutting in ahead of him on the road (*Nux vomica, Arsenicum*), with his blood pressure rising in proportion. Although this is a common occurrence, he not only feels personally insulted but also objects to the *principle* of the thing. He cannot tolerate the injustice of another breaking the rules and getting away with it. When this patient, child or adult, is asked what offends him in life the most, the reply will often be, "unfairness" or "injustice."

---

to humor her old father's whims. Thus her uncompromising (even though honorable) integrity brings on the tragic events of the play. Even the noble and devoted Edgar is *Natrum muriaticum* in his (partly self-imposed) martyrdom, silently enduring his father's injustices as he cares for him in his blindness; also the loyal retainer, Kent, who, though banished by Lear, remains faithfully at his side in disguise, attempting (unsuccessfully, of course) to protect him from further folly. Each character must play out his role alone and learn the hard way, unable to help the others or be helped. Misunderstanding thus prevails to the end, when it is already too late for mending.

Natrum muriaticum begins early in life to demonstrate his irre-pressible reforming urge by working on his parents, their tastes, values, attitudes (not least of all, toward himself), even religious beliefs, and going on from there to his teachers, friends, and acquaintances. He does not instinctively grasp, but must learn by experience, that most people want to live the way they are and be free to make their own mistakes, just as he does himself.

This came out in a college student under treatment for allergy to milk products. The prescription was a tossup between *Sulphur, Arsenicum,* and *Natrum muriaticum* until she mentioned her frustration at not being able to interest her parents in some semi-religious group therapy in which she was engaged and which involved shouting or screaming out her inhibitions. While this may have been an intrinsically worthwhile technique, it was obviously not one for her conservative and old-fashioned parents who were perfectly content with their life-style. Another constitutional type would have sensed the futility of such a course of action, but *Natrum muriaticum* pushes his reformist im-pulse to the point where others are bound to resist. Then he is hurt or offended and in an emotional deadlock. As the patient grew to tolerate milk better, so did she begin also to tolerate her parents' tastes. Subsequently, whenever she again voiced concern that her parents were not sufficiently liberated spiritually, and that it was her duty to rectify this situation, her physician took it as a sign that more potentized salt was needed.

This remedy has had an amusing impact on other patients as well. One young man with constant colds and sore throats during the winter and whose whole youth had been spent resisting parental guidance, was now expending much intellectual energy trying to persuade them to follow the teachings of his Indian guru. *Natrum muriaticum* in the 10M potency was prescribed for this and for the physical symptoms. He returned six weeks later to tell how wonderfully the remedy had acted and to announce that relations with his parents had never been better: "It completely altered my attitude! I now realize my error in trying to change them; I will never succeed, but I am serene about it . . . " The physician congratulated himself until the patient went on, "During the past weeks it has come to me in my meditations that in my next incarnation I am going to be a guru, and my parents will be disciples; then they will *have* to follow my teachings."

Thus *Natrum muriaticum*'s oft-encountered difficult or painful relationships with parents or other close family members stem in part from frustration at being unable to *reform* them. And parenthetically, the remedy is often needed by young adults who—in continuing re-enaction of their relations with their parents—seek out authority figures only to quarrel with them or overturn their authority once established.

The reforming instinct does not abate as *Natrum muriaticum* matures but is sublimated into reforming others on an expanded social or institutional scale. By nature he is a teacher, *full of passionate desire to impart information* and exhibiting an inordinate concern for the intellectual and spiritual welfare of others (a high percentage of teachers at all educational levels are *Natrum muriaticum*). The teacher (or preacher) in him comes out in such forms, as missionaries, social or pastoral counselors, legal-aid lawyers, unorthodox physicians who conscientiously and diligently instruct their patients in the holistic life style, and persons who work with the handicapped and underprivileged. The type is irresistibly drawn to the performance of "good works" and always eager to instruct others less fortunate or less enlightened than himself. Even if the work is emotionally draining and at times disappointing, he will persevere tirelessly if he thinks it will establish better communication among individuals and help them avoid the physical and emotional suffering to which he himself has been subjected. In fact, "helping others" is an almost religious imperative. Typically he will state, "I believe in God but I never go to church. I dislike the services and rites and won't join any religious group. I am not a joiner. I don't know how to pray, but I like to help others." His mind and ideals manifest a down-to-earth quality—the practical Martha as against the mystical Mary.

Although *Natrum muriaticum* is convinced that he can teach others how best to live and what to believe, he conveys more of a "Do as I say, not as I do" attitude (in contrast to *Lycopodium*'s "Be as I am and all will go well with you"). While seldom haughty or arrogant, he is more than a little self-righteous (along with *Lycopodium* and *Arsenicum*) and even intolerant. For this individual who is so concerned with the "Rights" and "Freedom" of humanity in general, and who generously puts himself out to champion these in some chosen form, actually has difficulty appreciating the "freedom" or "rights" of those with different values. The repression the young *Natrum muriaticum* so often feels around him is a projection of his own inability to tolerate another's viewpoint—or the least curb on his own freedom. Being subliminally authoritarian, he becomes righteously indignant at *any* opposition to his own ideas. The strong Democrat wishes that all Republicans would perish in one fell swoop, while the devoutly believing Republican cannot conceive why Democrats should be allowed to exist in the first place. Such feelings are held even by persons well enough educated to realize the advantages of the two-party system.

In fact, the tendency to self-righteousness can be one more reason for his difficulty relating to others. When they do not see eye to eye with him, they elicit the type's characteristic "reserved displeasure" (H. C. Allen). Thus he sets himself apart from a large portion of humanity. He will not waste time, even socially, with alien souls or with anyone of whom he does not thoroughly approve, preferring to stay home with a book or listening to "good" music. An enjoyable social occasion is an evening with a few close friends holding the same "right" values. When feeling insecure, or when the conversation is of no particular interest, he will simply withdraw ("taciturnity; avoids company": Hering). When the tone is frivolous, he may say nothing but will appear disapproving. *Arsenicum* may be similarly elitist but is less lonely in his self-imposed isolation. *Lachesis* can also be disapproving but associates with the objects of his disapproval. But when *Natrum muriaticum* conceives an aversion, he cannot tolerate that person's presence for a *single moment.* This almost hysterical antipathy can sometimes be justified by past history and is usually the result of complete disillusionment, but it can also arise instantaneously, after exchanging a few words with a stranger (also *Natrum carbonicum:* Borland).

While *Natrum muriaticum* may have difficulty relating socially in a spontaneous and unselfconscious way, or it leaves him drained, he readily adopts the role of helper or counselor. He is more at ease with those he can succor or instruct than with the privileged or with superiors—for he needs to be needed. This requirement of someone to instruct and advise, combined with his responsible nature and compassion for those in trouble, inexorably draws him to surround himself with unfortunates whose lives are filled with problems. Thus he plays the role of the substance from which the remedy originates. He is indeed the "salt of the earth," and, just as salt enhances the taste of food, so others' lives are enhanced by his giving of self. But the relationship is symbiotic. Without food salt cannot display its qualities. And the same is true for *Natrum muriaticum*: despite his introverted and loner tendencies, he needs people with whom to interact. And if, on the contrary, he cannot lend himself out, sustaining, instructing, and nurturing others, he dries up and withers emotionally, becoming "heavy," overly serious, emotionally numb, and proving the truth of the adage: "Too much salt makes a man dry."

Furthermore, his humanitarianism and reforming zeal have an egocentric aspect. Not only does he take profoundest satisfaction in guiding and helping others, but in so doing he is also trying to help himself. "Perhaps," he thinks, "by solving others' problems I will learn how to deal with—or forget—my own." In his emotional solitude, whether from voluntary withdrawal or imposed by circumstances, such as the loss or desertion of someone close, he sublimates his sorrow into benevolence towards others. These patients repeatedly emphasize that they can overcome their own hurt only by *depersonalizing* it—not by self-indulgence, entertainment, or fun, not by seeking out new companions or experiences, but by entering into a helping capacity: talking to the students they are instructing, the clients they are counselling, the friends they are comforting, or the patients they are treating. Thus *Natrum muriaticum*'s abstract love of humanity is often a substitute for the love which is lacking in his own life.

This whole picture is intensified by the fact that *Natrum muriaticum* in his "transitional stage" tends to *define himself* through helping others. Although this method carries validity, at some point he begins to lose himself by overidentification with them or taking on their problems, and finds himself once again thrown back on his own resources, having to delve deeper to discover his own identity. Finally, the ingrained stoicism that makes him determined not to be a victim of his own thwarted ideals or of others' wounding behavior, nor even to ask for help, can only be supported, and all these ends can only be achieved, by becoming a teacher, counselor or doctor.

In counseling he is encouraging, positive, optimistic, and unemotional, with none of his personal melancholy or minor-key modalities showing through; like the proverbial unmarried marriage counselor, he helps others attain a health and happiness that he may never experience. What is more, in this empathizing helping role he unconsciously takes the burdens from others and shoulders them himself. He knows he can bear them and prefers that to seeing another suffer. Yet it also affects him adversely. *Natrum muriaticum* illustrates the irony of the compassionate, nurturing type—he who contributes much to life must also suffer much.

Accordingly, he displays a great capacity for *vicarious suffering*, and this contributes to his bleak outlook. When he has no personal or professional reason to suffer, he identifies with the downtrodden, oppressed, or unrecognized portion of humanity; or he cultivates an obsessive preoccupation with (an unrelenting remembering of) the historic sufferings of his particular nation or race. More than one perceptive patient has said of himself, "Not only am I miserable, something in me is *determined* to be miserable. If there is nothing to be miserable about in my own life, I will find it in someone else's!"

Whatever the field of endeavor, *Natrum muriaticum* displays intense social consciousness and a powerful humanitarian impulse. Among writers, for example, the social reformer is sensed in the predominantly *Natrum muriaticum* Chekhov and Dickens far more than in Austen, Flaubert, Tolstoy, Virginia Woolf, Stendhal, Johnson, Dostoyevsky, or Henry James, just to name a few mentioned in this book.

Other types will work as conscientiously for humanity, but their motivations are different. We have already seen that *Arsenicum* derives satisfaction from hard work because it satisfies his perfectionist urge; *Sulphur* and *Lachesis*, with their colossal energy and creativity, hardly realize that they are working; *Lycopodium*, another hard worker, derives pleasure from sustained application to the task and satisfaction at a job well done. The benevolent *Sepia*, *Pulsatilla*, and *Calcarea* simply enjoy work with a philanthropic or altruistic dimension. *Phosphorus* derives energy from his love of performing and pleasing others. *Nux vomica*, even when directed by humanitarian impulses, is also motivated by determination to prove himself a well-rounded man. *Natrum muriaticum* is different from all of these. He works in part to sublimate his grief and overcome the pain of remembrance. But, equally important, the Puritan or Calvinist ethic is strong in him. Motivated by the sense of duty and sustained by righteousness, from work he derives *moral* satisfaction.

Finally, his talent for assessing people accurately contributes to his success as a teacher or counselor. While critical, he is a good judge of others' moral and intellectual capacities or potential. He easily detects pretense and sees through bluff or flattery. Contrary to *Sulphur* and *Lycopodium*, who have trouble distinguishing glitter from gold, *Natrum muriaticum* is quick to sense the low-key virtues and quiet strengths of those who possess them; he is also realistic about his own intellectual and artistic abilities (as is *Sepia*) and accurately assesses the extent of his influence over others.

Typical here is Abraham Lincoln who exhibited *Natrum muriaticum*'s fine judgment of people, as evidenced by his choice of cabinet members and other political appointees, including Ulysses S. Grant to lead the Union Army. Lincoln also embodied other characteristics of the remedy discussed in these pages. He lost his mother at an early age and never got over the bereavement. Although his stepmother was wonderfully supportive, the sadness which never really left him has traditionally been attributed to his mother's death. His personality— solitary ("the lonely man in the White House") and burdened with tragedy and grief—somehow made it all the more appropriate that his *Natrum muriaticum* shoulders should carry the weight of the Civil War.

The gawky in appearance and angular in manner Lincoln was also known for his love of a good joke and readiness to laugh. He seldom gave way to the chronic melancholy that was an essential part of his nature but instead found relief in the humorous stories he was constantly reading and quoting. The scene of Lincoln reading in his office at the height of the Civil War and laughing out loud is well known. When asked how he could laugh with so many men dying around him, he replied, "If I didn't find this vent for my sorrow, I would perish." The reserved Lincoln did not say such things lightly. Ironically, the author of the "Second Inaugural" and the "Gettysburg Address" then added that he would gladly trade all he had accomplished in life to write like the (now long forgotten) minor humorist he was reading.

Furthermore, Lincoln was famous for uxoriousness, despite the fact that his wife was difficult and at times impossible. She was vain, hysterical, wanting constantly to be the center of attention at public functions and in private; but the worse she behaved, the more patience and devotion he exhibited. He was so awkward with, and paid so little attention to, other women at White House functions that friends would ask him, "Why do you ignore them? Don't you find them attractive?" "On the contrary," was Lincoln's reply, "I find them too attractive."

At the same time Lincoln's sense of mission, his growing perception of the Civil War in religious, apocalyptic terms (*Sulphur*), his accurate presentiment of his own death (*Aconite,* the acute counterpart of *Sulphur*), his type of wit and the deep lines in his gaunt leathery face (*Lycopodium*), suggest that *Sulphur* and *Lycopodium* were the other sides of his nature.

Despite his good works, *Natrum muriaticum* frequently feels that he has failed in life. The remedy is prescribed for those who are *weary* from long striving and *disappointed* at the lack of recognition for their unremitting labors—who resemble the Prophet Jeremaiah crying in the desert, lamenting his own loneliness, his people's failure to heed his admonitions and teachings, his inability to find "a single just or honest man," and God's failure to reward his righteousness. Since God has betrayed him, he seeks deliverance from an ungrateful world.*

He may well take long to discover his true mission in life. He is the duckling who becomes a swan only in middle age after finally overcoming his "lack of independence" (Hahnemann) and passing through his "transitional stage"—or after attenuating somewhat his high ideals and becoming more realistic in his expectations. When *Lycopodium* or *Phosphorus*, having lived full and productive lives, are beginning to fall apart, *Natrum muriaticum* may just be finding that place to stand where, like Archimedes, he can move the world.

The ambitious individual seeks moral authority rather than material power or personal recognition. Some achieve it quite readily, a prime example being Charles Dickens whose *Natrum muriaticum* childhood colored his world outlook for life (as is revealed in both his biography and his fiction). He was able to arouse moral indignation against most of the social institutions and industrial conditions of Victorian England, and his influence for reform was thus immeasurable. More commonly,

---

* "Alas, alas, my mother, that you ever gave me birth. A man doomed to strife with the whole world against me . . . All men abuse me . . . I have never kept company with any gang of roisterers or made merry with them . . . For Thou hast filled me with indignation . . . Because I felt Thy hand upon me, I have sat alone. Why, then, is my pain unending, my wound desperate and incurable? Thou art to one like a brook that is not to be trusted, whose waters fail," and so on (*Jeremiah* xv: 10-18).

however, because *Natrum muriaticum* champions unpopular causes, he goes unrecognized. While morally right, he is out of step with the world. Either, like the early abolitionists, he trumpets his challenge before society is ready to respond or, like Don Quixote, fighting to resurrect the cause of the Knight Errant in Spain, he comes on the scene too late. Yet he himself believes that the rest of the world is out of step.

Even when attacking the existing order, he expects others immediately to salute the controversial or unconventional flag he has raised. He wants to criticize society freely ("for its own good") yet expects to be thanked for it. He feels aggrieved when it ignores him and continues in its erroneous path. Here he differs from other remedies. A *Sulphur* or *Lycopodium* espousing an unpopular cause expects opposition, may even welcome it, and is thus unaffected by nonrecognition, dismissing it with a shrug: "It's others' loss for not agreeing with me, not mine. I'll find someone else to support my views." *Arsenicum* enjoys pushing others around and hails their recalcitrance as a challenge. The determined *Lachesis* reformer is convinced that others are already on his side; he hardly notices when they are not. But *Natrum muriaticum*, always seeking approbation and taking everything personally, is well aware of others' lack of sympathy and morbidly sensitive to their disapproval.

Don Quixote

The nature's idealism, unconventional personality, self-righteousness, and reformist zeal are all beautifully portrayed in Cervantes' Don Quixote.*

This Spanish knight who is always tilting at windmills typifies the *Natrum muriaticum* who embraces some cause and proceeds to defend it against all enemies. If there are no enemies to fight, he will imagine them (windmills are hostile giants, peaceful friars or donkeys are villains seeking to abduct fair maidens, etc.). For he needs a grievance just as *Arsenicum* needs an anxiety. If he cannot find a legitimate one, he will conjure one up to fill the vacuum abhorred by nature. Thus

---

* His scholarly erudition on the subject of knight-errantry and his fixation on saving the world through this one great idea reveal a strong *Sulphur* side in Don Quixote as well. But we will concentrate on his *Natrum muriaticum* characteristics.

Don Quixote fantasizes that his fair mistress, Dulcinea (in reality a country wench who is unaware of his existence), has spurned him; he then undergoes fasting and self-flagellation, writes tragic verse, and indulges in the other classic responses to rejected love.

To view Don Quixote as a simple madman would be to misapprehend his character. He may be an enthusiast obsessed with an idea, but he has a firm grip on reality when he so chooses—for instance, recognizing wenches as wenches in spite of others' attempt to make him believe otherwise. It is just that, having once espoused an ideal, he is ready to play the role to the hilt. But in a typical *Natrum muriaticum* reversal of his original feelings, he suddenly abandons the role and denounces his former "cause" and passion. "My judgment is now clear and unfettered, and the dark cloud of ignorance has disappeared, which the continual reading of those detestable books of knight—errantry had cast over my understanding. Now I see their folly and fraud . . . I am now the sworn enemy of Amadis of Gaul and his innumerable brood . . . " and so on.

One aspect of his reforming zeal is a meddlesome officiousness. Nearly every time he volunteers his uncalled-for services as knight-errant, or seeks to defend a widow or orphan in their need, he makes matters worse than before. Typical is the scene where a shepherd boy is being flogged by his master for negligence while on duty; after Don Quixote interferes with the just punishment and retires quite pleased with himself for rendering this act of mercy, the poor boy is flogged doubly hard. *Natrum muriaticum*'s efforts to settle the disputes or alleviate the hardships of others sometimes take on this tinge of meddlesomeness. For instance, the patient who is crippled with painful arthritis will complain principally of frustration due to some family or work situation in which he is not directly involved. Others claim to be emotionally exhausted from trying to straighten out a sibling's marital troubles, depressed because a friend's son is imposing on his parents, or anxious because a thoughtless colleague is giving trouble to his employer. The victims themselves do not seem to be overly troubled (to *Natrum muriaticum*'s indignation), but this just makes him more determined to set things right. In such cases the physician may want to remind the patient that these matters are really not his concern. "Let others resolve their own problems. We are attempting to help *you*. Learn, like Voltaire's Candide, to cultivate your own garden before attempting to correct the injustices and inequities of the world" (this is the opposite of *Calcarea* or *Silica* whom the physician is tempted to advise, "Expand your field of vision. The world is larger than your own limited backyard").

A substantial part of Don Quixote's charm lies in his beautiful talk. He can be wise, amusing, informative, profound, but he talks of *nothing* but knight-errantry. He eats, sleeps and breathes this one subject. *Natrum muriaticum* can be eccentric in a similar way, if not always to the same degree. He talks only of the subject that interests him. He may discourse brilliantly on it but is still a "Johnny-one-note." Just as he is emotionally unequivocal, so he may be intellectually inflexible. His interests are intense, well-delineated, and one-sided. Even the best minds carve deep narrow grooves for themselves and remain in them. On the positive side this focussed determination overcomes all obstacles and contributes to his success. The negative side can be a Don Quixote-like imbalance.

The same onesidedness is encountered in his artistic tastes, which can verge on the bizarre. When asked what type of book he favors, the patient admits to reading *only* fiction or *only* history or *only* biography or *only* books relating to his particular field (he deepens his groove rather than widening it) or, these days especially, *only* books on health and self-improvement. The more immoderate types become enamored of a particular work (obviously a form of nonthreatening substitute love) and spend many months rereading it, sometimes dozens of times. "Why not?" they explain, "If one can listen to a piece of music innumerable times." By the same token, they may see the same movie over and over again.

Natrum muriaticum may try to diversify, acquiring knowledge outside his area of specific interest, but without true success. He cannot honestly enjoy or even appreciate whatever he is not attuned to at the moment and returns with relief to his tried and true favorites, upon whose emotional impact he can rely completely, as to close friends with whom he feels at ease. This contrasts with *Sulphur* who, unless he is a scholar, cannot bear rereading a book once he knows the plot or has grasped the overall idea; nor does he feel a need to see a movie more than once. He prefers something new which stimulates by its unfamiliarity.

Parallelling such one-sidedness in artistic tastes is one-sidedness in food and clothes. As mentioned earlier, he will eat the same food day in and day out for months or years on end, seeking security in a predictable monotonous diet and disoriented by any deviation from it (*Arsen-*

icum's repetitious diet is prompted more by love of order). And in clothes ("always made out of something *terribly* natural," as one sharp *Lachesis* observed) the *Natrum muriaticum* woman's familiar tweed skirt or blue sweater, the inevitable favorite bracelet or necklace are easily recognized; and the same sensible, comfortable (not to say too obviously practical), pair of shoes.

He also possesses a one-sided or eccentric memory. While he may forget in which century the Thirty Years' War occurred after just reading a book on the subject (*Calcarea*), his memory for what people *say* can be exceptional. He will recall whole sections of conversations held at social gatherings many years earlier; the physician remembers (apparently forever) the precise words of a patient recounting his symptoms. In fact, he is distressed when the patient contradicts himself: "But you said before . . . Now, you're telling me . . . which *exactly* is it?" That the patient might be in a different mood and view the situation from a different angle is disturbing to *Natrum muriaticum*, who sets inordinate store by consistency.

A woman in her early forties was suffering from food and environmental allergies, chronically blocked sinuses, anemia, headaches before, during, or after menses, constipation, and other symptoms—all of which had continued in a low-grade form for fifteen years. But she sought homoeopathic help only after developing heart symptoms: intermittent beats when lying down and periodic attacks of tachycardia (sometimes her whole body seemed to be shaking) for which she had once been hospitalized. This all made up a typical *Natrum muriaticum* picture, especially in the light of one key symptom—uncertain control of the bladder sphincter, causing urinary frequency and difficulty with retention when rising from the sitting position or walking, particularly in the morning (after 10 or 11 a.m. she was safe for the day). But the mental picture did not match: she was sociable, outgoing, with no visible neuroses, and never depressed; she was happy with her family and enjoyed her work as a primary-school teacher. She insisted that, apart from poor health, her life was happy and fulfilled in every way.

The physician, however, sensed that some *Natrum muriaticum* experience underlay this picture and proceeded to ask about her attitude toward people. She replied, "I am essentially tolerant, but one thing distresses me exceedingly: when a person expresses a certain feeling or opinion one day, then something quite different the next. It can be completely unimportant to me, such as whether he spent $3,000 on fuel last year or only $1,000, but for some reason it completely disorients me. I think to myself, 'How *can* he say that when last month he said the opposite?' I try to reason myself out of this aversion by remembering Emerson's saying, 'Consistency is the hobgoblin of little minds,'—but there it is. I am more tolerant of larger defects in people than of this one. Also, the fact that I seem to remember every statement, unimportant as well as important, made by anyone I care about, even without particularly wanting to, does not help matters much."

The constitutional picture was thus established, and the physician now probed more deeply. It turned out that twenty years earlier she had been much in love with an unsuitable man. Although the physical attraction was strong on both sides, their temperaments conflicted, and they decided not to marry. Despite her desolation at breaking up a romance of several years, she stuck by her decision. Her conscious mind had adapted to the loss, and she hardly ever thought of him, but her body and unconscious had neither forgotten nor forgiven; a few years later the *Natrum muriaticum* pathology emerged, and she began to accrue new sensitivities and symptoms every year.

The patient never dreamed, or at least could not remember them. But after receiving *Natrum muriaticum* 50M she began to dream of her former love and experienced a deep longing for him. Yet, as often as she reached out to him, she was never able to make contact (was he a *Lycopodium*?). It would then take her several days to get over the disturbing impression. In addition, the dreams were invariably forerunners of some physical ailment: a sinus attack, a migraine, heart symptoms.

With monthly, and then less frequent, prescriptions of *Natrum muriaticum*, as her physical health improved, the nature of her dreams began to change. She still dreamt of her past love but confronted him calmly and without longing. However, the dreams still presaged some physical relapse. The next stage in her dreams was a healthy indifference. As in her conscious state, she could now take him or leave him. Several years later, her rare dreams of him continued as presentiments of some physical breakdown, but a dose of the remedy averted or substantially attenuated whatever ailment was pending.

The case was long and difficult, with several remedies being needed to cure the patient once and for all. But *Natrum muriaticum* administered periodically in high potency kept the case progressing.

Sometimes the minor-key characteristics described in this chapter will be absent from the case. Either they have been modified by other aspects of the patient's constitution or the latter has simply been blessed with *Natrum muriaticum*'s cheerful happy traits rather than the burdensome and sorrowful ones. These individuals have often found happiness and serenity in some humanitarian work. But most of the time the *Natrum muriaticum* seeking medical advice or counselling will manifest the features presented here. If he does not exhibit them today, he may have overcome them in the past or may admit to a continuing struggle against festering feelings of misery and resentment, or a tendency to hang onto old injuries with bulldog-like tenacity.

The remedy can disperse the patient's tormenting *idées fixes* and soften his unbending pillar-of-salt personality, permitting greater subtlety of understanding and opinion; it helps him be less vulnerable, less defensive, and less inclined to self-condemnation. It makes him feel less of an outsider and less withdrawn, as he passes through the lonely transitional stage between separation from his past and discovering a new identity.

Every homoeopathic constitutional remedy performs psychotherapy while working also on the physical level, but in the introverted, repressed, morbidly sensitive or traumatized *Natrum muriaticum* this unblocking of emotions to allow the "vital force" to flow freely in the body — and carry away the accumulated and "condensed" bleak attitudes — is especially striking. After one dose, or several, of homoeopathic sodium chloride, individuals suffering from long-standing dejection or severe mood swings, or who are weighed down with cares, find themselves lighter, more self-accepting, less judgmental of others—more hopeful and open to the joyful aspects of life. Like Alexander's sword, which cut right through the Gordian Knot to make him ruler of Asia, this remedy can cut through the tangle of depression, insecurity, feelings of unworthiness and excessive self-absorption, making the patient master of himself.

Bibliography of works cited

Allen, H.C., *Keynotes of Leading Remedies*. Calcutta: Roy Publishing House, 1964.

Allen, Timothy F., *Encyclopedia of Pure Materia Medica*. Eleven Volumes. New York: Boericke and Tafel, 1874–1879.

Blackie, Margery G., *The Patient, Not the Cure*. London: McDonald and Jane's, 1976.

Boenninghausen, C.M.F., *Characteristics and Repertory*. Translated, compiled, and augmented by C.M. Boger, M.D. Parkersburg, West Virginia, 1905.

Boericke, William, *Materia Medica with Repertory*. Philadelphia: Boericke and Tafel, 1976.

Boger, C.M., *A Synoptic Key of the Materia Medica*. New Delhi: B. Jain, 1972.

Borland, Douglas M., *Children's Types*. London: The British Homoeopathic Association, n.d.

_____, *Homoeopathy in Practice*. Buckinghamshire: Beaconsfield Publishers Ltd., 1982.

Clarke, John Henry, *A Dictionary of Practical Materia Medica*. Three Volumes. London: The Homoeopathic Publishing Company, 1925.

Coulter, Harris L., *Divided Legacy: A History of the Schism in Medical Thought*. Three Volumes. Washington, D.C.: Wehawken Book Company, 1973, 1975, 1977.

_____, *Homoeopathic Medicine*. St. Louis: Formur, 1975.

Gutman, William, *Homoeopathy: The Fundamentals of its Philosophy, the Essence of its Remedies*. Bombay: The Homoeopathic Medical Publishers, 1978.

Hahnemann, Samuel, *The Chronic Diseases: Their Peculiar Nature and Their Homoeopathic Cure*. Two Volumes. New Delhi: Jain Publishing Co., 1978.

_____, *Materia Medica Pura*. Two Volumes. New Delhi: Jain Publishing Co., n.d.

_____, *The Organon of Medicine*. Calcutta: Roysingh and Co., 1962.

Hering, Constantine, *The Guiding Symptoms of Our Materia Medica*. Ten Volumes. Philadelphia: American Homoeopathic Publishing Co., 1879–1891.

Hubbard, Elizabeth Wright, *A Brief Study Course in Homoeopathy*. Bombay: Roy and Co., 1959.

Kent, James Tyler, *Lectures on Homoeopathic Materia Medica*. New Delhi: Jain Publishing Company, 1972.

_____, *Final General Repertory of the Homoeopathic Materia Medica*. Revised, corrected, augmented, and edited by Dr. Pierre Schmidt and Dr. Diwan Harish Chand. Second Edition. New Delhi: National Homoeopathic Pharmacy, 1982.

Nash, E.B., *Leaders in Homoeopathic Therapeutics*. Philadelphia: Boericke and Tafel, 1913.

Panos, Maesimund B. and Jane Heimlich, *Homoeopathic Medicine at Home*. Los Angeles: J.B. Tarcher, 1980.

Tyler, Margaret L., *Homoeopathic Drug Pictures*. Sussex: Health Science Press, 1970.

Vithoulkas, George, *Homoeopathy: Medicine of the New Man*. New York: Arco Publishing Inc., 1979.

Whitmont, Edward C., *Psyche and Substance: Essays on Homoeopathy in the Light of Jungian Psychology*. Berkeley, California: North Atlantic Books, 1980.

Remedies mentioned in the text and their common names

Aconitum napellus	Monkshood
Agaricus muscarius	Fly agaric
Argentum nitricum	Nitrate of silver
Arnica montana	Leopard's bane
Arsenicum album	Arsenic trioxide
Aurum metallicum	Metallic gold
Baryta carbonica	Barium carbonate
Belladonna	Deadly nightshade
Berberis vulgaris	Barberry
Bryonia alba	Wild hops
Calcarea carbonica	Calcium carbonate from the oyster shell
Calcarea phosphorica	Calcium phosphate
Calendula officinalis	Garden marigold
Capsicum	Cayenne pepper
Cantharis	Spanish Fly
Causticum	Hahnemann's tinctura acris sine kali
Chamomilla	Chamomile
Chelidonium majus	Celandine
China	See: Cinchona officinalis
Chionanthus virginica	Fringe tree
Cinchona officinalis	Quinine, Peruvian bark
Crotalus horridus	Poison of the rattlesnake
Ferrum phosphoricum	Phosphate of iron
Gelsemium sempervirens	Yellow jasmine
Graphites	Black lead, Plumbago
Helleborus niger	Christmas rose, Black hellebore
Hepar sulphuris calcareum	Hahnemann's calcium sulphide
Hydrastis canadensis	Golden seal
Hyoscyamus niger	Henbane
Hypericum perfoliatum	St. John's wort

Ignatia amara	St. Ignatius' bean
Kali carbonicum	Potassium carbonate
Lachesis trigonocephalus	Poison of the bushmaster
Lycopodium	Club moss
Medorrhinum	Gonorrheal virus
Mercurius vivus	Mercury
Mygale lasiodora	Black Cuban spider
Myristica sebifera	Brazilian ucuba tree
Natrum carbonicum	Sodium carbonate
Natrum muriaticum	Sodium chloride, Table salt
Natrum sulphuricum	Sodium sulphate
Nux vomica	Poison nut
Opium	Dried latex of the poppy
Phosphorus	Elemental phosphorus
Psorinum	Scabies vesicle
Pulsatilla nigricans	Wind flower
Ranunculus bulbosus	Buttercup
Rumex crispus	Yellow dock
Rhus toxicodendron	Poison ivy
Sabal serrulata	Saw palmetto
Selenium	Elemental selenium
Sepia	Ink of the cuttlefish
Silica	Pure flint
Spongia tosta	Roasted sponge
Staphysagria	Stavesacre, Larkspur
Sulphur	Elemental sulphur
Syphilinum	Syphilitic virus
Tarentula hispania	Tarantula
Thuja occidentalis	Arbor vitae, Tree of life
Tuberculinum	Tuberculosis virus